Coping With
Trauma-Related Dissociation

Coping With Trauma-Related Dissociation

Skills Training for Patients and Their Therapists

SUZETTE BOON

KATHY STEELE

ONNO VAN DER HART

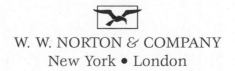

W. W. NORTON & COMPANY
New York • London

Note to Readers: Standards of clinical practice and protocol change over time, and no technique or recommendation is guaranteed to be safe or effective in all circumstances. This volume is intended as a general information resource for professionals practicing in the field of psychotherapy and mental health; it is not a substitute for appropriate training, peer review, and/or clinical supervision. Neither the publisher nor the author(s) can guarantee the complete accuracy, efficacy, or appropriateness of any particular recommendation in every respect.

Diagnostic Criteria in Appendix A reprinted with permission from the *Diagnostic and Statistical Manual of Mental Disorders*, Fourth Edition, Text Revision. (Copyright 2000). American Psychiatric Association.

For information about permission to reproduce selections from this book, write to Permissions, W. W. Norton & Company, Inc., 500 Fifth Avenue, New York, NY 10110

For information about special discounts for bulk purchases, please contact W. W. Norton Special Sales at specialsales@wwnorton.com or 800-233-4830

Manufacturing by Sheridan Books
Book design by Gilda Hannah
Production manager: Leeann Graham

Library of Congress Cataloging-in-Publication Data

Boon, Suzette.
   Coping with trauma-related dissociation : skills training for patients and therapists / Suzette Boon, Kathy Steele, Onno van der Hart. — 1st ed.
      p. cm. — (A Norton professional book)
   Includes bibliographical references and index.
   ISBN 978-0-393-70646-8 (hardcover)
   1. Dissociative disorders.   2. Psychic trauma—Complications.   3. Post-traumatic stress disorder—Complications.   I. Steele, Kathy.   II. Hart, Onno van der, 1941–   III. Title.
   RC553.D5B657 2011
   616.85'21—dc22   2010044302

ISBN: 978-0-393-70646-8

W. W. Norton & Company, Inc., 500 Fifth Avenue, New York, N.Y. 10110
   www.wwnorton.com
W. W. Norton & Company Ltd., 15 Carlisle Street, London W1D 3BS

To our patients, who have taught us much,
and are the true inspiration for this manual

CONTENTS

Preface   xi

Acknowledgments   xvii

A Personal Word to Patients   xix

Introduction for Patients   xxi

PART ONE
Understanding Dissociation and Trauma-Related Disorders

1. Understanding Dissociation   3

2. Symptoms of Dissociation   13

3. Understanding Dissociative Parts of the Personality   24

4. Symptoms of Posttraumatic Stress Disorder (PTSD) in Complex Dissociative Disorders   34

   Part One Skills Review   46

PART TWO
Initial Skills for Coping With Dissociation

5. Overcoming the Phobia of Inner Experience   51

6. Learning to Reflect   57

7. Beginning Work With Dissociative Parts   70

8. Developing an Inner Sense of Safety   82

   Part Two Skills Review   90

PART THREE
Improving Daily Life

9. Improving Sleep   97

10. Establishing a Healthy Daily Structure   111

11. Free Time and Relaxation   123

12. Physical Self-Care   137

13. Developing Healthy Eating Habits   149

   Part Three Skills Review   158

PART FOUR
Coping With Trauma-Related Triggers and Memories

14. Understanding Traumatic Memories and Triggers   165

15. Coping With Triggers   177

16. Planning for Difficult Times   187

   Part Four Skills Review   199

PART FIVE
Understanding Emotions and Cognitions

17. Understanding Emotions   203

18. The Window of Tolerance: Learning to Regulate Yourself   213

19. Understanding Core Beliefs   227

20. Identifying Cognitive Errors   236

21. Challenging Dysfunctional Thoughts and Core Beliefs   245

   Part Five Skills Review   254

PART SIX
Advanced Coping Skills

22. Coping With Anger   263

23. Coping With Fear   277

24. Coping With Shame and Guilt   287

25. Coping With the Needs of Inner Child Parts   301

26. Coping With Self-Harm   314

27. Improving Decision Making Through Inner Cooperation   323

   Part Six Skills Review   334

PART SEVEN
Improving Relationships With Others

28. The Phobias of Attachment and Attachment Loss   343

29. Resolving Relational Conflict   356

30. Coping With Isolation and Loneliness   365

31. Learning to Be Assertive   377

32. Setting Healthy Personal Boundaries   392

   Part Seven Skills Review   405

PART EIGHT
Guide for Group Trainers

33. Guide for Group Trainers   413

34. Introductory Session   434

35. Leave-Taking Sessions   437

Appendices

A. *DSM-IV* Diagnostic Criteria   443

B. Ground Rules for a Skills-Training Group   446

C. Participant Contract for a Skills-Training Group   449

D. Skills-Training Group Final Evaluation   451

References   455

Index   461

Coping With Trauma-Related Dissociation is the first manual developed for patients with complex developmental trauma disorders such as Dissociative Identity Disorder (DID) and Dissociative Disorder Not Otherwise Specified (DDNOS). The treatment of complex dissociative disorders has gained increasing acceptance because these diagnoses have been validated across numerous populations, and treatment approaches based on expert clinical consensus have shown consistent and significant promise (for treatment guidelines, see International Society for the Study of Trauma and Dissociation [ISSTD], in press). Studies to date, although methodologically flawed, indicate patients with a dissociative disorder benefit from treatment that "specifically focuses on dissociative pathology," with two thirds showing improvements in a range of symptoms that include dissociation, anxiety, depression, general distress, and posttraumatic stress disorder (PTSD) (Brand, Classen, McNary, & Zaveri, 2009, p. 652). Preliminary efforts to empirically validate these treatments have shown positive results (Brand, Classen, Lanius, et al., 2009), and further research is underway.

In the 1990s, skills-training books for traumatized and other psychotherapy patients began to emerge, but none were specific for individuals with a complex dissociative disorder. Many focused on a particular theoretical approach or techniques for problems related to but not specific for trauma, and thus have become useful additions to the treatment of traumatized individuals in general. Some were intended as an adjunct to individual therapy or for personal use, whereas others were designed for structured group settings.

These valuable manuals cover a wide range of topics, including safety, emotional regulation and affect phobia, social anxiety, addictions, self-harm, depression, anxiety, and relationship issues. Some of the prominent ones that have been particularly useful for many trauma survivors include dialectical behavior therapy for borderline personality (Linehan, 1993); systems training for emotional predictability and problem solving (STEPPS; Blum et al., 2008; Bos, Van Wel, Appelo, & Verbraak, 2010 also for borderline personality; short-term psychodynamic treatment of affect phobia (Mc-Cullough et al., 2003); and mindfulness and mentalization-based treatments such as acceptance and commitment therapy (ACT; Follette & Pistorello, 2007).

In the past decade, manuals that specifically address the treatment of trauma have emerged, a number of them empirically validated. Several are specific to PSTD, mostly based on cognitive-behavioral therapy (CBT) and prolonged exposure (for example, Rothbaum, Foa, & Hembree, 2007; Williams & Poijula, 2002). Other PTSD manuals have integrated CBT with additional modalities, including emotion regulation (for example, Ford & Russo, 2006: trauma adaptive recovery group education and therapy [TARGET]; Wolfsdorf & Zlotnick, 2001; Zlotnick et al., 1997); interpersonal and case management for trauma and addictions (*Seeking Safety*, Najavits, 2002); and an eclectic approach (*Beyond Survival*, Vermilyea, 2007). Cloitre, Cohen, and Koenen (2006) were the first to develop a psychotherapy manual specifically for complex PTSD in adult survivors of childhood abuse, based on CBT and attachment-interpersonal-object relations. In the Netherlands, a stabilization course for complex PTSD, "Vroeger & Verder" (Dorrepaal, Thomaes, & Draijer, 2008), was published, adapted from an original manual by C. Zlotnick et al., with some additional materials.

Some of these trauma-focused manuals are meant to specifically address the treatment of traumatic memories, but expert consensus indicates that patients with a complex dissociative disorder are at significant risk of being destabilized and may even decompensate when they are exposed prematurely to traumatic memories. The vast majority of these patients require a significant period of stabilization and skills building before they can successfully tolerate and integrate traumatic memories. In fact, the general clinical consensus for the treatment of chronically traumatized individuals, including patients with DID or DDNOS, is phase-oriented individual outpatient therapy, consisting of the following: (1) stabilization, symptom reduction, and skills training; (2) treatment of traumatic memories; and (3) personality integration and rehabilitation (Boon & Van der Hart, 1991; Brown, Scheflin, & Hammond, 1998; Chu, 1998; Courtois, 1999; Herman, 1992; ISSTD, in press; Kluft, 1999; Steele & Van der Hart, 2009; Steele, Van der Hart, & Nijenhuis, 2001, 2005; Van der Hart, Van der Kolk, & Boon, 1998; Van der Hart, Nijenhuis, & Steele, 2006).

The treatment guidelines for DID and DDNOS (ISSTD, 2011) and other publications by experts in the field provide an excellent overview of treatment approaches (for example, Kluft & Fine, 1993; Kluft, 1999, 2006; Putnam, 1989; 1997; Ross, 1989, 1997; Steele & Van der Hart, 2009; Van der Hart, Nijenhuis, & Steele, 2006). These publications also provide specific interventions. Nevertheless, therapists are still left to cull a hodgepodge of specific Phase I skills-based techniques from the literature and rich oral traditions of the field of dissociative disorders, leaving any given treatment at the mercy of the therapist's creativity and familiarity with the literature. In this manual, we have attempted to gather fundamental Phase I stabilization techniques for patients and their therapists, specifically tailored to address the dissociation that underlies and maintains many of their symptoms. Some of these skills include mentalization; mindfulness; emotion and impulse regulation; inner empathy, communication, and cooperation; development of inner safety; and cognitive, affective, and relational skills.

At the heart of the manual is approximately 30 years of clinical experience that each of the authors has had with patients who have DID or DDNOS, coupled with the magnificent and foundational work of many other colleagues who are pioneers in the field. It is well known that clinical innovations come from clinicians, not researchers (Westen, Novotny, & Thompson-Brenner, 2004), and until sufficient randomized controlled studies have been conducted on treatment of complex dissociative disorders, we are reliant upon this hard-won clinical wisdom. For the first time, this manual provides an operationalized treatment protocol that is subject to empirical validation for this most-in-need population which has been excluded from other studies on trauma treatments.

Development of the Skills-Training Manual

This manual is partly based on ongoing learning experiences with outpatient day treatment programs for patients with DID in the past decade in The Netherlands. These day programs usually ran daily during the week for a half to a full day, and they included adjunctive therapies, such as art and movement therapy. This distinguished them from the more cognitively oriented courses for borderline personality disorder. The nonverbal, experiential components of these treatment programs proved to be particularly destabilizing for many patients with complex dissociative disorders in the early stages of treatment. These modalities can reactivate traumatic memories and dissociative parts, which results in disorganization of the person as a whole, especially when the phobia of inner experience remains intense. These difficulties led one of us (S. B.) to develop a manualized course of limited duration, comparable to skills training such as dialectical behavior therapy (Linehan, 1993) and STEPPS (Blum et al., 2008; Bos et al., 2010), but specifically designed for patients with complex dissociative disorders.

An empirically validated Dutch stabilization course for patients with complex PTSD, developed by Ethy Dorrepaal, Kathleen Thomaes, and Nel Draijer (Dorrepaal, Thomaes, & Draijer, 2006, 2008), was the most important published source of inspiration for *Coping With Trauma-Related Dissoci-*

ation. As part of a research study, one of the authors (S. B.) conducted in 2005 a group for complex PTSD patients with an earlier unpublished version of this Dutch manual, *Vroeger en Verder* (Dorrepaal, Thomaes, & Draijer, 2006, 2008), and was greatly impressed with the results. However, patients with a complex dissociative disorder (DID and DDNOS subtype 1) were excluded, which further galvanized efforts to produce a manual specific for dissociative disorders. A positive experience with the Complex PTSD group was the impetus for the first author (S. B.) to develop a manual for patients with a complex dissociative disorder.

This manual has a comparable format to, and overlap in some themes in, *Vroeger & Verder* (Dorrepaal, Thomaes, & Draijer, 2008) and the *STEPPS* manual for emotion regulation in borderline personality disorder (Blum, Pfohl, St. John, & Black, 1992); it also has some similarities with other trauma-related skills manuals (Cloitre, Koenen, & Cohen, 2006; Harris, 1998; Najavits, 2001). What is unique about this manual is that it highlights ways for both the dissociative patient and the therapist to effectively work with an underlying dissociative organization of the personality as an essential part of coping with many of the well-known symptoms of chronic traumatization.

Over the past 6 years, several expert clinicians, including one of the authors (S. B.), have used an earlier version of the manual to conduct skills-training groups in The Netherlands, and more recently in Norway and Finland, resulting in further suggestions to improve the manual. Finally, over the past 3 years, the authors have collaborated intensively to refine and expand the manual. We have consulted with numerous other colleagues and some patients in an effort to receive a wide range of feedback and suggestions.

Although the manual was originally developed as a structured skills-based group treatment, we quickly came to realize that it can also be an invaluable adjunct to patients in individual therapy and can serve as a handbook for therapists. Thus, the manual can be used either for group or for individual purposes. And although this manual was developed specifically for patients with complex dissociative disorders, much of the content is also highly relevant for people with complex PTSD and trauma-related personality disorders.

Therapists who use the manual as part of individual therapy with patients should note that chapter 34, Introductory Session, and chapter 35, Leave-Taking Sessions, are for group use only.

All clinicians and patients should be cautioned that this manual is in no way a substitute for comprehensive treatment of dissociative disorders, nor for adequate training and supervision in the treatment of complex dissociative disorders. We strongly recommend that anyone using this manual become familiar with the updated International Society for the Study of Trauma and Dissociation Treatment Guidelines for DID and DDNOS (ISSTD Treatment Guidelines, 2011).

For more information on treatment of dissociative disorders, visit the Web site of the International Society for the Study of Trauma and Dissociation at http://www.isst-d.org or the Web site of the European Society for Trauma and Dissociation at http://www.estd.org.

For more information about *Coping with Trauma-Related Dissociation*, the authors, and specialized training for therapists, visit our Web site at http://www.copingwithdissociation.com.

ACKNOWLEDGMENTS

Many of our colleagues have made significant contributions to this manual, both through other training groups they have developed, and in offering ideas and suggestions. We especially mention Nel Draijer, Ethy Dorrepaal, and Kathleen Thomaes, who inspired us with their Stabilization Course, *Vroeger and Verder*, to develop this skills training. The teams and colleagues in the Netherlands who work with one of the authors (S.B.) have been invaluable in making contributions to the treatment of complex dissociative disorders and developing skills-training techniques. We would like to give special thanks to Sheri Miller, LCSW, and Kate O'Mullan, BA, for their helpful contributions to chapter 30, Coping with Isolation and Loneliness. We would like to thank Jolanda Treffers for her excellent preface for patients from the perspective of a survivor. She originally wrote this for our Dutch translation. We are glad that her text now will be included in all future translations and reprints.

Most of all, we would like to thank our patients, who had the courage to share themselves with us, who have worked tirelessly for healing, and who are our most important inspiration for the manual. Many participants of the courses run in The Netherlands in the past 6 years, as well as several in the United States, provided invaluable comments on earlier versions of the manual, thus helping us improve it. We are very grateful for your suggestions and comments.

This manual contains many techniques. It is impossible to trace the origin of some long-standing techniques, because they have often come from an oral history of psychotherapy traditions, and some are ubiquitous. We have done our best to credit those techniques, and we apologize if we have unintentionally failed to cite sources.

A PERSONAL WORD TO PATIENTS

Let's keep this just between us, but if someone had offered this book to me a few years ago, I would have run away screaming—if not on the outside, then certainly inside of me. I admit that this would not have been the best response given the situation, but hey, it was not unusual for me at that time to react differently from how I should have done. Back then, I felt like I was constantly pushing a wheelbarrow full of frogs down a bumpy, winding road. The frogs would not stay put; they croaked at the slightest movement and made the wheelbarrow lean over dangerously whenever I encountered a bump or a pothole on my way. It often took more strength than I thought I had to keep this wheelbarrow upright and to continue down the road.

The worst part, however, was that I didn't see anyone else struggling with such a peculiar load. I was ashamed of my wheelbarrow and did my best to make sure that nobody would notice it. After all, what could I answer if someone were to ask me how I came by so many frogs? To be honest, I hardly knew most of my frogs. I thought of them as green monsters and regarded them as no more than a burden that I had to bear. I did not even know how or when some of them had climbed into my wheelbarrow—or why.

Then one day, when I arrived at the biggest, deepest pothole in the road, I realized that I could no longer do this alone and that I needed help from someone else to keep the wheelbarrow upright on this stretch of the road. It took a lot of courage and a great deal of trust to dare ask for that help—trust in that other person, but even more, genuine trust in myself. I needed to believe that I *could* ask for such help, that I would *not* helplessly collapse if someone cast an eye on my many frogs, and that *together* we would find a way past, through, or over the biggest obstacles.

Trust is an important theme in this book. Again and again, you will read that you and all of your parts must learn to rely on each other, that it is important to connect with people you can count on, and that you can be sure of the support of your therapist. Of course, it is not at all easy to have or to feel such trust. However, that may be the most important (and most beautiful) lesson you can learn from this book: that there *are* people you can trust and that you are worthy of letting yourself be seen by them.

The authors of this book are such people. When you read what they have written, you will find that they have your very best interests at heart. They possess the knowledge, the experience, and the empathic skills to help you. I know, because I have worked through each and every topic in this book as part of my own process. Suzette Boon, Kathy Steele, and Onno van der Hart know what they are talking about. When I look back on the years I struggled with the topics they discuss in this book, I can only say that what they write is true. And, much more important, it helps.

I know my frogs now. If anything, they have turned from green monsters into dear green friends. They sit still when I want them to—and if the path becomes somewhat treacherous again at times, they are very willing to lend a hand and help push my wheelbarrow. They have considerably diminished in number, by the way, but that doesn't even seem important anymore. *Together*, the load was a lot easier to carry anyway.

In order to come to this point, I have had to learn many new skills. All of those skills are included in this book. I did not write the book, of course. Still, it *feels* like it's about me. That is probably exactly why I would have run away if someone had given it to me at the beginning of my therapy: It named that which I did not want to have named and it showed what I preferred never to look at. As I said above, it was not unusual for me at that time to react differently from how I should have done. With the wisdom that comes from hindsight, I would now accept it with both hands.

If this were indeed my book, I would dedicate it to my therapist—for the way she taught me how to trust her and for the trust she had in me. However, it is not my book. It belongs to *you*. And to *your* therapist. Now all you need to do is to take a deep breath, turn over the pages, and get to work. Believe in yourself, believe in all your parts, and believe in your therapist.

I know you can. I trust in you.

—Jolanda Treffers

INTRODUCTION FOR PATIENTS

This manual was developed for those of you who are struggling with complex trauma-related dissociative disorders, that is, dissociative identity disorder (DID) and dissociative disorder not otherwise specified (DDNOS, subtype 1). These disorders are often misunderstood by the public, and publications about treatment have been written primarily for mental health professionals. There is little reliable and practical help to be found, other than that which your therapists have been able to offer. Many of you have spent years in the mental health system before your core dissociative problems were recognized and treated. This manual offers you practical solutions to dissociative problems during the first phase of your treatment. We explain dissociation and other trauma-related symptoms in basic language, and we help you understand and work with dissociative parts of yourself in a rational manner. You will be introduced to essential ideas and themes useful to your healing from dissociation and trauma, and you will also learn practical skills to help you manage in daily life.

We strongly recommend that you use this manual only in the course of individual therapy or in a structured skills-training group run by trained clinicians, so that you will make the most of your experience and will receive adequate support. This manual is not intended to be used by yourself when you are not in therapy, although some content may be helpful. The manual may also be helpful to your loved ones who wish to understand and support you more effectively.

Each chapter includes an educational topic relevant to trauma and dissociation, as well as strategies to help you cope more effectively with your dissociation and other trauma-related problems. Homework assignments are included for every topic to help you practice your new skills. If you are using this manual in your individual therapy rather than participating in a group, you may ignore the agenda at the beginning of each chapter, as well as the entire Part 8, chapters 33–35, which are focused on group participation.

Some topics may not be relevant to you. Nevertheless, you may find some helpful tips in those chapters, so we encourage you to at least read about the topics before you decide to skip those chapters. Some topics may be too overwhelming or premature for you at this time. That is fine. Just skip those chapters and continue with those chapters that are right for you.

It is essential that you practice the homework exercises and modify them to your own needs as necessary. Reading the manual may be helpful, but it is no substitute for the consistent practice that earns you new skills. Make sure you collaborate with your therapist in your work in the manual.

It is essential for you to pace yourself in your work on this material. At any time you begin to feel overwhelmed, simply stop and practice grounding exercises and focus on the present moment, and consult your therapist, if needed. Healing takes time, and pushing yourself too hard can actually slow your progress. On the other hand, not pushing yourself at all to overcome avoidance of painful issues or to practice new skills also slows your healing. Find your pace, and if needed, ask your therapist to help you know when to push and when to slow down.

Participation in any of the exercises in this manual is voluntary. We have attempted to make the exercises appropriate for a wide range of individuals, but of course, not all exercises may be helpful or even right for you as an individual. Even though people with a dissociative disorder have much in common, they also have many differences. You will receive maximum benefit from the course if you can practice the exercises as much as possible, but you should also be aware of what is and is not helpful to you. Feel free to modify exercises for your benefit, to come up with some of your own, or to enlist the help of your therapist in additional ways to practice the various skills in this manual.

Throughout the manual you will often be asked whether you encountered any difficulties in completing your homework. Awareness of these obstacles is the first step in overcoming them. It is essential for you to take any difficulties to your individual therapist to receive further help and support.

Coping With
Trauma-Related Dissociation

PART ONE

Understanding Dissociation and Trauma-Related Disorders

Understanding Dissociation

AGENDA

- Welcome and reflections on the introductory session
- Exercise: Learning to Be Present
- Topic: Understanding Dissociation

  - Introduction
  - Learning to Be Present
  - Understanding Dissociation
  - The Origins of Chronic Dissociation
  - Dissociative Disorders

- Homework

  - Reread the chapter.
  - Practice the Learning to Be Present exercise twice a day, morning and evening, or an equivalent exercise that you and your therapist have agreed is best for you.
  - Complete Homework Sheet 1.1, Reflections on What You Have Learned.

Introduction

This manual focuses on helping you understand and cope with dissociation and the major dissociative disorders, as well as related experiences and problems. It is important from the beginning that you pace your work in this manual and also in your therapy according to what is tolerable for you at a given time. You may find that focusing on your dissociative symptoms may increase your anxiety temporarily; however, gaining an understanding of what is happening within you and learning more effective ways to cope will soon help you feel more relaxed and comfortable with your inner experiences. If you become too anxious at any time while working in this manual, stop for awhile and practice the Learning to Be Present exercise found later in this chapter or other exercises in this book that will help you become calmer and more grounded. You can always return at a later time to finish a chapter. You will begin by learning more about how to stay present. Once you have practiced the exercise suggested for being present, you can read about dissociation in the chapter.

Learning to Be Present

Being in the present, being aware of your surroundings and of yourself, is essential to learning, growing, and healing from a dissociative disorder. In the moment you are present, the past is behind you. Thus, before introducing any other topics, we begin with an exercise to help you focus on being present, because it is the foundation for all the work you will do in this manual and in your therapy, and because we know that when you have a dissociative disorder it can be a struggle to be present.

People with dissociative disorders encounter a number of problems that interfere with being present. When you are under stress or faced with a painful conflict or intense emotion, you may have a variety of ways to retreat from the present in order to avoid it. Although retreat may feel better in the moment, in the long run you will become increasingly avoidant of the present, which can make your problems worse.

There may be times when you feel spacey, foggy, or fuzzy. You may lose a firm connection with the present without even being aware of it, and only realize afterwards that you were not very present. Perhaps you become engulfed by negative images, feelings or thoughts from the past, or worries about the future such that you are so preoccupied in your own mind that you are not aware of the present. You may have times when you are aware of your actions, as though you are watching yourself, but do not feel you have control over them. It may seem as though you are present and not present at the same time! In addition, some people with complex dissociative disorders lose time, that is, they cannot account for what happened during significant periods of time in the present. And some people may "blank out" for periods and not be aware of anything. Other people retreat to fantasy or daydreams when life feels too stressful.

The following concentration exercise can help you focus your attention on the *here and now*. You can begin to learn to stop yourself from spacing out and eventually to overcome much of your dissociation by learning to stay present. Remember to gauge whether the following exercise is helpful to you, and if not, stop or modify it.

EXERCISE
LEARNING TO BE PRESENT

- Notice three objects that you see in the room and pay close attention to their details (shape, color, texture, size, etc.). Make sure you do not hurry through this part of the exercise. Let your eyes linger over each object. Name three characteristics of the object out loud to yourself, for example, "It is blue. It is big. It is round."
- Notice three sounds that you hear in the present (inside or outside of the room). Listen to their quality. Are they loud or soft, constant or intermittent, pleasant or unpleasant? Again, name three characteristics of the sound out loud to yourself, for example, "It is loud, grating, and definitely unpleasant."
- Now touch three objects close to you and describe out loud to yourself how they feel, for example, rough, smooth, cold, warm, hard or soft, and so forth.
- Return to the three objects that you have chosen to observe with your eyes. As you notice them, concentrate on the fact that you are here and now with these objects in the present, in this room. Next, notice the sounds and concentrate on the fact that you are here in this room with those sounds. Finally, do the same with the objects you have touched. You can expand this exercise by repeating it several times, three items for each sense, then two for each, then one, and then build it up again to three. You can also add new items to keep your practice fresh.

Examples

- **Sight**: Look around the room for something (or even someone) that can help remind you that you are in the present, for example, a piece of clothing you are wearing that you like, a particular color or shape or texture, a picture on the wall, a small object, a book. Name the object to yourself out loud.
- **Sound**: Use the sounds around you to help you really focus on the here and now. For example, listen to the normal everyday noises around you: the heat

or air conditioning or refrigerator running, people talking, doors opening or closing, traffic sounds, birds singing, a fan blowing. You can remind yourself: "These are the sounds of normal life all around me. I am safe. I am here."

- **Taste**: Carry a small item of food with you that has a pleasant but intense taste, for example, lozenges, mints, hard candy or gum, a piece of fruit such as an orange or banana. If you feel ungrounded, pop it into your mouth and focus on the flavor and the feel of it in your mouth to help you be more *here and now*.

- **Smell:** Carry something small with you that has a pleasant smell, for example, a favorite hand lotion, perfume, aftershave, or an aromatic fruit such as an orange. When you start to feel spacey or otherwise not very present, a pleasant smell is a powerful reminder of the present.

- **Touch**: Try one or more of the following touch exercises that feels good to you. Touch the chair or sofa on which you are sitting, or your clothes. Feel them with your fingers and be very aware of the textures and weight of the fabric. Try pushing on the floor with your feet, so that you can really feel the floor supporting you. Squeeze your hands together and let the pressure and warmth remind you that you are here and now. Press your tongue hard to the roof of your mouth. Cross your arms over your chest with your fingertips on your collar bones and pat your chest, alternating left and right, reminding yourself that you are in the present and safe (the butterfly hug, Artigas & Jarero, 2005).

- **Breathing**: The way in which we breathe is crucial in helping us to be present. When people dissociate or space out, they are usually breathing very shallowly and rapidly or hold their breath too long. Take time to slow and regulate your breathing. Breathe in through your nose to a slow count of three, hold to the count of three, and then breathe out through your mouth to a slow count of three. Do this several times while being mindful of how you breathe.

Notice whether there are already ways in which you ground yourself in the present.

Understanding Dissociation

In the following sections, you will learn about dissociation that developed from past trauma. This concept is based on years of careful observations and study (Boon, 1997; Boon & Draijer, 1993; Van der Hart & Boon, 1997; Van der Hart, Nijenhuis, & Steele, 2006), including historical research into the original 19th-century literature on the subject and the lessons of the late 20th-century pioneers in the dissociative disorder literature (for instance, Braun, 1986; Chu, 1998; Horevitz & Loewenstein, 1994; Kluft, 1985; Kluft & Fine, 1993; Loewenstein, 1991; Michelson & Ray, 1996; Putnam, 1989, 1997; Ross, 1989, 1997). *Dissociation* is a word that is used for many different symptoms, and at times, it is understood differently by various professionals. We will begin by explaining integration, which is what you strive for as a major part of your healing.

Integration

To understand dissociation, it is helpful first to understand a bit about its opposite, that is, *integration*. In the context of dissociative disorders, integration can be understood as the organization of all the different aspects of personality (including our sense of self) into a unified whole that functions in a cohesive manner.

Each of us is born with a natural tendency to integrate our experiences into a coherent, whole life history and a stable sense of who we are. Our integrative capacity helps us to distinguish the past from the present and to keep ourselves in the present, even when we are remembering our past or contemplating our future. It also helps us develop our sense of self. The more secure and safe our emotional and physical environment as we grow up, the more we are able to further develop and strengthen this integrative capacity.

Each of us develops typical and lasting ways of thinking, feeling, acting, and perceiving that are collectively called our *personality*. Of course, personality is not a "thing" that can be seen, or that lives and breathes, but rather is a shorthand term that describes our unique characteristic responses as complex, living systems. Usually, people function in a coordinated way so that they make smooth transitions between their response patterns to adjust and adapt to different situations, like shifting gears in a car. They can go from home to work and smoothly shift their thinking, feeling, decision making, and acting, yet still experience themselves as the same person. In this sense, our personality is stable and predictable. Yet, to be most effective in our lives, we are always subtly changing, adjusting, adapting, and reorganizing our personality as we learn and experience more. In this sense, our personality is flexible.

Sense of Self

Over the course of our development, we gradually learn to connect our life experiences across time and situations with our sense of self. We can then have a fairly clear perception of who we are, and we can place these experiences in our "life history" as an integral part of our autobiography. Each of us has a sense of self that is part of our personality and that should be consistent across our development and across different circumstances: "I am *me, I am myself* as a child, as an adolescent, as an adult, as a parent, as a worker. I am *me, myself* in good, in difficult, and in overwhelming circumstances. These circumstances and experiences all belong to *me*. My thoughts, behaviors, emotions, sensations, and memories—no matter how pleasant or unpleasant—all belong to *me*."

Dissociation

Dissociation is a major failure of integration that interferes with and changes our sense of self and our personality. Our integrative capacity can be chronically impaired if we are traumatized. It can also be disrupted or limited when we are extremely tired, stressed, or seriously ill, but in these cases, the disruption is temporary. Childhood traumatization can profoundly hamper our ability to integrate our experiences into a coherent and whole life narrative because the integrative capacity of children is much more limited than adults and is still developing.

Of course, not all failures in integration result in dissociation. Integrative failures are on a continuum. Dissociation involves a kind of parallel owning and disowning of experience: While one part of you owns an experience, another part of you does not. Thus, people with dissociative disorders do not feel integrated and instead feel fragmented because they have memories, thoughts, feelings, behaviors, and so forth that they experience as uncharacteristic and foreign, as though these do not belong to themselves. Their personality is not able to "shift gears" smoothly from one response pattern to another; rather, their sense of self and enduring patterns of response change from situation to situation, and they are not very effective at adopting new ways of coping. They experience more than one sense of self, and they do not experience these selves as (completely) belonging to one person.

Dissociative Parts of the Personality

These divided senses of self and response patterns are called *dissociative parts of the personality*. It is as though there are not enough links or mental connections between one sense of self and another, between one set of responses and another. For example, a person with a dissociative disorder has the experience that some painful memories of her childhood are not hers: "I did not have those bad experiences; I am not that little girl. She is scared, but that is not my fear. She is helpless, but that is not my helplessness." This lack of realization, this experience of "not me" is the essence of dissociative disorders.

The functions of each dissociative part of personality or self may range from extremely limited to more elaborate. The latter is especially true in cases of dissociative identity disorder (DID), which will be explained in more detail in chapter 3. Dissociation takes many forms, which we will discuss in the next chapter on symptoms. Many dissociative symptoms are common in people with dissociative disorders, but each individual may also have his or her own unique subjective experience of dissociation.

The Origins of Chronic Dissociation

Dissociation generally develops when an experience is too threatening or overwhelming at the time for a person to be able to integrate it fully, especially in the absence of adequate emotional support. Chronic dissociation among parts of the personality or self may become a "survival strategy" in those who have experienced early childhood trauma. To some degree, dissociation allows a person to try to go on with normal life by continuing to avoid being overwhelmed by extremely stressful experiences in both the present and the past. Unfortunately, it also leaves one or more parts of the person "stuck" in unresolved experiences and another part forever trying to avoid these unintegrated experiences.

It is important for you to know that in your journey toward understanding and coping with your dissociation, you do not need to focus immediately on the painful past. Rather, the first goal is to make sense of the dissociative aspects of yourself and to learn to deal more effectively with them so you can feel better in your daily life. Resolving the past comes after you learn to cope in the present both with your external and with your inner world.

There are biological, social, and environmental factors that make people more vulnerable to dissociation. Some people may have a biological tendency to dissociate or perhaps have organic problems with their brain that make it more difficult for them to integrate experience in general. Young children have less ability to integrate traumatic experiences than adults because their brains are not yet mature enough to do so. Their sense of self and personality are not yet very cohesive, and thus they are more prone to dissociation. And it has long been recognized that those without sufficient social and emotional support are more vulnerable to developing chronic trauma-related disorders, especially those who experience chronic childhood abuse and neglect. Finally, many families simply lack the skills to deal well with difficult feelings and topics; thus, they cannot help children who have been overwhelmed to learn effective emotional coping skills. Such skills are needed to overcome dissociation and resolve traumatic experiences. It is these skills, among others, that you will learn in this manual.

Dissociative Disorders

When people dissociate chronically in ways that disrupt their lives, they may be diagnosed with a dissociative disorder. There are several dissociative disorders, and it is important to know that these classifications cannot completely describe any individual; in fact, we are still learning about dissociation. There is general agreement, however, that the major complex dissociative disorders typically develop in childhood, and that they are the result of disruptions in the integration of the child's personality and sense of self, the effects of which continue on into adulthood.

At present, there are two classifications of diagnoses, and they differ to some degree from each other. One is the *Diagnostic and Statistical Manual of Mental Disorders* (*DSM*), which is currently in its fourth edition (American Psychiatric Association [APA], 1994), with the fifth in progress at the time of publication of this manual. Each new edition includes changes to the criteria for mental diagnoses based on further research and other developments in the mental health field. The *DSM* is the major classification system that is used in the United States and many other countries. The other classification system is published by the World Health Organization (WHO) and is known as the *International Classification of Diseases* (*ICD*). Some European and other countries primarily use the current 10th edition of the *ICD* (WHO, 1992). If we consider a continuum of trauma-related disorders, with posttraumatic stress disorder (PTSD) being the most basic, and developing in the aftermath of a traumatizing incident at any age, then complex dissociative disorders are a more pervasive developmental accommodation to trauma that originates in childhood, and they are further along the continuum.

This manual focuses on two particular dissociative disorders: Dissociative Identity Disorder (DID) and another dissociative disorder that is a kind of catchall category for people who have milder but similar symptoms of DID, called Dissociative Disorder Not Otherwise Specified, Type 1b (DDNOS) (see Appendix A). This latter disorder actually includes the majority of people who seek treatment for a dissociative disorder. The central difficulty in both disorders is a dissociation of the personality and self in which dissociative parts may take control of behavior or experience, or influence the person's behavior or experience from within. Of course, all dissociative parts compose the single personality of the person as a whole (International Society for the Study of Trauma and Dissociation [ISSTD], in press; Kluft, 2006; Putnam, 1989; Ross, 1997; Van der Hart et al., 2006).

You should discuss your diagnosis with your therapist if you have questions or concerns. Remember, diagnoses are not labels that make a statement about who you are. Rather, they are just ways to categorize broad experiences so that your therapist can help you. Most people with complex dissociative disorders first enter therapy with other complaints, such as anxiety, panic, depression, eating and sleeping difficulties, substance abuse, self-harm, suicidal tendencies, somatic problems, pseudoseizures, and relational difficulties. If the therapist does not adequately screen for an underlying dissociative disorder, such a person can spend much time in treatment without necessarily getting the relief that he or she needs. Usually these problems or symptoms will resolve when it becomes clear how they are related to an underlying dissociation of the personality, because dissociation can maintain these symptoms until it is addressed.

In this manual we have tried to offer practical help for you to cope with symptoms of dissociation that trouble you, rather than to focus on diagnosis. Of course, diagnosis is important, because it provides a map for you and your therapist to follow so that you get proper help. But because the diagnostic criteria change from time to time, and there are even legitimate disagreements about these criteria, it is probably most helpful for you to focus on what will aid you in resolving the dissociation that hampers your life, rather than to worry too much about your diagnosis.

Practice the exercise at the beginning of the chapter: Learning to be Present. Practice at least twice a day for a few minutes each time. You might try doing the exercise as soon as you get up and just before going to bed. You can also do this kind of exercise for a few moments wherever you are during the day.

Homework Sheet 1.1
Reflections on What You Have Learned

Reflect on what you have read in this chapter about dissociation.

• Notice and write down what may and may not fit your experience.

• Notice and write down any thoughts, emotions, concerns, fears, questions, or other experiences that come to your mind.

• Notice if you tend to want to avoid the topic, and if so, how you avoid.

CHAPTER TWO

Symptoms of Dissociation

AGENDA

- Welcome and reflections on the previous session
- Exercise: Learning to Be Present
- Topic: Symptoms of Dissociation

  ○ Introduction
  ○ Problems With Identity or Sense of Self
  ○ Experiencing Too Little: Dissociative Symptoms Involving Apparent Loss of Function
  ○ Experiencing Too Much: Dissociative Symptoms Involving Intrusions
  ○ Other Changes in Awareness
  ○ Expansion of the Learning to Be Present Exercise: Finding Your Own Anchors to the Present

- Homework

  ○ Reread the chapter.
  ○ Complete Homework Sheet 2.1, Recognizing Dissociative Symptoms.
  ○ Continue to practice the Learning to Be Present exercise twice a day, morning and evening (see chapter 1).
  ○ Complete Homework Sheet 2.2, List of Safe Anchors to the Present.

Introduction

Dissociation involves a wide array of symptoms, from mild to severe, from temporary to chronic. For those with dissociative disorders, symptoms are generally chronic and interfere with daily life, at least to a degree. Some dissociative symptoms are not only found in dissociative disorders but also in other psychiatric disorders. Among professionals there is an ongoing discussion about which symptoms should be considered dissociative, and which may be other, more common, symptoms related to changes in awareness and consciousness that everyone experiences to some degree. In this and the following chapter, we will describe the most important symptoms of dissociation.

Problems With Identity or Sense of Self

The majority of people with a dissociative disorder do not come to therapy with complaints about their identity or sense of self. Instead, they seek help for other problems, such as depression, anxiety, sleep problems, or relationship problems. But they also experience what seem to be strange and frightening symptoms that do not make sense, and which often lead them to fear they are "crazy." They often have few words to describe these inner experiences and may not share them unless asked because they are ashamed. In fact, these symptoms are usually related to the disowned actions of other parts of the personality or self. Once people understand their dissociative symptoms, they usually begin to feel more comfortable.

One of the major symptoms of dissociation is a *sense of involuntariness*, that is, a person is aware of thoughts, feelings, behaviors, memories, and events, and so forth, but these experiences do not seem to belong to him or her. These experiences have a quality of "not me." Some people have a sense of being "more than one person" or of having different "voices" or identities, some of which may have their own name, age, and other characteristics that are different from the person's experience of his or her own identity.

Each dissociative part of the personality has the potential to develop a relatively individual view of self, others, and the world, often with diverse thoughts, predictions, feelings and behavior from other parts, even if very limited. As a result, individuals with a dissociative disorder can be very confused about who they really are, what they think, feel, do, wish, or experience in their body. *Dissociative parts of the personality are not actually separate identities or personalities in one body, but rather parts of a single individual that are not yet functioning together in a smooth, coordinated, and flexible way.* In the next chapter we will describe dissociative parts of the personality in more detail.

The inner division of the personality can manifest in a range of symptoms that can be described in terms of experiencing "too little" or "too much."

Experiencing Too Little: Dissociative Symptoms Involving Apparent Loss of Functions

Some dissociative symptoms involve apparent loss of certain functions or experiences that, in principle, you should be able to own. Thus, you experience "too little." For example, you may have amnesia, the loss of ("too little") memory for important events or segments of your life. Or perhaps you may suddenly seem to lose a skill or knowledge that otherwise is a natural part of your life, such as being able to drive or manage money. Commonly, people who dissociate report that they suddenly are unable to feel an emotion or sensation in their body: They become emotionally or physically numb. These losses are not permanent or due to medical conditions, such as dementia or neurological problems. They are due to the activity of other parts of the personality that are rather separate from you.

These losses are only "apparent" because the function or experience that tends not to be available to you may actually be available to another part of yourself. For example, although you may not remember being afraid as a child, another part feels fear or terror whenever certain reminders of childhood events are evoked. You can see from this example that while you may experience too little (emotional numbness), another part of you may be experiencing too much, for example, overwhelming feelings. We will discuss symptoms of experiencing "too much" later in the chapter.

Dissociative Amnesia (Loss of Memory)

Everyone has natural amnesia for most of life prior to the age of 3 years because of immaturity of the brain, and people may not recall too much about the years before school. Of course, no one remembers everything that has happened to him or her, and everyone has a degree of normal forgetfulness and memory distortion. But generally people should have a fairly consistent recollection of their lives and the major events in their lives by the time they start elementary school, enough to be able to tell a flowing narrative about themselves.

Amnesia goes far beyond normal forgetfulness. It involves serious memory problems that are not caused by illness or extreme fatigue, by alcohol or other mind-altering substances, or normal forgetting. Amnesia falls on a continuum. People with a dissociative disorder may recall some aspects of an event but not other essential parts of it. In some cases all memory for certain events is unavailable for conscious recall. Some people with a dissociative disorder describe their memory as being like "Swiss cheese holes," "foggy," or "full of black holes." They may suspect that something happened, or may have even been told by others that something happened to them, but have no personal recollection of events and often feel afraid to think about them. People may have amnesia for longer periods of time during which normal life events took place, for example, a person may report being unable to remember anything from the fifth grade, or from ages 9–12.

People may not only have amnesia for the past but also for the present. This is called "time loss" and is a hallmark symptom of DIDs. People may find themselves in a place and have no idea how they got there, or they may report that there are hours or even days when they do not know what they have been doing. Or they discover that they have evidently done something (such as shopping or going to the library) but have no memory of doing so. They may meet others who recognize them, but have no recollection of ever meeting the other person. Some people find that others talk to them about a topic as though there had been some previous conversations about it, but they do not recall any conversations, and the topic does not seem familiar.

These symptoms, when they are not due to stressful inattention, are often related to the fact that one part is engaging in a behavior of which another part has limited or no awareness. Thus, there are parts that go shopping or to the library, while other parts are unaware of these actions, or in more extreme cases, parts that may have their own friends while other parts have never met these people. Frequent or prolonged time loss is much more common in DID than in DDNOS.

Time Distortions
People with a dissociative disorder often have related problems of *time distortion* (Van der Hart & Steele, 1997). They experience time passing by much too slow or fast; perhaps more time has passed than they thought, or an hour seems like an entire day. Some parts of the personality are often quite confused about where they are in space and time, believing they are still in the past.

Alienation or Estrangement From Yourself or Your Body (Depersonalization)
Many people normally experience temporary forms of depersonalization when tired or stressed, and it is a common symptom in many mental disorders. There is some discussion among professionals about whether some depersonalization symptoms are dissociative or whether they might be bet-

ter categorized as other kinds of changes in awareness (Boon & Draijer, 1993, 1995; Steele, Dorahy, Van der Hart, & Nijenhuis, 2009; Van der Hart et al., 2006). We describe these other changes of awareness in the last paragraph of this chapter.

Feeling estranged from yourself often involves dissociative parts of the personality, for example, one part of you may feel numb, blank, or foggy, but there may be another part that likely is overwhelmed. Or you may have the experience of watching yourself from outside your body, and see another part of yourself doing things as if you are watching someone else.

Some people with a dissociative disorder are able to know and recall what has happened in a situation, that is, they do not have amnesia, but they feel as if it did not really happen to them personally, as if it was a movie or a dream they were watching. Or they may know it happened, but they do not realize it happened to them, as though they were watching it happen to another person. In this way, they are able to continue to distance themselves from overwhelming experiences. Disconnection from emotions can make people feel as if they exist solely "in their head," as if they are dead inside, or like they are "wrapped in cotton," or feel like "cardboard" or "one dimensional." It seems as though they are not really in the present; they feel unreal, like they do not really exist or have any control over their actions. Some people also report a sense of being on automatic pilot or like a robot.

When people with a dissociative disorder are alienated from their body, they may be insensitive to physical pain or lack sensation in parts of their body. Some people report that they do not always properly register heat and cold, cannot feel whether they are hungry or tired, or feel numb in their body. Again, it is typically the case that other parts of the self do feel the physical pain, the hunger, or other bodily sensations.

There are many different symptoms of depersonalization, but in every case it seems to be a way of avoiding or attempting to regulate overwhelming feelings or experiences. Depersonalization symptoms may be temporary or chronic.

Alienation or Estrangement From Your Surroundings (Derealization)

In addition to alienation from yourself, you may also have the unsettling experience that your surroundings or people around you seem unreal. For example, your own house may appear to be unfamiliar, strange, or unreal, as though you are visiting someone else's house. Or a person you know well may seem strange and unfamiliar. The world may feel unreal as though you are in a dream or a play. Sometimes your surroundings may appear hazy, foggy, or distant. People's voices may sound very far away, as if down a long tunnel, even though they are close, or they seem far away visually even though they are right next to you. In people with a dissociative disorder, these symptoms of unfamiliarity or unreality may, at least some of the time, be related to parts of the personality that are living in trauma time, that is, they confuse the present with the past and thus do not experience the present as real or familiar. These parts may influence your perception of the reality to such an extent that you can become confused.

Experiencing Too Much: Dissociative Symptoms Involving Intrusions

Dissociative intrusions are those symptoms that occur when one dissociative part intrudes into the experience of another. Intrusions may happen in any arena of experience: memories, thoughts, feelings, perceptions, ideas, wishes, needs, movements, or behaviors. That is why so many different symptoms have a dissociative underpinning.

Possible dissociative intrusions include flashbacks of past traumatic events; sudden feelings, thoughts, impulses, or behaviors that come "out of the blue;" unexplained pain or other sensations that have no known medical cause; a sense of being physically controlled by someone else or other forces beyond your control; hearing voices commenting, arguing, criticizing, crying, or speaking in the background; or other jarring inner experiences that do not feel like your own. These experiences occur when a dissociative part of yourself enters your conscious awareness and you are privy to at least some aspects of what that part of you is experiencing. Such symptoms may wax and wane, depending on the circumstances and how much stress you are under.

At least in the beginning of therapy, it is often hard to know whether a symptom is dissociative, that is, related to a dissociative part of the personality. It is important for you to take your time in understanding the origin and meaning of your symptoms. One difficulty in recognizing dissociation is that people sometimes do not have words to describe their symptoms. It is important for you to practice being aware of and describing inner experiences, whether dissociative or not. This awareness will allow you to make more sense out of all of your experiences, and it will gradually help you cope more effectively with your inner experiences. The homework exercises at the end of the chapter are designed to help you become more aware of and more able to describe your dissociative experiences.

Other Changes in Awareness

Dissociation is strongly associated with other changes in awareness that are common in everyone and are also found in other mental disorders; thus, they are not unique to dissociative disorders. These symptoms may be easily produced by fatigue, illness and stress, and drugs or alcohol, and they are often only temporary. They include not feeling present; spacing out; being very forgetful and losing track of time; inability to concentrate or pay attention; being so absorbed in an activity (for instance, reading a book or watching a movie) that you do not notice what is going on around you; daydreaming; imaginative involvement; trance-like behavior, including "highway hypnosis"—driving so automatically that you do not recall much of your trip and sometimes miss your exit; time distortions; and low mental energy.

These symptoms may range from mild to severe, may be merely an aggravation, or may seriously impair a person's function, and they may be more temporary or more chronic (Steele et al., 2009; Van der Hart et al., 2006). People who have a dissociative disorder often suffer from many of these changes in awareness to a serious degree, in addition to symptoms related to dissociative parts of the personality or self. In fact, each dissociative part may experience variations of these problems with awareness, and the intrusion or interference of dissociative parts may also result in some changes in awareness.

EXPANSION OF THE LEARNING TO BE PRESENT EXERCISE: FINDING YOUR OWN ANCHORS TO THE PRESENT

You can expand the exercise from chapter 1, to be present in the here and now, and tailor it to your specific needs. Practice this exercise in your own home, finding anchors to the present in each room. Always begin this exercise when you are rested, preferably during the day, as light helps you stay more present. In fact, all new exercises should be practiced at times when you are at your best, because this is when you are most able to learn from them. Once you become more practiced, it will be easier to employ them when you are stressed.

> Walk around your home and in each room concentrate on the various things you can see, the sounds you hear, the smells you can smell, the things you might taste in the kitchen, the things you can touch or hold. What is important is that you find things that are neutral or pleasing to experience, that is, to see, hear, touch, and that connect you to the present. For example, look at a picture or poster on the wall, listen to music that you like, taste something pleasant from the kitchen, and so on. For each room, choose three things you can see, hear, feel, or touch. Consider whether you might want to make a written list of these anchors to have available when you need them, because people often forget to use their anchors when they are under stress. You may even ask someone to record a list of these things for you on audiotape, so you can listen to them when you feel stressed. The point is for you to concentrate on objects that help you to realize that you

are in the present, and for you to have these available when you need to ground and orient yourself in the present in your home. Thus, every room of your home should now have anchors, familiar places or objects that ground you and remind you to be present. When you are having a hard time, use these anchors repeatedly to help keep you, and all parts of you, in the safe present.

You might even want to buy a little something for yourself that reminds you of being in the present and give it a special place in your home, for example, a photo, a stone, a statue, anything that may help you or parts inside to connect to the present. Every time you look at it or pick it up, you remind yourself that this object is from the present and you are here and now with it. Some parts of your personality may find different items more important or helpful for grounding than you do. And some may not like something you choose. For example, some parts who experience themselves as younger may want to have something that adult parts may believe is childish. Yet it is often these young parts that have the most trouble staying present and need help in doing so. Try to be inclusive and respectful, so that all parts of yourself get what you need to feel safe and comfortable.

Note: As you search for anchors to the present in your home, you may come across items that remind you of painful experiences in the past. For the time being, put these away if you are able. You can find specific suggestions about how to avoid or reduce these traumatic reminders in chapter 15. Some objects may trigger painful experiences for one part of you, but not for another; thus, it is important to take into account the needs and feelings of all parts as best you can when deciding whether to remove or avoid certain items.

Homework Sheet 2.1
Recognizing Dissociative Symptoms

1. What was it like for you to read about dissociative symptoms?

    a. Describe your thoughts, emotions, and/or physical sensations as you read about the symptoms. For example, did you feel relief, confusion, fear, shame?

    b. Describe whether and how some of these symptoms may fit your experience.

2. Circle any two dissociative symptoms that you may have noticed in the past week:

- Sense of fragmentation or division of self or personality (may include some awareness of dissociative parts)
- Amnesia in the present
- Alienation from yourself or your body
- Alienation from your surroundings
- Experiencing too little: loss of functions
- Experiencing too much: intrusions
- Other changes in awareness

3. Describe your experience of each of these two symptoms and how they affected your functioning at the time.

4. What have you done in the past that has helped you deal with these dissociative experiences?

5. What dissociative symptoms would you most like help with?

Homework Sheet 2.2
List of Safe Anchors to the Present

Reread the instructions for finding anchors in your home.

1. Make a list below of anchors in each room of your home (for example, bedroom, bathroom, living room, and kitchen). Notice your experience when you think of these anchors.

2. Make a list of anchors in other places where it is important for you to stay present, for example, in the car, in your therapist's office, or at work or school.

CHAPTER THREE

Understanding Dissociative Parts of the Personality

AGENDA

- Welcome and reflections on previous session
- Discussion of homework
- Topic: Understanding Dissociative Parts of the Personality

    o Introduction
    o The Inner World of the Dissociative Individual
    o The Meaning and Functions of Specific Types of Parts of the Personality

- Review of exercise on Developing Personal Anchors
- Homework

    o Reread the chapter.
    o Continue to practice the Learning to Be Present exercise.
    o Complete your list of anchors.
    o Complete Homework Sheet 3.1, Identifying Dissociative Symptoms.
    o Complete Homework Sheet 3.2, Recognizing Dissociative Parts of Yourself.

Note: This chapter contains a significant amount of material. If you are using this manual in a group setting, it may be helpful to take more than one session to cover the content.

Introduction

People with a complex dissociative disorder have a dissociative organization of their personality that is comprised of two or more dissociative parts, each having (at least somewhat) different responses, feelings, thoughts, perceptions, physical sensations, and behaviors. The inner world of these individuals involves interactions among various parts of the personality, whether or not within conscious awareness. Everyone's personality, as we noted before, is a complex dynamic system that, like all systems, involves continuous actions and reactions, with parts of the system interfacing for better or worse. Dissociative parts may take control or influence the person as a whole to a greater or lesser extent. As we have noted, these parts, no matter how separate they are experienced, are not other "people" or full "personalities," but rather are manifestations of the way in which your single personality is organized. You are still one person, although we understand that you may not always feel that way.

The Inner World of the Dissociative Individual

Images of the "Inner World" of Dissociative Parts

Many people with a dissociative disorder (though not all) visualize an inner space or world in which their parts reside, and they may also visualize an image of a particular part. They may describe inner scenes such as hallways with doors, houses with rooms, or particular scenes in which parts "live," such as a child huddled in the corner, or a teenager with stringy hair who looks very angry. These images are helpful because they can be changed therapeutically to increase inner safety and communication. For instance, rooms may have intercoms installed for better communication, or the image of a warm blanket or stuffed toy might be added to the picture of a child huddled in the corner to increase a sense of safety and comfort.

The Basic Functions of Parts of the Personality

Although each person may have some unique features of his or her dissociative parts, there are some typical underlying similarities in the basic functions of parts. When people have been traumatized, their personality is generally organized into at least two types of parts based on functions. The first type of part is focused on dealing with daily life and avoiding traumatic memories, while the second type is stuck in past traumatic experiences and focused on defense against threat (Van der Hart et al., 2006).

The part(s) of the personality that function in daily life often comprise the major portion of the personality. Most people with DDNOS have only a single part that functions in daily life, while those with DID have more than one. This type of part usually avoids dealing with or even acknowledging other parts, though it may be influenced by them in various ways, which we will discuss below. This part may avoid situations or experiences that might evoke traumatic memories. Such avoidance originally helps people cope with daily life while keeping painful (past) experiences at bay. However, over time, it results in a life that becomes increasingly limited.

While the part of the personality that copes with daily life is avoidant, at least one other and usually more than one other part remain "stuck" in traumatic memories and think, feel, perceive, and behave as though these events are still happening (at least to a degree) or are about to happen again. These parts are typically stuck in repeating behaviors that are protective during threat, even when they are not appropriate. For example, some parts fight to protect even when you do not need such protection in the present, others want to avoid or run away even though you are safe, some freeze in fear, and others completely collapse. These parts are often highly emotional, not very rational, limited in their thinking and perceptions, not oriented to the present time, and are overwhelmed. They primarily live in trauma-time, that is, they continue to experience the traumatic past as the present, and hold emotions, beliefs, sensations, and so forth that are related to traumatic experiences.

Awareness of Parts for Each Other

Dissociative parts may have varying degrees of awareness for each other. Some are not aware at all of other parts or are only aware of a few other parts. One part may be aware of another, but not vice versa. Some may be aware that other parts exist but do not understand the meaning of those parts. Even when parts are aware of each other's existence, they often are not in agreement about issues that are important to the person as a whole. One of your goals in using this manual is to learn to develop skills for reaching agreements among parts—which is different from forcing other parts to comply with you or ignoring their needs.

The Influence of Parts on Each Other

Regardless of the degree to which parts are or are not aware of each other, they do influence each other. Any part may intrude on and influence the experience of the part that is functioning in daily life without taking full control of functioning, an experience referred to as *passive influence* (Kluft, 1987) or *partial intrusion* (Dell, 2002). In the previous chapter we discussed briefly some of these intrusion symptoms. You can be influenced by other parts in your thoughts, feelings, body sensations, perceptions, urges, or behaviors. For example, while in a store, people with a dissociative disorder may hear an inner voice that says, "Get out, get out, it's not safe in here! You have to go home!" even though they know that nothing is wrong. This is more than a wish, but rather a desperate inner voice that comes from another part of the personality that may be visualized as a terrified young child. Perhaps such individuals might also hear or sense other inner voices that tell the child part to shut up or that complain about how stupid they are to go shopping because they do not need anything.

Such people may then feel confused, ashamed, and afraid of what is happening inside themselves and might feel a sense of impending doom, as though something terrible is about to happen. And all the while, they remain aware that they are simply in a store where everyone else is going about their business quite normally. In addition, they may hear or sense interactions among several inner parts so they feel like a bystander to a conversation or argument in which they are not included.

These intrusions have a different quality than the normal distress some people without a dissociative disorder may experience in a crowded store ("*This store is crowded and I am eager to finish and leave*"). Instead, it is as though a person with a dissociative disorder has (at least) two completely different minds that do not understand each other or are conversing about completely different topics. These intrusions may seem so bizarre or alien that you might have worried that you are insane, but this is not the case. Even though you may not fully understand yet, other parts of you have their own agendas, their own perceptions, thoughts, feelings, wishes, needs, and so forth for good reasons. Your challenge is to learn about and accept them without judgment, even if you do not agree with them. Only from that point of understanding can you make changes that support all parts in working together more smoothly.

Executive Control

In some cases, especially in DID, one dissociative part may take full control of your behavior in the world. The process of one part taking over from another, often an involuntary event, is called *switching*. If you experience switching, you may lose time when another part of you is in control. Or perhaps you are aware of what is happening, but it is as though you are watching and have no control over your behavior. For example, one person lost time whenever she was in a crowded store. She "came to" in her car with all her groceries but could not remember buying them. Another person experienced watching herself in the store as though she were walking behind herself or seeing herself from above, outside her body, wondering why she was being so slow in shopping. She reported being back in her body once she returned to her car.

Most dissociative parts influence your experience from the inside rather than exert complete control, that is, through passive influence. In fact, many parts never take complete control of a person, but are only experienced internally. Frequent switching may be a sign of severe stress and inner conflict in most individuals. However, for some patients with DID, switching in daily life is common.

Elaboration and Autonomy of Parts

Parts of the personality may have a very wide range of elaboration of their characteristics, and autonomy, that is, a sense of being separate from other parts (Kluft, 1999, 2006; Putnam, 1997; Ross, 1997; Van der Hart et al., 2006). Some may have their own names, ages, sex, and preferences, but not all of them. But each part does, at the least, have a set of relatively limited memories, perceptions, thoughts, emotions, and behaviors. A few parts may become quite elaborated, with a much wider range of actions, skills, and more complex sense of self, particularly in individuals with DID. For example, a part may be active at work and also in social situations, requiring very complex emotions, thoughts, behaviors, and sense of self, while another part may only cry without words and feel afraid. This latter part has a very limited repertoire of experiences, behaviors, emotion, thoughts, and perceptions. Of course, most people with dissociative disorders have a single main part of the personality that is quite separate and complex, and which functions in the world. As a general rule, the more parts, that is, the more fragmented the personality, the more rigid and limited is the experience of many (not all) such parts. The more active a part, the more interactions with other people and with other parts, the more this part may extend its own life history and activities. Parts also vary in their degree of autonomy, that is, the degree to which they are able to act on their own outside the control of other parts, including gaining full or executive control (Chu, 1998; Kluft, 1999, 2006; Putnam, 1997; Ross, 1997; Van der Hart et al., 2006).

Number of Parts

People sometimes wonder how many parts they may have. The actual number is not important in itself. It is significant only in that the greater the fragmentation of the personality, the lower the person's integrative capacity tends to be. This usually means that people who have "more" parts may need to work more in therapy on increasing their capacity to integrate their experiences.

The Meaning and Functions of Specific Types of Parts of the Personality

Parts of the personality have their own unique characteristics based on their functions within the person as a whole. Their characteristics, such as age, gender, emotional range, beliefs, and behaviors indicate what still needs to be integrated for the whole person. For example, a very young child part who calls for her mother likely holds longings for love and care that the person as a whole has found overwhelming, shameful, or otherwise unacceptable. Because parts of the personality are representations, they may take an infinite variety of forms, limited only by a person's experience and creativity. For example, a strong male part in a female individual protected her when she was vulnerable in a frightening situation, thus avoiding the realization that she was actually helpless. Another person described a part as a bird. That part could eventually be understood as a part that, in her imagination, tried to fly away and escape when experiences were overwhelming. Thus, the characteristics of a part are informative but are not the important focus of therapy, and they should not be taken literally. It is the *meaning and function* of what they represent that is essential for you (and your therapist) to understand.

Parts of the Personality With Functions in Daily Life

As noted earlier, people with DDNOS have one major part of their personality that functions in daily life, while those with DID have more than one part active in the world, for example, parts that go to work or take care of children. In extreme cases of DID, parts that function in daily life are not aware of each other. More commonly, there is some awareness, at least for many individuals, but also a degree of avoidance. And most parts that function in daily life are phobic of parts stuck in trauma-time.

Parts of the Personality That Hold Traumatizing Experiences

There are several typical types of parts of the personality that are stuck in trauma-time. These parts are representations of common conflicts and experiences that tend to be difficult to integrate. Please note that the following descriptions are general and that the examples that are given may not fit for you. It is important that you accept your own inner experience as it is and not try to make it fit any descriptions in this manual.

Young parts. Most people with a dissociative disorder who experienced childhood trauma will have parts of the personality that experience themselves as younger than the person's actual age: adolescents, child parts of primary school age, and even toddler or infant parts. It is as though these parts are stuck in various developmental time periods of the past. They often hold traumatic memories, distressing, painful emotions or sensations, but sometimes also have positive memories. They typically hold unresolved feelings of longing, loneliness, dependency, and need for comfort, help, and safety, and also of distrust and fear of rejection or abandonment. These parts will be discussed more thoroughly in chapter 25.

Of course, it is completely natural and understandable that people who have been neglected or abused have these experiences of need. At the same time it is common for other parts of themselves to find these normal needs repulsive or dangerous, because they have had negative past experiences with expressing what they want or need. Thus, some parts of the personality reject "needy" parts and have the belief that it is better to have no needs and to be completely self-reliant. This sets up a typical inner conflict between parts that need and parts that are fearful or repulsed by those needs.

Helper parts. Some people with a dissociative disorder, but certainly not all, have "helper" parts in their inner world that take care of the well-being of other parts, an inner form of regulation that can be a resource and basis for learning further self-soothing skills. Sometimes helping parts are modeled on a kind person from the past or on an appealing character from a book or movie or television. These parts are the traumatized child's attempt to soothe and comfort himself or herself. For some people, the major part of the personality who functions in daily life can learn to be quite empathic and helpful for inner parts as well.

Parts that imitate people who hurt you. Usually there are parts of the personality that hold anger and rage that are unacceptable or very frightening to other parts. Some may resemble people from the past who were abusive. These parts shame, threaten, or punish other parts inside, or they may direct their anger to other people in the outside world. Although the behavior of these parts can be quite frightening or shameful, as well as unacceptable, it is important for you to understand that these parts have good reason to exist and are representations, and thus not the same as the people who hurt you. They originally developed to protect you by containing many distressful experiences of anger, helplessness, and sometimes guilt or shame. Furthermore, their function often is to prevent other parts behaving in a way that, in the past, evoked fear or shame. Over time it is important to appreciate why they exist, even though their "methods," that is, their behavior and attitudes, may not be acceptable. Your fear and shame about these parts must be overcome in order for you to heal. These parts, like all parts of yourself, need to become part of an internal "team" that collaborate and represent you as the whole person and your own history. And once they do so, you will be surprised at what tremendous help they will be to you. These parts are further discussed in chapter 22.

Fight parts. Some angry parts are stuck in a fight defense against threat. They have the explicit function of protecting the individual by means of fight responses, either toward other people or toward parts inside that in some way evoke a sense of threat. Fight parts often believe that they are strong, have not been hurt, and are capable of carrying out strong aggressive reactions to perceived threat or disrespectful behavior. Often they view themselves as a "tough" child or teenager or a large, strong man.

Ashamed parts. Shame is a major emotion that maintains dissociation (see chapter 24 on shame). Some parts of the personality are especially avoided and reviled because they hold experiences, feelings, or behaviors that you, or some parts of you, have labeled as shameful or disgusting. You will need to be especially empathic and accepting toward these parts of yourself.

A central problem for people who have a dissociative disorder is that parts of the personality avoid each other and their painful memories and experiences, or they tend to have strong conflicts with each other. In the literature this has been described as *phobia of dissociative parts* (Van der Hart et al., 2006). Parts typically feel fearful, ashamed, or repulsed by other parts. In particular, dissociative parts that function in daily life want as little as possible to do with dissociative parts that are fixed in traumatic experiences. Parts stuck in trauma-time often feel abandoned and neglected by the parts that try to move on without them in daily life.

These ongoing inner conflicts can be painful and frightening, and they cost a person with a dissociative disorder a tremendous amount of energy. As we said before, all parts need to learn to accept and cooperate with each other. After all, in order to adapt and be at our best, we must learn to accept ourselves and all our aspects. Only in acknowledging and accepting are we able to make positive changes in ourselves.

However, we are aware that getting to know yourself and working more cooperatively internally can be a long and difficult process. You cannot expect yourself to immediately function differently when parts have spent a lifetime avoiding each other or being in conflict. Please remember that you will need much patience and self-acceptance in this work and go at your own pace. Remember to be empathic and accepting of yourself as a whole person.

The following exercises that help you to stay in the present can be useful to the parts stuck in the past, especially finding "anchors" in the present.

Homework Sheet 3.1
Identifying Dissociative Symptoms

1. Circle two dissociative symptoms that you may have had in the past week:

   o Sense of fragmentation or division of self or personality (may include some awareness of dissociative parts)
   o Alienation from yourself/not feeling real
   o Alienation from your surroundings
   o Experiencing too little/loss of function, for example, amnesia
   o Experiencing too much/intrusions

2. Describe your experiences of these symptoms and how they affected your functioning at the time.

3. What have you done in the past that has helped you deal with these dissociative experiences?

Homework Sheet 3.2
Recognizing Dissociative Parts of Yourself

There are various ways in which you can notice parts of yourself. For example, consider the following:

- You have lost time and you discover that something has been done that only you could have done, yet you have no memory of it.
- You hear yourself talking, but it seems as though the thoughts or words you hear are not your "own" and you have no control over what you say.
- You experience yourself as outside your body, as though you are looking at someone else.
- You have body sensations that do not feel they belong to you or that seem to come "out of the blue" and do not fit with your present situation. Sometimes these sensations are accompanied by feelings of fear or panic.
- You have thoughts or emotions that you experience as sudden, not appropriate to the situation, or as not belonging to you.
- You hear voices in your head that talk to you or to each other.
- You find yourself in a place and have no idea how you got there.
- You feel your body, your movements, or behaviors are not within your control.

1. Describe one example of noticing the (inner or external) actions of another part of yourself. How did you become aware of this part?

2. Describe what you understand about your own internal organization of parts. For example, how do parts of yourself seem to interact, if at all? Which parts do you avoid or are avoided by other parts of you? What emotions are held in parts of yourself? Are there parts you feel more comfortable with? Less comfortable? Do some of your parts communicate with each other?

CHAPTER FOUR

Symptoms of Posttraumatic Stress Disorder (PTSD) in Complex Dissociative Disorders

AGENDA

- Welcome and reflections on previous session
- Homework discussion
- Break
- Topic: Symptoms of PTSD in Complex Dissociative Disorders

    o Introduction
    o What Is PTSD?
    o What Are the Symptoms of PTSD?
    o DID and DDNOS as Complex Posttraumatic Stress Disorders
    o Optional Reading: Complex PTSD and Dissociation

- Homework

    o Reread the chapter.
    o Complete Homework Sheet 4.1, Identifying PTSD Symptoms.
    o Complete Homework Sheet 4.2, My Coping Skills for PTSD Symptoms.
    o Complete Homework Sheet 4.3, Repeat Practice: Learning to Identify and Cope With Dissociative Parts of Yourself.
    o Practice the Stress Reduction and Healing exercise from this chapter at least once a day.

Introduction

Trauma-related disorders have extensive overlap in symptoms, so it is possible for a person to fit several diagnostic categories. This does not mean more is wrong with you; rather, it speaks to the fact that descriptions of trauma-related disorders are not very precise and have a lot of overlap. In this chapter we will discuss some of the most basic and common symptoms of trauma-related disorders, those of posttraumatic stress disorder (PTSD). Dissociative disorders are considered to be more complex forms of PTSD that arise when traumatizing events affect a child's normal personality development, and in fact, many PTSD symptoms involve dissociation. Thus, it is likely that you have had or currently experience some symptoms of PTSD. Once you understand these symptoms, you can work to overcome them with some practical skills.

What Is PTSD?

PTSD involves a set of symptoms that arise after a traumatizing event (or many events). These symptom groups include avoidance, intrusion of traumatic memories, and physiological dysregulation. These symptoms will be discussed further later on in this chapter. Posttraumatic stress symptoms develop some time after a traumatizing event. For example, PTSD is commonly seen in many victims of war, rape, and natural disasters. People with PTSD often also experience depression, substance abuse, and physical complaints. Some professionals have proposed a diagnosis called Complex PTSD, which is a category that fits somewhere between PTSD and dissociative disorders (Herman, 1992; Pelcovitz, Van der Kolk, Roth, Mandel, Kaplan, & Resick, 1997; Van der Hart, Nijenhuis, & Steele, 2005). If you like, you may read more about that proposed diagnosis in the optional reading material at the end of the chapter.

What Are the Symptoms of PTSD?

Basic symptoms of PTSD include three core groupings:

- Intrusions of traumatic experiences (for instance, flashbacks, nightmares)
- Avoidance, numbing, and detachment
- Hyperarousal (startle reflex, anxiety, fear, agitation)

Intrusion Symptoms

- Flashbacks, that is, reliving some or all of a traumatizing event as though it is happening in the present. Flashbacks can involve images, smells, sounds, taste, emotions, thoughts, and physical sensations.
- Nightmares of traumatizing events or of similar content
- Hallucinations, delusions, or illusions that are related to traumatizing events
- Severe, recurring anxiety reactions or panic, with heart palpitations, rapid breathing, sweating and trembling, and sense of impending doom
- Feeling paralyzed with fear or wanting to run away

These reactions mainly occur in situations that remind (trigger) you of a past traumatizing event, or rather some part of yourself that is "stuck" in that original situation, that is, living in trauma-time (Van der Hart, Nijenhuis, & Solomon, 2010). Thus, that part responds to these reminders with the same sense of overwhelming threat as was the case in the past.

Avoidance Symptoms

- Strong efforts to avoid any thoughts, feelings, or situations that might evoke traumatic memories, for example, by focusing too much on work, excessive cleaning, staying too busy, using drugs or alcohol, or spacing out
- Amnesia, that is, inability to recall some or all of significant aspects of traumatizing events
- Emotional numbness
- Inability to enjoy life or feel love
- Feeling as though you are on automatic pilot
- Isolation and avoidance of other people
- Reluctance to talk about traumatic experiences

Hyperarousal Symptoms

- Persistent physical symptoms of tension: tenseness, agitation, restlessness, impatience, and feeling constantly on the alert
- Jumpiness, easily startled, and hypersensitivity to what is going on around you
- Irritability, outbursts of anger or rage
- Emotional outbursts
- Serious difficulty falling asleep or frequent waking
- Concentration and attention problems

Our bodies and minds are innately prepared to deal with emergency threat situations by automatically shutting down certain activities and enhancing others. For example, digestion is slowed down, heart rate and breathing increase, blood rushes to the brain and limbs, and our muscles tense to prepare for running away or fighting. We shift from a "normal, everyday" state in which we love, learn, work, and play, to one of high alertness that involves hypervigilance, fight, flight, and/or freeze. Activity shifts from the parts of our brain that help us think through complex problems to the parts of the brain that help us react in life-threatening situations during which there is probably not enough time to think about options. These automatic actions can help us survive threat in the same way that animals of prey use them to survive a predator. Unfortunately, when dissociation occurs, parts of the personality can become stuck or fixed in being hyperaroused. When these parts are activated, you will experience symptoms of hyperarousal.

Hypoarousal Symptoms

Although hypoarousal symptoms are not currently included in the symptoms of PTSD, there has been increasing awareness and acceptance of the fact that some people experience a kind of dissociative shutdown in response to trauma, rather than hyperarousal (Lanius et al., 2010). In fact, most people with PTSD alternate between these two physiological conditions, both of which many experts consider to be dissociative. We humans are very much like mammals in our reactions to danger. In addition to hyperarousal, we—like our animal cousins—have a line of defense that involves hypoarousal. It is an automatic, unconscious physiological strategy to help ensure survival when there are no other options available. Heart rate and breathing slow drastically, muscle tone becomes limp, and our mind and bodies go into a kind of deep hibernation. We conserve energy by going into this automatic state of "collapse," sometimes called "death feigning" in animals. Opossums do this when they "play dead."

Symptoms of posttraumatic hypoarousal include the following:

- Emotional numbness
- Physical numbness, inability to feel pain
- Blank mind, unable to think or speak
- Profound detachment
- Inability to move or respond
- Extreme drowsiness and even temporary loss of consciousness

Just as with hyperarousal, hypoarousal reactions may be due to the intrusion of a part of the self that is chronically in this physical condition. Usually these parts are triggered when hyperaroused parts can no longer be effective or become exhausted.

DID and DDNOS as Complex Posttraumatic Stress Disorders

DID and DDNOS are considered to be complex trauma-related disorders on a continuum with PTSD. Thus, most people with a complex dissociative disorder have a degree of chronic posttraumatic stress symptoms. Each part of the personality may be stuck in a particular group of PTSD symptoms. For example, some parts that are fixated in traumatic memories are chronically hyperaroused, while others are extremely shut down (hypoaroused). Some parts, usually those functioning in daily life, are avoidant and emotionally constricted, or sometimes are irritable and impatient, depressed, and have nightmares and other intrusive symptoms. The work you accomplish with this manual will help you develop a strong foundation for resolving these posttraumatic stress symptoms.

STRESS REDUCTION AND HEALING EXERCISE

When you have posttraumatic stress symptoms, it is important to learn how to reduce your stress and feel calmer and more present. The exercise that follows, or a variation that you create yourself, may be helpful to you.

You will need a *stress ball*, also sometimes called a *squeeze ball*—a small soft ball that fits in the palm of your hand and which you can squeeze. These are very inexpensive and are readily available in a wide variety of stores or online. You will also need a small object to hold in your hand that represents healing and calm for yourself. Perhaps this may be one of your anchoring items, which you developed earlier, or a rock, a stuffed animal, a book—whatever you can hold in your hand and that feels right to you.

Find a position that feels comfortable, preferably sitting or standing, both feet on the floor. If you are standing, place your feet slightly apart, in line with your shoulders and keep your knees slightly bent, that is, do not lock your knees. Begin the exercise by holding a stress ball in your nondominant hand (for the right-handed person, this is the left hand and vice versa). Concentrate your attention on your nondominant hand.

Squeeze the ball as hard as possible while you imagine that you are letting all the tension and unpleasant feelings converge from all over your body and begin to flow toward your arm, down your arm, down into you hand, and then flow through your hand into the ball. You can visualize the ball as working like a magnet, drawing all the tension towards it, through your shoulder and your arm, your hand and fingers. Watching the ball and noticing your squeezing motions may help you stay focused and present. When the ball is saturated like a sponge with your tension and unpleasant feelings, you can open your hand and let go of the ball, allowing all your tension to be held in the ball, away from you. As soon as you let go of the ball, the tension leaves it and dissipates into the air, disappearing from the room. You can practice this exercise several times until you feel that all negative tension has been released out of your body. You might remind all parts of yourself that they are also welcome to use the ball to release their tension, too.

When you feel calmer and less stressed, let go of the ball one last time and turn your attention to your dominant hand (that is, the hand that you use most often; for most people, this will be the right hand), and follow the suggestions below.

Choose an object that you can easily hold in your hand, and which symbolizes a sense of well-being or healing for you, perhaps one of your anchors to the present. Hold this object in your dominant hand. Imagine that this object holds all the well-being and healing that you need: a sense of safety and contentment, of peace and calm, of mental and emotional clarity, free of tension and conflict. Now allow these feelings of well-being and healing to radiate warmly and gently from the object through your hand, your arm, your shoulder, all through your body. Allow it to gently flow through your body, your mind, and your heart. All parts of you can take in this well-being and healing in their own way, in a way that works for them. With each breath in, allow more well-being and healing to flow through you. With each out breath, let any remaining tension go.

Whenever you wish to remind yourself of this sense of well-being, your dominant hand can automatically recall the feeling of the object, its shape and texture, its temperature and color, and you can fully experience those positive feelings and sensations of well-being and healing once again. As you practice more, your dominant hand can almost automatically close as though holding the object of your healing, and at any time you wish or need, you can once again experience that sense of well-being and healing.

Homework Sheet 4.1
Identifying PTSD Symptoms

Check or underline any PTSD symptoms that you might have recently experienced. If you are not currently experiencing any symptoms, circle those you have had in the past.

Intrusion Symptoms

- Flashbacks, that is, reliving some or all of a traumatizing event as though it is happening now. Flashbacks can involve images, smells, sounds, taste, emotions, thoughts, and physical sensations.
- Nightmares
- Hallucinations, delusions, or illusions that derive from traumatizing events
- Severe, recurring anxiety reactions or panic
- Feeling paralyzed with fear or wanting to run away

Avoidance Symptoms

- Strong efforts to avoid any thoughts, feelings, or situations that might evoke traumatic memories, for example, by focusing too much on work, excessive cleaning, staying very busy, using drugs or alcohol
- Amnesia, that is, inability to recall some or all of significant aspects of traumatizing events
- Emotional numbness
- Inability to enjoy life or to feel love
- Feeling as though you are on automatic pilot
- Isolation
- Unwillingness to talk about your experience, shutting yourself off from others

Hyperarousal Symptoms

- Persistent physical symptoms of tension: tenseness, agitation, restlessness, lack of patience, and feeling constantly on the alert
- Jumpiness, easily startled, and hypersensitivity to what is going on around you
- Irritability, episodes of rage or crying
- Difficulty falling asleep or frequent waking
- Concentration and attention problems

Hypoarousal Symptoms

- Physical numbness, inability to feel pain
- Blank mind, unable to think or speak
- Profound detachment
- Inability to move or respond
- Extreme drowsiness and even temporary loss of consciousness

Homework Sheet 4.2
My Coping Skills for PTSD Symptoms

You have probably been living with trauma-related symptoms for a large part of your life, and you have likely already discovered certain things that can be of help. For example, perhaps you call a friend, write or use art, take a walk, go shopping, meditate, or exercise. Make a list some of the helpful ways you have learned to cope with these symptoms. You can add more strategies as you learn them over time.

1.

2.

3.

4.

5.

Homework Sheet 4.3
Repeat Practice: Learning to Identify and Cope With
Dissociative Parts of Yourself

This homework sheet is meant to help you practice more of what you learned in chapters 2 and 3.

1. Describe an experience of noticing a part of your personality (this may be some inner experience, such as hearing a voice, or a situation in which another part was active in the world).

2. What was your reaction to this part of you? (For example, what did you think, feel, sense, or do?)

3. What might help you become more accepting of this part? (For example, you might try understanding why this part of you feels a certain way, or know that you can get help in working with this part from your therapist.)

Optional Reading: Complex PTSD and Dissociation

Some clinicians who work extensively with PTSD have found that many trauma survivors who experienced chronic interpersonal traumatization tend to have more problems and symptoms than those who only have PTSD and who have experienced a single trauma. They thus proposed a new diagnostic category, sometimes referred to Complex PTSD or disorders of extreme stress, not otherwise specified (DESNOS; Herman, 1992; Pelcovitz et al., 1997). This diagnosis is not yet included in the *DSM* or *ICD*. People with complex dissociative disorders typically suffer from at least some of the symptoms of Complex PTSD described in the next section. As noted earlier, this proposed diagnosis falls somewhere in the middle of a continuum of trauma-related disorders, between PTSD and the currently recognized dissociative disorders in *DSM-IV*. For those with a dissociative disorder, various parts of the personality may have these symptoms, and they may be experienced by you, the person as a whole.

Symptoms of Complex PTSD

Complex PTSD consists of six symptom clusters, which also have been described in terms of dissociation of the personality (Van der Hart et al., 2005). Of course, people who receive this diagnosis often also suffer from other problems as well and diagnostic categories may overlap significantly (Dorrepaal et al., 2008). The symptom clusters are described next.

Alterations in Regulation of Affect (Emotion) and Impulses

Almost all people who are seriously traumatized have problems in tolerating and regulating their emotions and urges or impulses. However, those with Complex PTSD and dissociative disorders tend to have more difficulties than those with PTSD because disruptions in their early development have inhibited their ability to regulate themselves. The fact that you have a dissociative organization of your personality makes you highly vulnerable to rapid and unexpected changes in emotions and sudden impulses. Various parts of the personality intrude on each other either through passive influence or switching (see chapter 3) when you are under stress, resulting in dysregulation. Merely having an emotion, such as anger, may evoke other parts of you to feel fear or shame, and to engage in impulsive behaviors to stop or avoid the feelings.

Changes in Attention and Consciousness

People with Complex PTSD suffer from more severe and frequent dissociative symptoms, as well as memory and attention problems than those with simple PTSD. In addition to amnesia due to the activity of various parts of the self, people may experience difficulties with concentration, attention, other memory problems, and general spaciness. These symptoms often accompany dissociation of the personality, but they are also common in people who do not have dissociative disorders. For example, almost everyone can be spacey, absorbed in an activity, or miss an exit on the highway. When various parts of the personality are active, by definition, a person experiences some kind of abrupt change in attention and consciousness.

Changes in the Perception of Self

People who have been traumatized in childhood are often troubled by guilt, shame, and negative feelings about themselves, such as the belief that they are unlikable, unlovable, stupid, inept, dirty, worthless, lazy, and so forth. In complex dissociative disorders there are typically particular parts that contain these negative feelings about the self while other parts may evaluate themselves quite differently. Alternations among parts thus may result in rather rapid and distinct changes in self-perception (Van der Hart et al., 2005).

Changes in Relationships With Others

It is especially hard to trust other people if you have been repeatedly abused, abandoned, or betrayed as a child. Mistrust makes it very difficult to make friends, and to be able to distinguish between the good and bad intentions in other people. Some parts do not seem to trust anyone, while other parts may be so vulnerable and needy that they do not pay attention to clues that perhaps a person is not trustworthy. Some parts like to be close to others or feel a desperate need to be close and taken care of, while other parts fear being close or actively dislike people. Some parts are afraid of being in relationships, while others are afraid of being rejected or criticized. This naturally sets up major internal as well as relational conflicts.

Somatic (Physical) Symptoms

People with Complex PTSD often have medically unexplained physical symptoms such as abdominal pains, headaches, joint and muscle pain, stomach problems, and elimination problems. These people are sometimes most unfortunately mislabeled as hypochondriacs or as exaggerating their physical problems. But these problems are real, even though they may not be related to a specific physical diagnosis. Some dissociative parts that are stuck in past experiences that involved pain may intrude such that a person experiences "unexplained" pain or other physical symptoms. And more generally, chronic stress affects the body in all kind of ways, just as it does the mind. In fact, the mind and body cannot be separated. Unfortunately, the connection between current physical symptoms and past traumatizing events is not always so clear to either the individual or the physician, at least for a while. At the same time, we know that people who have suffered chronic trauma are much more likely than the average person to suffer from serious medical problems. It is therefore very important that you have physical symptoms checked out, to make sure you do not have a problem for which you need medical help.

Changes in Meaning

Finally, chronically traumatized people lose faith that good things can happen and people can be kind and trustworthy. They feel hopeless, often believing that the future will be as bad as the past, or that they will not live long enough to experience a good future. People who have a dissociative disorder may have different sets of meaning in various dissociative parts. Some parts may be relatively balanced in their worldview, others may be despairing, believing the world to be a completely negative, dangerous place, while other parts might maintain an unrealistic optimistic outlook on life.

PART ONE
SKILLS REVIEW

You have learned a number of skills in this section of the manual. Below you will find a review of those skills and an opportunity to develop them further. As you review, we encourage you to return to the chapters to read them again and repractice the homework a little at a time. Remember that regular, daily practice is essential to learn new skills.

For each skill set below, answer the following questions:

1. In what situation(s) did you practice this skill?
2. How did this skill help you?
3. What, if any, difficulties have you had in practicing this skill?
4. What additional help or resources might you need to feel more successful in mastering this skill?

Chapter 1, Learning to Be Present Exercise

1.

2.

3.

4.

Chapter 2, Developing and Using Anchors in the Present

1.

2.

3.

4.

Chapter 4, Stress Reduction and Relaxation Exercise (With Stress Ball)

1.

2.

3.

4.

PART TWO

Initial Skills for Coping With Dissociation

Overcoming the Phobia of Inner Experience

AGENDA

- Welcome and reflections on previous session
- Homework discussion
- Break
- Topic: Overcoming the Phobia of Inner Experience

  - Introduction
  - Understanding the Phobia of Inner Experience
  - Why People Develop a Phobia of Inner Experience
  - The Need to Overcome the Phobia of Inner Experience

- Homework

  - Reread the chapter.
  - Complete Homework Sheet 5.1, Becoming Aware of Avoiding Inner Experience

Introduction

Our inner experience is that which we think, feel, remember, perceive, sense, decide, plan, and predict. These experiences are actually *mental actions*, or mental activity (Van der Hart et al., 2006). Mental activity, in which we engage all the time, may or may not be accompanied by behavioral actions. It is essential that you become aware of, learn to tolerate and regulate, and even change major mental actions that affect your current life, such as negative beliefs, and feelings or reactions to the past that interfere with the present. However, it is impossible to change inner experiences if you are avoiding them because you are afraid, ashamed, or disgusted by them. Serious avoidance of your inner experiences is called *experiential avoidance* (Hayes, Wilson, Gifford, & Follette, 1996), or the *phobia of inner experience* (Steele, Van der Hart, & Nijenhuis, 2005; Van der Hart et al., 2006). In this chapter you will learn about the phobia of inner experience and build a foundation of skills to overcome it.

Understanding the Phobia of Inner Experience

Most people think of phobias as a fear and avoidance of something external such as spiders, heights, or flying. But some people can be equally terrified of a feeling like rage or sadness, of a thought or wish, or a prediction that if they try something new it will fail, or even of physical sensations such as the rapid heart beat and difficulty breathing that accompany panic. Such a phobia of inner experience may involve shame or disgust in addition to fear (Hayes, Follette, & Linehan, 2004; Van der Hart et al., 2006). The phobia of inner experience is a serious problem, contributing to ongoing psychological stress and inhibition of pleasant or spontaneous activities (Kashdana, Barrios, Forsyth, & Steger, 2006).

For example, people may be intensely ashamed of feeling rage, because they believe that emotion could only belong to a "bad" person, or because they fear the consequences of expressing it. They feel enraged, and instead of being able to deal with the anger, they increase their misery by giving themselves negative labels: Their misery has thus become compounded. Subsequently, they avoid anger and situations that might evoke anger, and any time they begin to feel angry, they recoil in shame and disgust. Other people may have intense fantasies of being cared for, yet feel very afraid, ashamed, and disgusted by these wishes, because they have negative beliefs that being "needy" or "dependent" is weak and not normal, again creating more inner distress and preventing them from accepting important needs.

Many individuals with a dissociative disorder are afraid of inner voices that come from other parts of themselves. They label themselves as "crazy" and feel ashamed and afraid of these voices. Such feelings are sometimes intensified if they have been labeled psychotic or "crazy" by mental health professionals or others who did not understand the dissociative nature of the voices.

Some inner experiences may feel so threatening that almost any means of avoidance or escape may be used, no matter how destructive. Perhaps you avoid your inner experience by working too much, so you do not have to pay attention to yourself, as Marilyn Van Derbur, a survivor of child abuse, noted: "That was my *survival mechanism*, staying so busy there was not time to have unthinkable memories surface" (2004, p. 45). Other avoidance behaviors might include using drugs or alcohol or other addictive behavior, increasing self-criticism, withdrawing from others, or blaming others for your inner problems. Of course, each dissociative part of yourself is a part of your inner experience that you likely avoid, even to the point of not feeling or knowing it is "your" experience.

Avoidance can be conscious or unconscious. We will begin by helping you be more aware of the ways in which you avoid inner experience in conscious ways. Once you become more comfortable in noticing how you consciously avoid your inner experience, you gradually can begin to feel more secure to focus on some inner experiences of which you may not yet be aware. For example, you may become more aware that you cringe and feel fear when you hear an inner voice, but you may not yet know much about why that voice exists or what that part of you experiences.

Why People Develop a Phobia of Inner Experience

Generally the phobia of inner experience develops for three different reasons. First, many people who were traumatized early in life did not get much help in learning how to understand and cope with typical intense inner experiences such as overwhelming emotions. They received too little help and reassurance from caretakers. Thus, they feel easily overwhelmed, simply because they do not understand these experiences and feel they are not controllable.

Second, people tend to evaluate their inner experience as "good" or "bad." They go on to label themselves in the same way: "Anger is bad and dangerous, so if I feel anger, I must be bad and dangerous;" "Only people who are unlovable and worthless feel shame; so if I feel shame it means I am a failure and unlovable." Of course, we all want what is good and pleasant, and we want to avoid what is painful, just as we want to be good people, not bad ones. But our inner experiences are not what make us good or bad; they are just a natural part of everyone's internal world.

Finally, certain inner experiences serve as reminders of past traumatic experiences or as signals that something terrible is about to happen. For example, when people, or some dissociative parts of themselves, feel anxious, the emotion and physical sensations may immediately remind them, even if only on an unconscious level, of the fear they felt when they were being hurt in the past. They thus try to avoid feeling anxious so as not to be reminded of unresolved traumatic memories. Others might perceive an inner experience as a signal that something is about to go wrong. For instance, a person who feels sadness may believe or merely sense that this emotion precedes an overwhelming experience of despair, lack of comfort, and aloneness. Thus, sadness is avoided to prevent the other expected and really difficult experience from occurring. The painful paradox is that what is fearfully anticipated and avoided would not likely take place if the present feeling of sadness is accepted and calmly experienced.

The Need to Overcome the Phobia of Inner Experience

It is completely understandable that you might want to avoid certain inner experiences that are related to past traumatizing events. Yet healing requires you to work with these inner experiences in order to understand and change them. And you cannot change that which you avoid or do not know. Although it may be difficult, it is essential for you to learn how to accept, understand, regulate, and cope with all of your inner experiences.

Inner experiences have good reason to exist and should not be judged as "good" or "bad." Everyone has internal experiences; some are more congruent with who you want to be, others less so. Some are more comfortable, others are not. Some are more under your control, others occur spontaneously. All humans have this wide range of inner experiences. Everyone gets angry, feels afraid, ashamed, or incompetent at times. If you are able to tolerate those feelings and their accompanying thoughts and sensations, you can begin to learn to sit back and understand a bit more about them, and thus what to do about them. Otherwise you remain a captive of your inner experience, with *it* in control of *you*.

Your work in your therapy and with this manual can help you learn to accept your inner experiences without judgment, including dissociative parts of yourself. In fact, this entire manual is geared toward helping you begin to overcome your phobia of various aspects of your inner experience and to feel less vulnerable and more comfortable as a whole person. You will learn much more about how to approach your inner experiences in the next chapter.

Homework Sheet 5.1
Becoming Aware of Avoiding Inner Experience

Each day this week try to notice a time when you consciously avoid some type of inner experience. You do not have to make yourself stop avoiding it, but just notice what you are avoiding and under what circumstances you avoid it. For example, perhaps you want to avoid a feeling of anger, a thought that things are hopeless, or the sound of a dissociative part crying or criticizing you.

Name one inner experience (emotion, thought, sensation, memory, fantasy, etc.) of which you are a little afraid or ashamed. Imagine that you put your fear or shame on a scale of 1 to 10, with 1 being very little and 10 being very much. Choose an experience that is closer to 1 or 2, so that you will not get overwhelmed.

Complete the following questions for each day of the week:

1. What inner experience did you avoid or want to avoid?

2. What were your beliefs or concerns about what might happen if you allowed yourself to accept that inner experience?

3. What did you do to avoid the experience?

4. What help or resources do you imagine you might need in order to be less avoidant of this inner experience?

Example
  1. I avoided feelings of sadness, I don't like to cry and I can't think when I am crying. There is a part of me inside that cries all the time. I hate hearing it. I just want to get away from that sound and feeling.

2. If I give in to being sad, I am afraid I will get so depressed that I cannot work. I'd like to get rid of that crying part of me. Nobody likes a crybaby.
3. I just worked and worked and kept busy all week so I didn't have time to think about it or feel anything.
4. I need help to feel safer with being sad. I am so afraid that I will never stop crying.

Sunday

Monday

Tuesday

Wednesday

Thursday

Friday

Saturday

CHAPTER SIX

Learning to Reflect

AGENDA

- Welcome and reflections on previous session
- Homework discussion
- Break
- Topic: Learning to Reflect

  ○ Introduction
  ○ Reflection: Empathic Understanding of Yourself and Others
  ○ Example of Reflective Functioning
  ○ Problems With Reflection for People With a Complex Dissociative Disorder
  ○ Retrospective Reflection
  ○ Tips for Developing Reflective Skills

- Homework

  ○ Reread the chapter.
  ○ Complete Homework Sheet 6.1, Learning to Reflect.
  ○ Complete Homework Sheet 6.2, Reflecting on Your Inner Experience in the Present.
  ○ Continue practicing the Learning to Be Present and Developing Your Anchors exercises from chapters 1 and 2.

Introduction

The empathic understanding of yourself and others involves the ability to reflect, also known as *reflective functioning.* This skill is defined more generally as the ability to consider our inner experience and make sense of it. A specific type of reflective functioning, called *mentalizing,* is the ability to accurately infer our own motivations and intentions, as well as those of others (Fonagy & Target, 1997). Reflection is an essential skill in learning to overcome the phobia of inner experience. In this chapter you will learn how to reflect on your own experience as well as how to reflect accurately on other people's intentions toward you.

Reflection: Empathic Understanding of Yourself and Others

Reflection helps us understand our own reactions rather than just being in the middle of them, and reflection supports us in changing automatic reactions to chosen responses. It also helps us more accurately predict what another person might be feeling, thinking, and what he or she is likely to do next in a relationship. When we can understand and predict ourselves and others, we naturally feel more secure and more "in sync" with those for whom we care. In other words, reflective skills involve the capacity to make sense of our own minds and the minds of others (Allen, Fonagy, & Bateman, 2008; Fonagy, Gergely, Jurist, & Target, 2002).

Most animals simply react to emotions and impulses. Their emotions direct their behaviors: Anger evokes fight or attack, hunger evokes a search for food, fear evokes freezing or running away, and so forth. With a very few exceptions—such as some primates, elephants, and dolphins—animals do not seem to have self-awareness. But as humans with self-aware minds, we have the opportunity to add richness to our experience by understanding the meaning of our mental activities, challenging narrow beliefs, and changing how we respond to what we hold in mind, and to what we believe others are thinking, feeling, or perceiving. We take in what we perceive and make sense of it based on our accumulated experiences, knowledge, and beliefs, and on our needs and goals.

Reflection helps us understand the nature of feelings, our patterns of thoughts, our emotional reactions, and our habitual movements, so that we can change them and act in ways that are more effective. Reflection also helps us realize that other people also have their own minds and their own needs and goals, which may involve quite different perceptions, thoughts, feelings, motivations, and intentions than we have. Of course, we cannot "read" people's minds by assuming we know what is there, but we can make some fairly accurate predictions based on our experience of that individual person. We can weigh different alternatives and points of view.

Example of Reflective Functioning

Imagine that you are startled by someone walking into the room unexpectedly, and you react with terror and panic, convinced you are going to be hurt. This reaction is not reflective, but rather automatic, that is, *prereflective* (Van der Hart et al., 2006). If you can reflect, you are not just stuck in this terror, in the grip of your feeling, and behaving fearfully. Rather you are able to step back from the situation a bit and observe that your fear is not proportional or even appropriate to what is happening. Instead of just feeling or thinking without awareness, you notice what you feel and think, how you experience those feelings and thoughts in your body, and perhaps why you feel and think a certain way. This is reflective functioning. You can learn to acknowledge and accept the feeling, having some empathy for yourself: *"I am feeling very afraid right now. Let me take some breaths and slow myself down. It's OK that I have this feeling even though I know I am safe."* You can learn to observe that the person who entered the room has no expression of malice, and in fact, is not even focused on you. You remind yourself that this person is known to you and would not hurt you. You can consciously relax your body. You can give yourself time to sort out why you might be feeling so very scared. Is it something from the past? Is there a dissociative part of yourself that is reacting without much awareness of the present? You can work on calming yourself down and using the fearful experience to learn more about your patterns of emotion, thought, and behavior.

Problems With Reflection for People With a Complex Dissociative Disorder

Reflective functioning is a learned skill. Children learn it over time when their caregivers are sufficiently attuned to their feelings and needs, and it can help them be curious about their mind and how it works. Unfortunately, these reflective skills are often absent to a large degree in dysfunctional and abusive families, where caregivers typically do not have these skills to pass on to their children. So you may not have had much experience with self reflection or reflecting on others. But like any skill, reflection can be learned. However, it is not always easy: Reflection takes more energy and mental work than automatic reactions, especially as you are just beginning to learn. But be patient and persistent, and it will become a natural part of your coping.

Reflective Functioning Can Be Impeded by Dissociation

As we explained in previous chapters (chapters 2 and 3), people with a complex dissociative disorder experience a division in their self or personality and, as a result, have conflicting and alternating experiences and perceptions of themselves and others. They may be influenced by wishes, needs, emotions, thoughts, and so forth, that emerge from other parts of self, and they may be relatively unaware of these parts. Thus, their inner experience seems arbitrary, inconsistent, and confusing, making reflection more difficult than usual. As we explained earlier, people may be very phobic of their inner experiences, including dissociative parts of self. This phobic reaction can seriously hamper their ability to reflect.

Revisit the earlier example about being startled by someone coming into the room unexpectedly. Imagine that you were so frightened that you dissociated and lost time as soon as someone walked in the room, and you became aware again only after the person left. You might then have no idea what happened and be afraid that perhaps something bad had occurred. The very fact that you do not remember frightens you, increasing your fear reaction. Perhaps you found yourself huddled in a corner and cannot recall how you got there, or you have a strong urge to run away and hide that does not make sense to you as an adult. Various parts of yourself may be activated; you may hear crying in your head, or yelling about what a coward you are, or a voice that urges you just to get back to work and not think about it. You may begin to have flashbacks of past traumatic experiences. Perhaps you experience contradictory feelings, impulses, thoughts, and so much inner chaos in your head that you find it hard to think at all, much less reflect on what is happening and how best to respond. These are some of the added burdens of dissociation when learning how to reflect.

The materials in this manual begin to help you overcome your dissociation through regular reflection. In this chapter you will begin to learn how to reflect on your own inner experiences, including the ways in which you interact (or avoid interacting) with dissociative parts of yourself. You will also learn more about how to reflect about other people so that you are able to "read" their intentions more accurately. In fact, you will be using reflective skills in every chapter of this book, and in therapy, so you will have a lot of practice! At first, you will learn to reflect in retrospect, that is, you may only be able to reflect on a situation after the fact. Gradually it will become a more natural skill that you employ in the moment.

Just like everyone else, you will be able to reflect most easily when you feel relatively safe, relaxed, calm, and free from distractions. You also need to learn to become more curious about yourself, for example, why you always respond to criticism by freezing, and explore the possibility of physically responding differently. You can never know everything about yourself; no one can. The first step is just accepting your experience as it is, without judgment or urgent need to change or avoid it. You do not need to know everything about yourself all at once, and in fact, uncertainty is a very normal part of everyone's experience.

Retrospective Reflection

As noted earlier, you first learn reflection by looking back at an experience. In the following section, you will find some examples of retrospective reflection that will help you understand more about how to use it for yourself, including all parts of you, and for other people.

Example 1: Using Reflection With a Chronic Reaction to an Emotion

We all develop automatic (conditioned) reactions based on past experience. For example you, or parts of yourself, may have learned to automatically isolate from others when you feel sad, because you believe you will be ridiculed or hurt when you are vulnerable (this likely involves core beliefs; see chapter 21). You may or may not realize that you are sad; you just withdraw. And perhaps you may not even be especially aware of becoming more isolated. You just stop spending time with others. Perhaps you do not even notice that you feel sad, but you hear a persistent crying or keening in your head that greatly disturbs you, or just have an uneasy sense that something is not right.

Reflection helps you notice that you feel sad, to recognize the physical sensations of sadness, and notice the thoughts that accompany the feeling. You may or may not know why you (or parts of you) are sad, but you can accept that it is what you are feeling in the present. If you hear a sad or crying voice, you do not avoid it, but try to understand and help that part of you, or perhaps ask other parts to help. The sad part of you may then feel comforted and understood, the voice quiets, and you feel calmer. You notice that you are isolating yourself, and that this may not be the best solution. You learn early signs of your tendency to withdraw so you can do something different. You call a friend to have dinner, even though it takes energy. You remind yourself that connection with others helps sadness. You can work with isolated parts of yourself to help them learn to feel safer with people. You are now learning to be more in charge of your experiences by understanding all parts of yourself better and by taking all their needs and points of view into consideration. You are learning to reflect on your own inner experience, make sense of it, and use it to help you feel better.

Example 2: Using Reflection with a Dissociative Part of Yourself

You often hear the voice of an inner part of yourself that makes negative comments about what you are doing, or says that you are stupid. You react by being afraid of that part, and even of hearing the voice, and ashamed because you believe what it says is true (at least on some level). Sometimes your reaction to the voice is so painful that you engage in some destructive behavior to make it stop, such as using alcohol or drugs, physically hurting yourself, or overeating. This cycle may go on and on. You may label yourself as crazy because you hear this voice and you feel very ashamed (see chapter 24).

Reflective skills can help you observe the process of what happens when you hear this voice, and to change your reaction to it, and eventually to change the entire interchange between you and that critical part of you. You can begin to notice what you feel as you hear that voice: perhaps crazy, or afraid, or ashamed, or frustrated. You notice when you hear that voice, you stop talking in therapy and perhaps have a panic attack. Every time you hear that inner criticism, you notice that you cringe, your body gets tight, your head hangs down, and you do not want to move. When you can notice your tendency to react without doing so immediately, you can then begin to respond differently. You can be curious about why that voice is there (you may have always assumed it is there just to speak the "truth" about yourself, but there are likely other reasons). You could begin to dialogue with the part whose voice you are hearing. You could ask that part of you to help, and begin to work to develop inner empathy and cooperation, as you will be learning through this manual. You can empathize with yourself about how painful it is to always feel criticized, scared, less than others, hopeless. You can empathize with how hard that part of you works, yet never seems to get satisfactory results. You could take some deep breaths, hold your head up, and put your shoulders back. You have options to respond to the voice that you did not have before.

In the same way that we use our ability to reflect to better understand ourselves, we also use reflection to understand the minds of other people, that is, to make sense of their motivations and intentions.

Example 3: Using Reflection to Understand Other People

You call a friend to invite her out to dinner. She does not return your call. You assume she has not responded because she does not want to be your friend anymore or that you are not important to her. You decide you do not want to have anything to do with her.

These prereflective beliefs about why your friend did not call back are typically based on your past experiences and on your ongoing fears of being rejected, long before you could even think of the many possibilities of why she might not have returned your call. They are a kind of implicit and inaccurate reflection, a reaction based on a reaction, your own reactions (from the past) rather than on really understanding your friend. And you may have contradictory thoughts and feelings about your friend coming from parts inside—some wanting to continue the relationship, some feeling she is not worth having as a friend, some believing she is dangerous—confusing you even more. However, it turns out that your friend's phone was out of order, and she did not receive the message.

You have a tendency to react the same way each time you feel rejected: You withdraw, feel hurt, and assume that people do not like or want to be around you. But reflective skills allow you to explore many possibilities of your friend's intentions toward you. We will start with the one that you probably assumed, and then move to other possibilities that allow for reconnection and relational repair.

- Your friend does not like you or care enough about you and she intentionally chose not to call you back (intentionally hurtful; the reason you assumed).
- She was sick, or out of town (unable to respond to you, and not intentional).
- She did not expect a call from you and did not check her messages (not intentional).
- She intended to call you back, but forgot to respond because there was a crisis at work or in her family (unintentional, and not because you are unimportant or she does not care, but still hurtful).
- She forgot to call you back because she tends to be scattered, forgetful, and not very reliable (in this case, her own issues have created a problem, but still it was not intentional, although hurtful).
- She *did* call you back, but when you did not answer the phone, she did not leave a message (not intentional, but irritating!).

Reflective skills can also help you sort out your own experience and those of other parts of yourself. You might say something like, "*Of course, I am disappointed that she didn't respond to me. It is only natural that I would first assume that she didn't like me or was mad at me. But I can understand that perhaps there might be other reasons she did not call back which have nothing to do with me. I feel sad that it is so hard for me to trust others, and that I always tend to assume people don't like me. It feels very lonely and shameful to feel I am not likable. Perhaps next time, if someone doesn't respond to my first call, I will take the risk to call again.*" You might have an inner dialogue with parts of yourself that may have had different interpretations of and feelings about the situation, empathizing with each one, but also reminding all parts of you that there are many possible motives and intentions behind the behavior of others. It is always helpful to get more information before jumping to conclusions.

Tips for Developing Reflective Skills

To be reflective, you will be learning how to gradually have more awareness of the present moment, of all parts of yourself, and of other people.

Be in the Present

It is impossible to reflect on your inner experience if you avoid or are not aware of it. Likewise, it is hard to reflect on your current situation if you do not feel present. Reflection begins with being as present in the moment as much as you are able, which takes consistent and concentrated practice. Use your anchors for the present (practice the exercises on anchors in chapters 1 and 2).

Notice Your Inner Experience Without Judgment

Take time to turn your attention inwardly to your thoughts, feelings, sensations, and other parts of yourself. If you do not understand what you notice, do not judge yourself; just do the best you can and move on. If you do not notice anything, do not judge yourself; simply note that you do not notice anything and move on. It helps for you to be curious about yourself, about what is going on inside, and why you think or feel or behave in particular ways.

Even though you may try to understand your mind and that of others, some of your perceptions, assumptions, or beliefs may be inaccurate (you will learn more about inaccurate thoughts and beliefs in chapters 21, 22, and 23). Your reflection may be limited by past experiences that are no longer relevant to the current situation (for example, having a prereflective belief that your therapist is going to yell at you in anger, because your parents did so, even though your therapist has never yelled) or by inaccurate beliefs and predictions (for example, believing you are crazy and will "be put away" because you hear inner voices). In fact, each part of you likely has a particular set of reactions to other people, many of them inaccurate. Notice these beliefs and thoughts, as well as the feelings and behavioral tendencies that accompany them. Write them down so you can reflect on them more easily.

Notice Similarities and Differences

It helps for you, and all parts of you, to notice similarities and differences—in your inner experience, in others, in situations. That is, you can begin to separate the past from the present, your inner fears or beliefs from external realities. You can notice that you react similarly each time you feel lonely, rejected, sad, or angry. You can notice that you have patterns of reactions that go back to your past history, that have become automatic. You can begin to notice what is different about the current circumstances that might call for a different response from you (for example, your friend will never hit you, so you need not expect it).

Be Empathic

You must be empathic with yourself, including all parts of yourself, each toward the others, and also empathic with other people's foibles and struggles. You can develop the capacity to "walk in the shoes" of another and of different parts of yourself (for instance, noticing yourself with empathy when you feel angry, incompetent, or ashamed). Over time, you will be able to recognize all parts of yourself as you. And you will learn much more about successfully developing and maintaining secure and safe relationships with others.

Homework Sheet 6.1
Learning to Reflect

Reflect in retrospect on a minor situation in which reflective skills might have been helpful. Use the aforementioned examples as a guide.

• Briefly describe the situation as you perceived it at the time.

• What were your thoughts, feelings, sensations, predictions?

• What did you do in this situation?

• If you are aware that any other parts of yourself were involved in the situation, whether directly, or by having an inner, private reaction, please describe those reactions.

• Describe ways, if any, in which dissociative parts of yourself affected your behaviors and decisions in that situation.

• Was your reaction (for example, your feelings, thoughts, sensations, or behavior), or that of other parts of yourself, a familiar pattern? If so, please describe the pattern.

• Notice in retrospect ways in which you or other parts of yourself might have reacted not only to the situation but to your own feelings, thoughts, or behaviors. For example, feeling ashamed of feeling jealous, and criticizing yourself for being jealous.

Homework Sheet 6.2
Reflecting on Your Inner Experience in the Present

1. Notice your current inner experience, including any thoughts, feelings, sensations, or other parts of yourself. Try to acknowledge and accept those experiences with interest and without judgment. Notice any possible negative reactions that may occur during this exercise, for example, thinking that this is a stupid exercise or being convinced that you cannot succeed in learning the skills in this manual. You may write down what you notice.

2. Reflecting about another person's intentions and motivations. Choose a person with whom you are acquainted but not very close, and whose behavior has bothered you at some point in time. Describe the behavior and in what ways it bothered you or other parts of yourself.

    a. Describe what you thought and felt about yourself and the other person.

    b. Describe what you imagine the other person thought and felt.

    c. Imagine and list possibilities, even if you do not agree with them, about why that person might have acted in that particular way.

d. Can you feel empathy for that person and for yourself? If so, please describe your experience of feeling empathy (for example, your thought and feelings). If not, describe what you did think and feel (without judgment).

CHAPTER SEVEN

Beginning Work With Dissociative Parts

AGENDA

- Welcome and reflections on previous session
- Homework discussion
- Topic: Beginning Work With Dissociative Parts

  ○ Introduction
  ○ Initial Dilemmas in Working With Dissociative Parts of the Self
  ○ First Steps in Working With Dissociative Parts of the Self
  ○ Forms of Inner Awareness and Communication
  ○ Techniques for Inner Communication

- Break
- Homework

  ○ Reread the chapter.
  ○ Complete Homework Sheet 7.1, Stages of Awareness and Acceptance of Dissociation.
  ○ Complete Homework Sheet 7.2., Recognizing Dissociative Parts of Yourself.
  ○ Complete Homework Sheet 7.3, Practicing Inner Communication.
  ○ Consult with your therapist as needed for help with working with parts of yourself.
  ○ Continue to practice the Learning to Be Present exercise and practice your reflecting skills.

Introduction

Connecting with yourself and reflecting on your experiences are essential tasks in which you must engage every day in order to function at your best. The more you know and understand about yourself—all of you—the better decisions you can make to improve your life. Every day you need to make many choices and compromises. All people sometimes have conflicting thoughts, wishes, needs, and feelings. This is no different for individuals with dissociative disorders, except that their inner experience happens to be organized as relatively compartmentalized or divided parts of the personality that have their own "minds," so it is harder for you to be aware of inner conflicts or to resolve them. You must learn to take into account the various needs and feelings of dissociative parts that seem as though they do not belong to yourself. In this chapter you will learn some basic approaches to understanding more about parts of yourself and how to work with them.

Initial Dilemmas in Working With Dissociative Parts of the Self

Cooperating with various parts of yourself is sometimes more easily said than done because there is so much avoidance and conflict that keeps dissociative parts separated. We previously mentioned that many people initially find it difficult to accept their diagnosis, in part because they have a strong avoidance, that is, a *phobia for dissociative parts of the personality* (Van der Hart et al., 2006). Others find it a great relief to finally be understood. People with dissociative disorders often make comments such as: "*That (part) isn't me!*" or "*That voice doesn't belong to me!*" or "*I don't want anything to do with those voices or those other parts!*" These attitudes are quite understandable and are the result of confusion about, or fear or shame of the experiences contained by other parts.

People also fear losing control to other parts because some parts may have such different or unacceptable emotions and behaviors. For instance, some parts want to come to therapy, while others would rather avoid it or believe that there is no need for it. Some parts want to focus on work, while others find work boring and would rather have fun or stay in bed. Some parts want to have a close relationship, while others are terrified of being close. Some parts are focused on daily life, while others are stuck in the past. The more you tend to avoid these conflicts and dissociative parts of yourself, the more difficulties you are likely to have in daily life. The less collaboration among parts, the more inner conflict you have.

First Steps in Working With Dissociative Parts of the Self

When you have a dissociative disorder, there are several stages of realization about how your personality and self are organized and function. In your homework in this chapter you will find a description of these stages, which range from complete unawareness or avoidance to complete acceptance. First, you must learn to acknowledge dissociative parts, and accept the sense of being and feeling fragmented. It is typical for you to need support to overcome your fear or shame of other parts of yourself. Then you can decide how you might be able to make conscious efforts to communicate internally with parts.

The first dialogues among parts should be focused on building internal communication and cooperation solely toward improving the quality of everyday life. These inner dialogues include the following:

- Learning to deal with triggers, that is, stimuli that evoke (aspects) of traumatic memories (see chapters 15 and 16)
- Increasing internal and external safety
- Working together in therapy
- Cooperating to complete daily life tasks

Traumatic memories, emotions, or sensations generally should not be shared among parts at this point. That work is for later, when you feel more calm and steady, and parts have more empathy toward each other, are working together well, and are better able to cope with emotions.

Finally, it is important to realize that various parts actually have often been cooperating for years for mutual aid or protection without your conscious awareness. Sometimes this happens almost automatically (for instance, one part automatically takes over from another part in a particular situation, or some parts that are very troubled are inactive while you are at work). Other times it is a deliberate, conscious choice.

When parts of yourself are not cooperating with each other, when they do not function in a coordinated and effective way, and when they each emphasize different priorities, then inner conflict, chaos, and confusion can ensue. The first step toward resolution is to help all parts of yourself to focus on what you are doing in the present, especially in relation to therapy and daily life tasks.

Forms of Inner Awareness and Communication

Cooperation among parts of yourself requires you to learn to accept and then communicate with all of you. We will now focus on basic inner communication.

Gradually Acknowledge and Accept Parts of Yourself

When you have not been very reflective in your life, you are not accustomed to paying attention internally. Becoming aware of parts of yourself is one of the early tasks toward the end of acknowledging and accepting yourself as a whole person, with all your thoughts, emotions, your body, and your behaviors. We have already discussed some ways in which you can begin to notice parts of yourself in Homework Sheet 2.3. Acknowledging and accepting yourself is not always easy, even for people who do not have a dissociative disorder. It can be complex and sometimes daunting at first. But each time you are aware of a part of yourself, you can also begin to be aware of how you think and feel about that part of you. Those thoughts and feelings are extremely important to your therapy work.

Once you notice parts of yourself, you can begin to accept them without judgment. When you are less judgmental, you feel less afraid or ashamed, less threatened. And when you feel less anxious, you may become more curious about parts of yourself, how they function, and how you can work together more effectively.

Listen to and Communicate With Parts of Yourself

Once you are able to acknowledge and accept parts of yourself, you can then learn to communicate, which involves listening and sharing. Many people with a dissociative disorder hear inner voices that represent various dissociative parts. They are able to carry on internal conversations. Others may experience this a little more indirectly, by "sensing" or having a kind of strange "knowing" about what parts are trying to communicate. In learning to communicate with another part, others find it helpful to imagine talking to a real person, though, of course, parts of yourself are *not* other people. The imaginal exercise is just a way to develop a better sense of other parts of you. Some people find it effective to write from the perspective of each part. It is important for you to find your own way of communicating that is comfortable for you. Listening to and talking with the voices in your head instead of trying to make them go away will ultimately be the fastest and most effective way of healing.

But initially you may find inner communication difficult. Do not hesitate to ask your therapist to help you during these initial attempts. Everyone finds it helpful to set aside a specific, quiet, calm time each day for inner communication. At first, you are likely quite naturally afraid or ashamed of parts of yourself, and you may want to avoid communication. And some parts may also want to avoid you. Sometimes it may seem as though all parts of you are talking at once. People describe this as a chaotic noise or incessant murmur in their head which is overwhelming and confusing, making it hard to think. Generally this experience occurs when you (or other parts of you) are feeling especially anxious, threatened, or ashamed.

A common difficulty in the beginning is inner threats when you try to communicate with parts of yourself. Usually this comes from a dominant, highly critical part of you. Such parts, as noted in early chapters, are only trying to protect you by reacting with the limited and rigid patterns of response that are familiar to them. These parts need help to learn more effective and empathic ways of protecting you and dealing with fear, anger, and shame. It is easiest, if possible, to start inner dialogue with a part of yourself with which you feel most comfortable.

One way to start communication is to find common ground upon which all parts can agree. For example, it is highly likely that all parts of you want to feel better, no matter how they seem to feel or act. Usually every part can agree with this goal, even though they are not likely to agree on how to achieve it in the beginning. But it is a place to start.

When daily life is going more smoothly, we all tend to feel better. One of your first objectives is to focus on learning to help all parts of you become more cooperative and communicative about daily life. You might have inner discussions, for example, about how to work together to get to appointments on time or to complete chores more efficiently, or how to best use your leisure time. You may not be able to communicate with every part of yourself immediately. This is normal and expected. It may take some time for all parts of you to feel comfortable and safe enough to allow more communication.

Techniques for Inner Communication

Following are some alternatives to "inner dialogue" that might be helpful to try.

Written Forms of Communication

Try writing to parts of yourself, introducing your therapy as an avenue of healing, and sharing your good intentions. Emphasize that even though you are scared or ashamed, you still want to make the effort to get to know all parts of yourself in a paced way. You are willing to try. Also emphasize that traumatic memories should be contained for the time being, until parts begin to feel more safe and comfortable with each other and are able to work together more effectively in daily life. Many people like to write on the computer. It is faster and the file may be deleted quickly if you are worried that someone might read what you have written. What is most important is that you begin to learn to tolerate knowing a little more about parts of yourself in the present.

Talk Inwardly

Another way of communicating or making contact is "talking inwardly," in other words, having a one-sided conversation with parts of the personality, even if you are not yet ready for them to communicate back to you. You can use this technique if you seem agitated, anxious, confused, or afraid inside. You do not always need to know immediately the reason for your inner turmoil or which part(s) is having trouble to be able to help. Just quietly talk inwardly to all parts of yourself, calming and reassuring these parts of you that you are safe, that you are willing to learn to care for yourself more effectively, that you are getting help. Remind all parts of the present by looking around and noticing your surroundings. Use your anchors in the safe present from the first two chapters. The goal is to connect to parts of yourself and let them know you are willing to pay attention and help.

Inner Meetings

Some people may be ready to conduct "inner meetings," in which parts come together internally to discuss issues. Some may find this too overwhelming or not fitting. We describe the details of this technique in chapter 27, if you feel ready to practice it at this point in time. It is essential to take your time and go at your own pace.

Homework Sheet 7.1
Stages of Awareness and Acceptance of Dissociation

Below you will find a list of steps toward acknowledging, accepting, communicating, and cooperating with parts of yourself. You should work at your own pace and not expect to be able to accomplish all these steps at once. Circle all statements that apply to you now. Later in the course of therapy, you can revisit these steps to check your progress.

- I do not want to accept that I have dissociative parts.
- I am aware that some parts exist with which I am not in communication.
- I am aware, but avoidant of (some of) my parts.
- I accept the existence of (some of) my parts.
- I am beginning to communicate with (some of) my parts.
- I can negotiate and collaborate about some issues in daily life with (some of) my parts.
- I take into account the needs of (some) parts of myself.
- I understand and accept the functions of (some of) my parts.
- I feel empathy for (some of) my parts.
- I am able to help (some of) my parts feel more safe and comfortable.
- I have regular communication with (some of) my parts to discuss issues of daily life.

Homework Sheet 7.2
Recognizing Dissociative Parts of Yourself

There are various ways in which you can notice the presence of another part of yourself. Read the following examples and see if they fit your experience. Below the examples, describe one experience of becoming aware of a part of yourself.

- You have lost time and discover that you have done something of which you have no memory, yet you know you must have done it.

- You hear yourself talking, but it seems as though the words you hear are not your "own."

- You experience yourself outside your body, as though you are looking at someone else from a distance and you cannot control your actions.

- You have thoughts, emotions, sensations, memories that you experience as not belonging to you.

- You hear voices in your head that talk to you or to each other.

- You find yourself in a place and have no idea how you got there.

- You feel your body, your movements, or actions are not within your control.

Homework Sheet 7.3
Practicing Inner Communication

Record your attempts at inner communication each day this week.
Answer these questions for each day of the week.

1. Describe what you said or did to establish empathic communication with a part of yourself.

2. Describe the response of that part of yourself.

3. What, if anything, made it difficult to communicate?

4. What if, anything, helped you communicate?

Sunday
1.

2.

3.

4.

Monday

1.

2.

3.

4.

Tuesday

1.

2.

3.

4.

Wednesday

1.

2.

3.

4.

Thursday

1.

2.

3.

4.

Friday

1.

2.

3.

4.

Saturday

1.

2.

3.

4.

CHAPTER EIGHT

Developing an Inner Sense of Safety

AGENDA

- Welcome and reflections on previous session
- Homework discussion
- Topic: Developing an Inner Sense of Safety

  ○ Introduction
  ○ Developing an Inner Sense of Safety

- Break
- Exercise: Experiencing an Inner Sense of Safety
- Homework

  ○ Reread the chapter.
  ○ Practice the exercise Experiencing an Inner Sense of Safety each day.
  ○ Complete Homework Sheet 8.1, Developing an Inner Sense of Safety and Safe Places.

Introduction

Being safe in the external environment is a major initial goal in therapy for traumatized people who are still threatened in their present-day life. In chapters 28–31 we will address the subject of choosing safe people in your life and of setting limits when you do not feel at ease with someone. If you are not safe in your current external environment, it is imperative to discuss this serious problem with your therapist, so you can get help. However, even though many traumatized people are (relatively) safe in their environment, they still do not feel safe. Thus, a major goal in therapy is to establish a sense of inner safety, of being safe with yourself, all parts of yourself, with your inner experiences. An inner sense of safety, also referred to as a *safe state* (O'Shea, 2009), is the awareness of feeling relaxed and calm in the present moment, when there is no actual threat or danger.

Developing an Inner Sense of Safety

Inner safety is strongly related to being able to be present in the here and now, and in feeling secure in at least one or two trusting relationships with other people. When young children grow up in the context of safe and trusting relationships, where they are provided a safe environment, they naturally develop an inner sense of safety. Many people with a history of early traumatization have not had many opportunities to experience a safe environment or safe relationships, and therefore they have been unable to develop a sense of inner safety and security. Thus, it may be hard for them to even imagine what it feels like to be safe. They may know cognitively that their current environment is safe, and yet they do not feel safe or comfortable at all, as though something terrible is going to happen any minute. And even when their present situation is safe, some parts of them remain stuck in trauma-time, unable to experience the safe present. In addition, traumatized individuals often do not feel safe with their own inner experiences, that is, with some of their own emotions, thoughts, sensations, and other actions of dissociative parts. Subsequent avoidance of inner experience makes it hard to stay present, and it sets in motion an inner cycle of fear, criticism, and shame, adding yet more to a lack of inner safety.

Even if you cannot imagine feeling totally safe, probably there have been times when you have felt less unsafe than others, and you can begin learning about safety from that point. If the concept of "safety" seems too foreign to you, you may think instead of a pleasant and calm place, a place where you feel understood and accepted, or perhaps a place where you are alone and know you will not be disturbed.

Next we describe ways to create a sense of inner safety, including imagery of safe places in which you and other parts of you can find safe and calm refuge from the stresses of daily life and from your painful past, until you are able to heal more fully.

Being in the Present

First, we will focus on developing an inner sense of safety in the present. It is essential to help all parts of yourself feel calm and relaxed once you are able to determine that the *present moment* is actually safe externally. You can train yourself to consciously let go of inner tension, to allow all parts of you to notice this moment of safety and well-being, of relaxation and inner quiet, even though at first these moments may be few and far between. Some parts of you may find it easier to experience an inner sense of safety than others. For some parts of you, finding that state is easier with someone whom you trust; for others it may be when you are alone, when you are with a beloved pet, listening to your favorite music, or outdoors in a special, quiet place in nature.

Most certainly, an inner sense of safety can only be experienced when your environment is actually safe. And even if there are situations that feel threatening in the present, there are still moments when you are actually safe. It is in these moments that you can begin to focus on developing an inner sense of safety.

A sense of safety can occur when all parts of you can agree to at least temporarily let go of inner conflicts and criticism and to focus on the present moment. This may be difficult to achieve and may not last long in the beginning, but you will find that all parts of you appreciate this state, and the more you practice, the easier it will become.

Developing Imaginary Inner Safe Places

Inner safe spaces are images of places where you can be safe, relaxed, and cared for. These images have been shown to be helpful to many people, not just those with dissociative disorders. This type of imaginal activity is well known to produce a feeling of relaxation and well-being in those who use it regularly. If your inner experience feels so jarring, unsafe, and frightening, as it often does in individuals with dissociative disorders, the ability to imagine these spaces becomes especially important and helpful.

When you have a dissociative disorder, some parts of you remain stuck in trauma-time and thus do not experience a sense of safety. They may be on high alert for potential danger and thus unable to relax enough to feel safe. And individuals with a dissociative disorder typically experience a vicious cycle of rage, shame, fear, and hopelessness inside that contributes to a lack of inner safety. Some parts are angry and critical, while others are hurting, afraid, or ashamed. There are often strong conflicts among these different parts. The more parts express their pain, the angrier and more hurtful other parts become, because they cannot tolerate what they consider to be "weakness." The more angry and critical parts are toward other parts, the more these parts suffer. This creates an endless loop of inner misery and lack of safety.

When you are able to create one or more imaginary safe places for parts of you that are in pain or afraid, this opens the door to the possibility of alleviating this negative loop. Angry parts feel some relief once they learn that terrified or hurting parts are quieter when they feel safer. Thus, you are able to reduce conflict by helping both types of parts simultaneously. Once you are able to develop an inner imaginary safe space, all parts of you can experience it and have it available anytime you need or want. For example, when some parts of the personality are overwhelmed, and you need to accomplish an important task, these parts may go to the safe place to rest while you complete your task. Such parts may feel calmer in an imaginary safe place until such time that they can focus on their healing during therapy. Or they can remain undisturbed in some situations that might trigger painful past experiences, such as going to a doctor or being in a meeting at work in which there is conflict.

Some people find that one imaginary place is sufficient for all parts of themselves, while others feel the need for different places that match the differing needs of parts. And of course, inner safe places should always be paired with efforts to ensure your safety with other people and in the world. You cannot have an inner sense of safety without actually being safe!

Examples of Imaginary Inner Safe Places

- Pleasant outdoor places such as lakes, meadows, streams, pools, islands, forests, mountains, oceans
- Structures: Tree houses, huts, porches, mountain and beach cottages, safe homes
- Rooms especially adapted to the needs of each part
- Safe cave or cavern
- Spacecraft
- Your own special planet
- Submarine or underwater home
- Hot air balloon
- Although technically not spaces, some people like the image of protective covering: space suit, suit of armor, invisible force field, invisible cloak (for more of this type of imagery, see "The Store" exercise in chapter 14).

You may want a safe (or quiet) place for all parts of yourself together, or some parts may want their own place. Pay close attention to what various parts of you want or need. Remember that imagination is limitless and can be continually adapted as your needs change.

If you cannot imagine a place, do not hesitate to ask your therapist to help you. Sometimes it helps to draw one or to find a picture of a place that you like. And as we noted earlier, start with a feeling of being less unsafe than at other times. You can make a list of all the comfort measures you would like to have in your safe place. Also remember that a prime rule is not to criticize or judge parts for what they imagine, and for what they want or need, even if you do not agree. Perhaps not all parts of you can yet participate; that is fine. Just start where you are able.

A safe place should be a private place that only you know about, and that no one else can find or intrude upon without your permission. If you feel especially unsafe, you can imagine that your place is surrounded by a fence, a wall, a special invisible field, or an alarm system. You are in charge of whether you allow other people there. You can also negotiate with all parts to respect each other's places and not intrude or "visit" without permission.

Your safe place can protect you or particular parts of yourself from any overwhelming stimuli in the present, and it should be comfortable and pleasant. It is a place in which you feel your needs for safety, comfort, rest, and so forth are fulfilled. Feel free to add anything you want in this place to improve your sense of comfort, well-being, and safety. You can imagine comfortable beds; your favorite foods, games, and movies; and animals that you like. Your place can be populated with animals or other people, or no one but yourself. You can have people nearby, but not too close. This place is yours to construct, and yours alone.

Any part of you may go to a safe place at any time. Some parts may voluntarily go to a safe place when there has been some inner collaboration and agreement that this might provide temporary relief or containment. However, never try to shut away or hide parts to get rid of them! Prisons are not safe places, and trying to avoid parts in this manner will only heighten your inner sense of being unsafe. It is important for all parts of you to see the value of a sense of safety and the use of safe places, and to do their best to cooperate together to create this healing image.

A literal safe place at home is also important for many people. You can create a special room or corner of a room that represents your safe place. You may add items to this place that represent safety and calm to you. Choose colors and textures that are pleasant or quieting, objects that have a positive meaning to you, photographs of people who care about you, or of places that you find pleasant.

EXERCISE: EXPERIENCING AN INNER SENSE OF SAFETY

Using the section above and Homework Sheet 8.1 as guides, you can practice developing an inner sense of safety and a safe space now. In group, you can help each other as desired, and you may use your group trainers as resources as well.

Homework Sheet 8.1
Developing an Inner Sense of Safety and Safe Places

1. Practice feeling an inner sense of safety or calm.

   a. First, describe a situation in which you can experience a moment of inner safety and/or calmness. Would it be at home alone, with another person, outside in nature, listening to music?

   b. Next, allow yourself and all parts of you to experience that inner sense of safety. Describe your experience of it, that is, your thoughts, emotions, sensations.

   c. Notice what, if anything, disrupts your inner sense of safety and describe it below. Is it a thought, a feeling, a sensation, a shift away from being present? Is it another part of you that is not yet able to share in this sense of safety in the current moment?

   d. Imagine that experience of inner safety now and notice again what it feels like.

   e. Try to create moments of inner safety every day. Regular practice improves your ability to create your inner sense of safety.

2. Describe, if you feel comfortable, your safe place. If you do not want to share it, try to describe what you feel like when you are in that place. Describe what is helpful about your safe place to you, or other parts of yourself.

3. If other parts of you need their own unique safe place, work on creating those images. Pay close attention to what those parts want or need in terms of safety and comfort. If you feel comfortable doing so, describe those places here.

4. If you have difficulties in developing an inner sense of safety or safe places, please describe what has interfered below. You are encouraged to get help from your therapist with these temporary difficulties.

PART TWO
SKILLS REVIEW

You have learned a number of skills in this section of the manual. In this section you will find a review of those skills and an opportunity to develop them further. As you review, we encourage you to return to the chapters to read them again and repractice the homework a little at a time. Remember that regular, daily practice is essential to learn new skills.

For each skill set below, answer the following questions:

1. In what situation(s) did you practice this skill?
2. How did this skill help you?
3. What, if any, difficulties have you had in practicing this skill?
4. What additional help or resources might you need to feel more successful in mastering this skill?

Chapter 5, Overcoming a Phobia of an Inner Experience (Thought, Sensation, Emotion, etc.)

1.

2.

3.

4.

Chapter 6, Reflecting on an Inner Experience

1.

2.

3.

4.

Chapter 7, Inner Communication With Parts of Yourself About Current Issues in Daily Life (Not Your Past History)

1.

2.

3.

4.

Chapter 7, Developing Empathy Toward a Part of Yourself

1.

2.

3.

4.

Chapter 7, Cooperation Among Parts of Yourself to Accomplish a Common Task or Goal in Your Daily Life

1.

2.

3.

4.

Chapter 8, Developing a Sense of Inner Safety and Safe Places

1.

2.

3.

4.

PART THREE

Improving Daily Life

Improving Sleep

AGENDA

- Welcome and reflections on previous session
- Homework discussion
- Exercise
- Break
- Topic: Improving Sleep

  - Introduction
  - Types of Sleep Problems
  - Factors That Contribute to Sleep Problems
  - Improving the Quality of Sleep
  - Tips for Dealing With Specific Sleep Problems

- Homework

  - Reread the chapter.
  - Complete Homework Sheet 9.1, Sleep Record.
  - Complete Homework Sheet 9.2, Making Your Bedroom a Pleasant Place for Sleep.
  - Complete Homework Sheet 9.3, Developing a Sleep Kit.
  - Complete Homework Sheet 9.4, Developing a Bedtime Routine.

Introduction

People with complex dissociative disorders almost always suffer from periods of disturbed sleep for a variety of reasons. Some of these may be physiological; others are related to the activity of various dissociative parts. They may even have an underlying sleep disorder. Thus, it is important to discuss your sleep problems with your primary care doctor. The less you sleep, the more tired you are. This increases your chance of struggling in daily life because you have less energy and are more prone to become emotionally vulnerable and to have difficulties with thinking. In this chapter we will discuss types of sleep problems and how to improve your sleep, including how to cope with nighttime flashbacks and nightmares, and with parts of yourself that may be disruptive during the night.

Types of Sleep Problems

It is important for you, your therapist, and your doctor to know what types of sleep problems you experience in the present, and what you have struggled with in the past. Of course, sleep problems may vary over time and even have different causes over time. Following is a list of common sleep problems in people with dissociative disorders. Check the ones that are currently a problem for you.

- Difficulty falling asleep
- Difficulty staying asleep
- Frequent waking
- Very early morning waking
- Excessive sleepiness (for instance, falling asleep during the day)
- Disturbed sleep–wake patterns (for instance, sleeping in the day and being awake at night)
- Nightmares
- Night terrors
- Sleepwalking
- Teeth grinding
- Bedwetting
- Restless legs
- Panic during the night
- Sleep apnea (short episodes of not breathing during sleep; often associated with obesity)
- Feeling that you have not slept deeply or well, and subsequently feeling tired

- Activity of dissociative parts during the night
- Postponing bedtime due to being afraid of going to sleep or getting in bed
- Flashbacks as you fall asleep or awaken
- Illusions and hallucinations as you fall asleep or awaken
- Severe difficulty waking up or being roused by someone else
- Narcolepsy (sudden, uncontrollable episodes of deep sleep during waking hours). Narcolepsy should be distinguished from episodes of collapse, as described previously in the manual, and must be diagnosed with a sleep study.

Factors That Contribute to Sleep Problems

There are numerous causes of or contributing factors to sleep problems in those with dissociative disorders. Often more than one factor is involved, making it important to receive a comprehensive assessment for serious sleep difficulties.

Traumatization

It is harder to sleep well when you are traumatized. When it gets dark and quiet, your mind sometimes starts to work overtime. If you tend to avoid traumatic memories, you are more vulnerable to having them emerge once you are no longer preoccupied with work or other activities. Because some traumatizing events may have occurred at night, in the dark, or in bed, many people are afraid of the dark or dread going to bed. These fears may be prominent in parts that live in trauma-time. You, or certain parts of you, may also feel more alone, vulnerable, or unprotected in the dark or when you are sleeping. You, or parts of you, can become more jumpy, fearful, and hyperalert; therefore, you may sleep more lightly and awaken often during the night.

People with a dissociative disorder often suffer from trauma-related nightmares, night terrors, flashbacks, or nighttime panic attacks. Thus, they tend to avoid going to bed or only sleep once it is light outside. Sleepwalking, crying, moaning, shouting, or fighting while asleep are not uncommon. A few may have bedwetting on occasion. Although this may be embarrassing, it is important to understand that some dissociative parts of the self may experience themselves as very young and terrified. Such parts may be too afraid to get out of bed to go to the bathroom, or they may be so terrified that you urinate involuntarily. If this happens, do not be hard on yourself. Just change your bed linens and continue to work on grounding, inner empathy, and reassurance about present-day safety for those parts of yourself. The more you can reassure and comfort all parts of yourself, the fewer problems you will have at night.

Struggle for Time Among Dissociative Parts

People with a complex dissociative disorder, especially DID, may have an internal struggle for control among parts of themselves. Parts may want or demand specific time for themselves, feeling that they do not have enough time for their own activities. This may become a major problem, interrupting not only daytime activities but also sleep. Sometimes dissociative parts may be more active at night, when the main part of the personality is more fatigued and less "on guard." Some dissociative parts may only be active during the night. The following morning you may feel exhausted and not understand why. You may find evidence of activities that you have done, such as using the computer, eating, cleaning, or drawing. Sometimes parts stay busy because they dread going to sleep or are afraid to close their eyes. They may fear losing control or having nightmares.

Other Emotional Problems

Sleep disturbances are common in those who experience moderate to severe anxiety or depression. Many traumatized individuals experience both. This additional biological contribution to sleep problems can best be addressed with a combination of medication, therapy, and healthy lifestyle changes.

Excessive Stimulation

Drinking too much caffeine or alcohol, or using drugs or tobacco can have an adverse effect on your sleep. Heavy exercise or eating, reading stimulating books, or watching exciting or disturbing movies before bed can also affect your sleep. Some people may not be aware that other parts are engaging in these behaviors. If you lose time in the present and suspect this possibility, please discuss it with your therapist.

Lack of Stimulation

On the other hand, sleeping or resting too much during the day, being too sedentary, and inadequate exercise can also lead to poor sleep.

Improving the Quality of Sleep

With a few adjustments in lifestyle and some inner empathy, communication, and cooperation, you can improve your sleep.

Making Your Bedroom a Pleasant Place for Sleep

Make your bedroom, or the place where you sleep, a safe and comfortable place for all parts of yourself. Set an agreeable temperature in your bedroom: A bit cooler is usually preferable. Make sure you have sufficient light to be able to get your bearings if you wake up during the night, for instance, a night light or dim lamp. It is helpful for your bedroom to be relatively uncluttered and for your bed linens to be fresh. If you wish, spray a nice fragrance in your room before sleep. Use the anchors you developed in the exercise from chapters 1 and 2 and have them in full view in your bedroom, to remind you of being in the present. Ensure that all parts of yourself have anchors that are helpful to them. Also create a "sleep kit" for yourself (see Homework Sheet 9.3). Remove items from your bedroom that may be triggering. These could be objects or colors that remind you of the past, but they could also be certain sounds or smells. Some people find it helpful to take out everything from their room that would be a distraction from sleep, including televisions, radios, and video games. Others find it helpful to have background noise, such as soft music or the TV, in order to sleep. However, if you need noise, a steady, droning "white" noise is preferable for sleeping, such as a fan.

If you, or parts of you, feel afraid during the night, make sure your home is as secure as possible, for instance, lock the doors and install a security system if you feel the need. Some people feel safer with a pet in the house. Have your local emergency phone number preprogrammed into your phone, and keep your phone by your bed. These are common-sense precautions, but they may also provide an extra feeling of security for parts of you.

Preparing All Parts of Yourself for Sleep

Take the time to communicate with all parts of yourself so that you have maximum awareness of your concerns and needs about sleeping. It is essential that internal agreement is made about a regular time for you (all parts of you) to sleep each night. Some parts may be active during the night because they perceive it as "their time," when you are not burdened by the responsibilities of daily life. This activity is a sign that you are not giving yourself sufficient personal time during the day. If you can communicate and negotiate with these parts and allow for some regular personal time during the day, you may see a drastic decrease in activity during the night.

Some parts may have preferences about sleeping that other parts do not share. Please be respectful of all parts of yourself, and pay attention to everything that comes to your mind about improving your sleep. For example, you may have a strong desire to keep a stuffed animal on the bed, but as an adult, this makes you uncomfortable. If there are parts of you who experience themselves as younger, you may need to address their needs compassionately and find compromises that are acceptable for all parts. Remember that parts can be stuck in the past and experience themselves as young, and your job as an adult is to help those parts of you feel secure and safe in the present.

Establishing Sleep Routines

Everyone finds it helpful to have a regular time to go bed and to get up. Set a time that is reasonable for going to sleep and aim to go to bed around that time every night. It can be helpful to engage in restful and relaxing activities before bed, activities that are not too stimulating. For example, read a nice book, watch a funny TV program, listen to your favorite music, take a relaxing bath or shower, or a have a caffeine-free drink and small healthy snack. Make a regular routine of activities that slowly wind you down toward sleep.

Some people like to imagine younger parts of themselves gathering around for a story, or imagine tucking them in to bed. One person liked to hug a pillow as though she were hugging a child, as she talked to her young self inside: *"Don't forget that I am taking care of you and that you are safe."* Make sure that you, in your own way, communicate with all parts of yourself to remind yourself that you are safe and it is OK to go to sleep.

Most people prefer to wear something when they are sleeping—pajamas might provide a feeling of safety and protection. Avoid sleeping in your daytime clothing, because it may not be comfortable, and changing into pajamas is a nice ritual that reminds you it is now bedtime.

If you have a TV in your bedroom and you need the sound to help you sleep, make sure you do not watch programs that might be upsetting to you or to parts of yourself. The point is to determine what helps you get to sleep and stay asleep on a regular basis. Some people prefer music, as long as it is relaxing and soothing. Others enjoy recorded nature sounds, such as the ocean or the wind in the trees. If you like to read and it helps you go to sleep, do so quietly in bed for a while, but make sure what you are reading is pleasant and not overly stimulating. If you read to avoid going to sleep, then try not to take a book to bed with you. Try a short relaxation or meditation exercise before going to sleep. One nice meditation is to reflect on three or four things for which you are especially grateful in your life.

Tips for Dealing With Specific Sleep Problems

If You Cannot Slow Down Your Thoughts

- Check with all parts inside. Ask whether some part of you needs to communicate inside. If so, ask that part whether it can wait until the next day. It is important to be able to temporarily delay worry and thoughts that interfere with much needed sleep. Find out whether parts of you need something to be different in order to get to sleep. Be attentive to and respectful of all parts of yourself.

• Distract yourself.

○ Count sheep (or your favorite animal), or count backward slowly from 100 and stay focused on that mental activity, as silly as it may sound. It keeps your mind from straying into problem areas that would keep you awake. Each time you lose track of the count, bring yourself back and start at the beginning.

○ Imagine a big STOP sign each time you start thinking about something. After you see the stop sign, refocus your attention on breathing slowly in and out. Breathe in to the count of three, hold for a count of three, and breathe out to a count of three. Repeat several times, just focusing on your breathing.

○ When you cannot get your mind off your problems when you lie down, imagine your thoughts flowing past you in a stream, and one by one, they flow past you, and down the stream. You know they are there, but you have no need to do anything other than observe them flow through your mind.

○ Some people find it helpful to get up and write down what is bothering them, with an internal promise that they will deal with it the next day.

○ Imagine putting your problems in a safe container (computer file, bank vault, box, etc.) for the night. You can return to them at the right time the following day.

○ Imagine one of the following:

▪ A warm, white light that envelops you such that you feel utterly relaxed and safe

▪ A beautiful balloon that you inflate. As you blow air into the balloon, imagine blowing all your tension and problems into the balloon. When you feel more relaxed, tie the balloon and allow it to float up into the sky. If you wish, you may keep it on a string.

▪ Leaning back against a very safe and caring person

▪ Use one of the additional relaxing imagery exercises in chapter 11.

If You Cannot Sleep After a Reasonable Amount of Time

• Turn the clock away so you cannot keep checking the time. You will only become obsessed with the time if you cannot get to sleep, which will make the problem worse.

- Remind yourself that there will be times when you cannot sleep. You have always been able to function the next day. If you cannot sleep tonight, then you may take something to help you sleep the following night. Your body will eventually sleep.
- Stop trying to make yourself go to sleep. Get up and go to another room (or another part of the bedroom), do something quiet to distract yourself (for instance, read a book or watch a TV program that is not too exciting, listen to peaceful music, do some stretching exercises), and go back to bed when you feel sleepy. Do this as often as necessary during the night.

If You Wake Up After a Nightmare

- If you wake up at night after a disturbing dream or nightmare, or feel anxious and panicky, it is important to be able to calm down and comfort yourself and other parts that are anxious. Work with yourself and your therapist to develop various ways to help yourself.
- The first step is always to get your bearings in the present. Use all the anchors to the present you have put in your bedroom. Talk to yourself quietly and tell yourself out loud where you are.
- Turn on the light and get out of bed. Perhaps have something to drink and find something to distract you.
- Splash cool or cold water on your face, hands, and the back of your neck. This will help you get more present and awake.
- Consciously slow your breathing. Try some breathing exercises.
- Do some gentle stretching exercises to help your body reorient to the present.
- If you have a pet, spend a little time petting or cuddling with him or her.
- If you have physical symptoms, such as a bad taste in your mouth, or pain or discomfort, be mindful in talking to yourself inwardly as you do things to soothe yourself (for instance, brush your teeth, have a noncaffeinated drink, suck on a mint or hard candy, massage painful muscles): *"I am in the present now. Whatever happened to me is over. I am safe. My mouth, my legs, my body, etc., are in the present. I am doing all I can to help all parts of myself."* Try to be aware of any internal sense of what might help.
- Some people find that it helps if they write down a distressing dream or image and then put it away, tear it up, or bring it to therapy. The idea is not to go further into the experience, but to contain it by putting it on paper and leaving it until a more appropriate time.
- You might try "changing" your nightmare. Add a supportive or strong

person to the dream, invent a way out of the situation, or give yourself special powers to overcome any sense of powerlessness or fear in the dream. Your therapist may be able to help you with this kind of technique.

• Some people wake up from a nightmare and find they are unable to move. Although this is extremely uncomfortable and even frightening, it will not last for very long. It is simply the state of being paralyzed by fear. If this happens to you, make sure you have some anchors to the present visible from every angle from the bed: on your left, your right, even on the ceiling. Even though you cannot yet move, you can begin to see the anchor and gradually perceive you are in the present. This perception will help your body shift out of that paralysis mode. Try starting with a tiny movement, for instance, blinking your eyes, and just barely twitching your toe or little finger. When you can do this, then move the opposite toe or finger. Then make a slight movement with your hand or foot, then your arms or legs. Continue slowly and patiently until your entire body has become more able to move.

Using Sleep Medication Appropriately

If you have persistent sleep difficulties in spite of trying these solutions, make sure you are checked by your physician. There may be medical reasons for your sleep issues. Sleep disorders often accompany trauma-related disorders. Ask your doctor about whether you may need a sleep medication. Check with your doctor before you take any nonprescription medications or herbs, because they may interfere with your prescribed medications. Many sleep medications are addictive; thus, they should be taken only as prescribed. They cannot be mixed with other types of sedatives or with alcohol or drugs. Often, it is sufficient to use medication for a couple of nights to get yourself in a routine and then stop taking them until the next time you have trouble.

Homework Sheet 9.1
Sleep Record

Use the record below to record your sleep difficulties during the following week.

	What time did you go to bed?	What time did you wake up?	What difficulties, if any, did you have with your sleep during the night?	How did you try to help yourself if you had trouble sleeping?	What is the total number of hours you slept?
Monday					
Tuesday					
Wednesday					
Thursday					
Friday					

	What time did you go to bed?	What time did you wake up?	What difficulties, if any, did you have with your sleep during the night?	How did you try to help yourself if you had trouble sleeping?	What is the total number of hours you slept?
Saturday					
Sunday					

Homework Sheet 9.2
Making Your Bedroom a Pleasant Place for Sleep

1. Check to make sure your bedroom feels comfortable for all parts of you. Describe your thoughts, emotions, and sensations when you look around the room.

2. List anything you can and want to change in your bedroom to make it more comfortable. What would you or parts of you like to change?

3. Describe any inner conflict about your bedroom.

4. Notice any items that might trigger you. Remove or change them if you are able. If it is not possible to remove or change them, post a little note that says something like, "*All is well here and now,*" to remind you of the present. Also, intentionally notice the difference in the context for the item in the present. For example, "*This bed reminds me of my bed as a child, but it is in my room, with my linens, on my floor. It is just a bed, and beds cannot hurt or scare. It is just a thing.*"

Homework Sheet 9.3
Developing a Sleep Kit

Develop a "sleep kit," a real or imagined box full of items that can help to reassure and calm you and all parts of you and bring you back to the here and now. You can use your sleep kit before you go to bed or if you awaken during the night feeling anxious or triggered. Your kit might include relaxing and soothing music or sounds, anchoring items, a special pillow or blanket, a night light, a favorite piece of clothing, a doll or stuffed animal, a wonderful book, photographs of people who care for you, or of safe and relaxing places, a list of people you can call if needed during an emergency, a list of pleasant experiences, or even a pet that helps you feel safe. Remember that it is important to take into account the needs and preferences of all parts in developing your sleep kit. List your sleep kit items below.

Homework Sheet 9.4
Developing a Bedtime Routine

1. Describe what helps you and all parts of yourself to unwind and prepare for bed.

2. List activities you know you should *avoid* before bedtime.

3. Describe a routine that you have or would like to establish once you get in bed (for instance, a short meditation, breathing exercises, imagery, reading a nice story).

4. Describe the best way for you to check in with all parts of yourself at bedtime, and remind yourself that you are safe and it is now time to sleep safely and comfortably (for example, talking inwardly, asking inside, imagining all parts in a circle or curled up in nice beds).

5. Are you willing and able to go to bed and get up at approximately the same time every day? List your approximate bedtime and wake time. If you are not willing or able, please describe the reasons below. Obstacles to a regular sleep routine are important to address.

CHAPTER TEN

Establishing a Healthy Daily Structure

AGENDA

- Welcome and reflections on previous session
- Homework discussion
- Exercises
- Break
- Topic: Establishing a Healthy Daily Structure

  - Introduction
  - Problems With Daily Structure for People With a Complex Dissociative Disorder
  - Reflections on Developing a Healthy Daily Structure
  - Keeping Track of Time
  - Tips for Keeping Track of Time
  - Developing Healthy Work Habits
  - Reflections on Developing a New Healthy Daily Structure

- Homework

  - Reread the chapter.
  - Continue working on your sleep kit and bedtime routine if needed.
  - Complete Homework Sheet 10.1, Your Current Daily Structure.
  - Complete Homework Sheet 10.2, Developing a Realistic and Healthy Daily Structure and Routine.

Introduction

A daily and weekly structure, with a balanced distribution of work, activity, and leisure, is of great importance for everyone. A satisfying life includes knowing how to enjoy working but also how to enjoy and use to best advantage your leisure or free time. Everyone does best with a daily structure that is consistent, but not too rigid. Structure helps people keep track of time and of what they are doing, so they can be more attentive and able to concentrate, and less worried or confused about what comes next. Structure may help reduce the risk of intrusion of, or switching among, parts of the personality; it may also help reduce the risk of prolonged flashbacks or sinking into depression. Everyone has the need to start and complete certain tasks in a timely manner, to manage a household, and to make relatively balanced choices about how he or she spends free time.

Daily and weekly structures should include a regular time to get up and go to bed, regular and healthy meals, necessary chores (for instance, shopping, cooking, paying bills, cleaning), time for relationships and social contacts, personal ("me") time, inner check-ins, physical exercise, fun, and other safely stimulating activities, and so forth. In this chapter we will focus on tools for establishing a daily structure, including keeping track of time, healthy work habits, and using your leisure time to best advantage.

Problems With Daily Structure for People With a Complex Dissociative Disorder

The establishment of a daily structure is often difficult for individuals with a dissociative disorder for a number of the following reasons:

- Disrupted time sense and an often chaotic and conflicted inner world.
- Dissociative parts may fight for time and have many conflicting wishes, needs, and preferences about how to spend time.
- As a consequence, different parts may begin certain activities but cannot finish because other parts interfere or shift to another task.
- Difficulty concentrating and completing tasks.
- Problems with impulse control and difficulty finishing a task that does not easily hold your attention, for instance, cleaning, paying bills, studying.
- Structure and routine were often not something that was modeled for you as a child, so you never learned how to develop and keep a healthy structure and have not experienced its benefits.
- You may have created an excessive and rigid structure, incessantly go-

ing from one activity to the next, never taking a rest, exhausting yourself (see also discussion that follows).

Finding a balance in your daily structure may present a big challenge. Too much structure and busyness may be a way for you to avoid feeling or knowing more about yourself or your inner world. And perhaps it may be an attempt to feel competent by doing "everything" or to prevent other parts from taking over from you. But excessive busyness can deplete you more than you might be aware.

On the other hand, if you have too little structure, problematic symptoms can increase dramatically. Perhaps it is difficult for you to decide exactly what you would like to do, or you have no idea what you want or need to do, and thus plan nothing for the day. You may notice that you have a more difficult time on totally unstructured days, especially on the weekends. You may start and stop a number of different tasks without finishing anything. This "start-stop" behavior, often due to the interference of parts, leaves all parts of you burdened by yet more unfinished business, depleting your energy further. Or perhaps you feel unmotivated to do anything, and just sit, watch TV, play computer games, or sleep.

For people with DID, some parts may be active at the expense of others, so that they lose time and do things that they were not intending to do, for instance, painting or watching TV instead of completing tasks that need to be done, such as cleaning the house. And without inner communication and cooperation, the activities and plans of some parts may overlap and interfere with those of other parts of yourself. Then you may find yourself overcommitted, adding to a sense of being overwhelmed and conflicted.

Reflections on Developing a Healthy Daily Structure

Make a list of your basic daily tasks, for example, work or volunteer time, taking care of children, cleaning, shopping and other errands, cooking, laundry, paying bills, taking care of pets, gardening or yard work, and so on. If more than one part of you is engaged in these tasks, set aside some quiet time to communicate and coordinate a reasonable schedule. The following questions may be important as part of your inner reflection:

- Are there specific tasks that cause inner problems among parts? For example, is a part triggered by caring for children, or overwhelmed by the many choices presented to you in the grocery store, or too impulsive to deal with spending money?
- If there are inner problems evoked by a certain task, which seem the

easiest to solve? Begin with that problem and as you gain more confidence and practice with inner communication and cooperation, you may move to the next problem. Remember to be patient: You cannot change everything at once, and no one expects you to do so.

- Do you or parts of you have a tendency to have too much structure and exhaust yourself? If so, see if you can notice why, for example, avoiding feelings or memories, feeling pressured to achieve, afraid to stop, and so forth.
- What might be the benefits to you and other parts of you if you were more flexible with your daily structure? For example, better capacity to tolerate emotions, permission not to work so hard, and the like.
- What activities are important for you as a whole person? Negotiate with parts inside to plan a set number of activities each week that is comfortable and reasonable to you and all parts of you, not too many and not too few. If you are overly active and busy, make sure you plan for down time between engagements. And be sure to plan for the time it takes to get from one place to another without having to rush.
- Do you or parts of you have too little structure? If so, see if you can determine why. For example, some people are too depressed or tired to provide themselves with structure to do anything; others may not know where to start or how to use structure, and so on.
- What might parts of you need in order to develop more structure? For example, more support from other people or from parts inside, some suggestions for structure, and so forth.
- Would you be willing to push just a little to do one or two activities each day?
- If you decide to develop a new structure or routine, do not criticize yourself or other parts if you are not able to keep it all the time. Just try again! You do not have to be perfect to be successful. For most people, it takes several months (and sometimes even more) to make a new routine become a more automatic habit.

Additional Tips

- Everyone needs time for relaxation and pleasure. Make time for yourself and for parts of yourself every day, preferably during the day or in the early evening, not at bedtime (see chapter 11).
- Everyone needs time for personal reflection and inner deliberation. Some people with a dissociative disorder find it helpful to have an inner meeting with parts of themselves to discuss daily routines, plans, and so forth (see chapter 27).
- Engage in some type of physical exercise every day (cycling, walking,

or some other form of activity). Try to go outside every day and get 15 to 20 minutes of sun.

- Try to have contact with other people at least several times a week, especially if you live alone. Isolating yourself is often a habit that is not helpful. Be aware of when you want to isolate and intentionally make plans with friends or acquaintances instead, or just walk around where people are nearby, for example, in a park or a mall.
- If you tend to lose yourself in an activity, try setting an alarm to stay aware of time. Virtually every personal electronic device now has reminder alerts that can be set.
- If you are living with someone else, you will both benefit by having clear and fixed arrangements about who does which chores. Fuzzy arrangements and lack of clarity can cause irritation and resentment. You may need to be assertive to make sure you have personal time for yourself and your parts, and to make sure the tasks are distributed fairly.
- Many books and Web sites are dedicated to offering practical tips for organization, routines, and structure. Make use of these as needed. Personal organizers, trained individuals who help with your daily organization, are also available in most areas.

Keeping Track of Time

A sense of time is essential to maintain structure and routines, but when you have a dissociative disorder, an accurate time sense and adequate time management are often problems. It is as though some parts of you do not live in time and even have trouble understanding the concept of time (Van der Hart & Steele, 1997). Time can seem too fast or too slow, gaps of lost time make it hard to keep track of the day, time may not be experienced at all, and time sense may differ among various dissociative parts. All these problems with a sense of time lead to confusion. In addition, many people with a dissociative disorder have trouble with time management due to problems with executive functioning, that is, with planning, organizing, sequencing, and prioritizing abilities.

Tips for Keeping Track of Time

- Use a diary, a calendar, or a planning board, or all three (even if you feel there is inner conflict about planning). Keep your calendar in a place where you will see it every day. Mark off days as they pass so you can easily find the day and date.

- If you have DID and lose time, written communication may help all parts of you begin to coordinate a single schedule. Invite parts to use the same planning tool. And the more you have inner agreement about a schedule, the better you will be able to keep it. Try to plan one week at a time.
- Put important reminders on your calendar, for instance, due dates for bills and taxes, appointments, and errands to run during the week.
- Wear a watch, so you can keep track of hours. Preferably use a watch that has an alarm, so you can set it as a reminder for appointments or tasks. Some people prefer to use their cell phone to track time instead of a watch; that is fine, too, but a watch on your wrist is a visual reminder to check the time, perhaps more so than your phone.
- When you have an appointment, set a reminder alarm for 15 minutes before you should leave to make it on time. For example, if it will take you 30 minutes to drive to your therapist, set your alarm to remind you that your appointment is in 45 minutes. Do not allow yourself to get involved in another task before you leave.
- Keep a list of things to do and appointments posted on your refrigerator or calendar, which you will see every day.
- Put a colored hair band around your wrist to remind you that you need to do something.
- If you tend to lose lists, keep them in a single notebook used only for that purpose and keep the notebook in the same place at all times. Make an agreement among parts not to hide or destroy the notebook.
- Before going to the store, make a list of what you need that is agreeable to all parts of you, so you need not spend hours shopping or overspend. Only buy what is on your list; then leave.
- If you have trouble remembering when and if you have taken your medication (if you take any), buy a weekly pill organizer box, available at any pharmacy. Each week, put your medications in the appropriate box, and you can check the box to see whether you have taken them. Set an alarm to take your medication, if necessary.
- If you have DID, you may find some part of you is able to keep good time and can remind you.

Developing Healthy Work Habits

Whether people go to a job each day, or whether they work at home, raise children, or volunteer, they all need healthy work habits. This includes the ability to concentrate and focus, organize one's work, start and stop activities on time, and balance work with other important life priorities. People who work too much set up a lifestyle of chronic exhaustion, rigidity, and imbalance, which makes them more vulnerable to switching, flashbacks, and periods of poor functioning. People who are unable to work generally do not feel very worthwhile and may be unable to take care of themselves financially. The resulting stress can lead to increased symptoms and difficulties.

People often have particular dissociative parts that deal with work, while other parts may be unaware of work. Some parts may sabotage or interfere with work or projects, or prefer to play instead of work. And parts living in trauma-time may become triggered by various situations at work, such as an angry or irritated boss.

Dissociative parts that are focused solely on work typically are not sufficiently aware of your body to know when you are tired or stressed; thus, they tend to overdo. On the whole, such parts may not be particularly interested in "cooperation" and slowing down but are often only focused on a work goal that needs to be accomplished. This is hardly surprising, because such parts likely use work as a protection against the intrusion of painful memories or the realization of a painful past, or against dealing with other dissociative parts that might not be appropriate at work.

All people need to feel successful at their work, whatever it is, because success helps us feel competent and good about ourselves. It is thus understandable that people with dissociative disorders do not want to take the risk of losing that area of competence and thus are reluctant to decrease the barriers that protect parts that are able to work. But as noted earlier, overworking prevents you from having to cope with and confront your inner world. Thus, "staying busy" and forcing yourself to do more and more is a very common form of unhealthy coping. To heal, you must develop inner collaboration to balance yourself in life and cope more effectively.

Reflections on Developing a New Healthy Daily Structure

- Reflect on how you would like to ideally and realistically spend your time. Please note if there are conflicts among parts of you about how to spend time.
- What are your priorities about which activities you would like to spend your time (for instance, work, being with friends, play, reading)?
- When do you need more or less structure? Weekends? Evenings? Daytime? Holidays?
- Are there particular times of day that are especially hard for you? If so, imagine what changes you could make in your routines and structure to help you (see chapter 16 on planning to cope with difficult times).

- Consider how much time you can or should spend on work or tasks in a given day.
- Notice how your time is distributed among work/chores, and leisure/social time, play and rest, and personal ("me") time.
- Reflect on how to give yourself meaningful private time for tending to your inner needs (including those of other parts of you). This should include time for inner reflection and contact with parts of yourself. How might you structure that time to be fair and agreeable to all parts of yourself?
- Consider which activities give you energy or drain you of energy. Try to cooperate with all parts of yourself to set a realistic daily pace, given your energy level and the amount of energy your activities give or demand of you.
- Take into account other ways to balance your life, for example, exercise, socializing, getting out of the house, enjoying a hobby.

Homework Sheet 10.1
Your Current Daily Structure

Describe your current daily structure and routines so you assess what is working well for you and what might need to be different. Include the approximate amount of time you spend in each of the four categories listed below. You do not have to go into detail.

1. Work / tasks / chores / appointments / meals
2. Leisure and social time, for instance, hobbies, being with friends or family
3. Personal time for yourself, including inner reflection and communication with parts
4. Do nothing; that is, watch mindless TV, surf the Internet, play video games, stare at the wall, sleep, and so on

Sunday

Monday

Tuesday

Wednesday

Thursday

Friday

Saturday

Homework Sheet 10.2
Developing a Realistic and Healthy
Daily Structure and Routine

Now describe a realistic and healthy structure and routine that you would like to develop in the next few months. Before you begin, you may want to refer back to the earlier section on reflections for helping you develop your new structure and routine. Remember to change only one thing at a time so you will not become overwhelmed or discouraged.

1. Work / tasks / chores / appointments / meals
2. Leisure and social time, for instance, hobbies, being with friends or acquaintances
3. Personal time for yourself, including inner reflection and communication with parts
4. Do nothing; that is, watch mindless TV, surf the Internet, play video games, stare at the wall, sleep, and so on

Sunday

Monday

Tuesday

Wednesday

Thursday

Friday

Saturday

CHAPTER ELEVEN

Free Time and Relaxation

AGENDA

- Welcome and reflections on previous session
- Homework discussion
- Topic: Free Time and Relaxation

  - Introduction
  - Problems With Free Time and Relaxation for People With a Complex Dissociative Disorder
  - Tips for Resolving Inner Conflicts About Relaxation and Free Time
  - Tips for Managing Free Time
  - Learning to Safely Relax
  - Relaxation Exercises

- Homework

  - Reread the chapter.
  - Practice the relaxation exercises.
  - Complete Homework Sheet 11.1, Developing a Relaxation Kit.
  - Complete Homework Sheet 11.2, Exploring Inner Obstacles to Leisure Time and Relaxation.

Introduction

We all need time to safely relax and do what we like. An essential part of your healing is learning to make use of free time for relaxation, rejuvenation, fun, and new interests. Learning, laughing, having fun, and being curious all help maintain balance and perspective in daily life. In the same way as with balancing work, people with dissociative disorders need to find the right distribution of their free time, including personal time to communicate and work with inner parts. However, for traumatized individuals, a number of factors may impede the use of what should be healing relaxation and leisure time.

Problems With Free Time and Relaxation for People With a Complex Dissociative Disorder

You may find that you avoid free time, relaxation, or leisure activities, even though other people generally find them to be rejuvenating and essential. Such unstructured times may present an opportunity for the inner turmoil and distress that you avoid to rise up into your awareness. And perhaps you have developed negative beliefs and fears about free time or relaxation. Thus, you may encounter some of the following difficulties:

- If you try to relax, you may be afraid of losing control, becoming overwhelmed, or of having other parts of you take control.
- Various parts may have different needs and wishes about leisure time, resulting in conflicts about how you should spend your free time. And at times, some part might believe that a particular activity, such as relaxing, is dangerous and thus inhibits other parts from engaging in it. Ongoing conflicts may sometimes result in a "stalemate" in which you do not do anything at all.
- Free time (for instance, weekends, holidays) may trigger memories of painful past experiences, making it more difficult to enjoy your time in the present (see chapter 16).
- You may have inner feelings or voices that prohibit pleasure, enjoyment, or play. Perhaps these messages are shame based, coming from a belief that you do not deserve to feel good or that you are lazy. Or they may be based on a fear that you will "get in trouble" or that "bad things always happen when you are feeling good."
- You, or some parts of you, may be afraid to "let down your guard." That is, you feel a strong need to be on high alert all the time and thus find it impossible to relax. In fact, attempts to relax may actually increase a feeling of being vulnerable or unsafe.

The most effective way to deal with inner conflicts about how to spend your free time is to reflect on the inner concerns, beliefs, and needs of all parts of yourself. And then, as with all other inner conflicts, steadily learn to empathize, negotiate, and cooperate about your leisure time. Of course, it is important to be realistic and reasonable about what you are able to do: Work, play, relationships, and relaxation must be balanced and within your capacity as a whole person. For example, you cannot stay up having fun all night and expect to go to work and be at your best the next day. Nor can you work excessively long hours each day and expect yourself to have quality time for inner reflection and care for inner parts of yourself. Always consider your commitments, budget, and energy level in planning your free time.

Tips for Resolving Inner Conflicts About Relaxation and Free Time

If you experience some of the conflicts described earlier or in Homework Sheet 11.2 (at the end of this chapter) about free time and relaxation, try some of the following suggestions to help you resolve them:

- Take time to reflect on why you might be having difficulties with free time or relaxation and make a list of these obstacles.
- Do not judge yourself about these conflicts; just notice them.
- Prioritize as best you can from the least to the most difficult conflicts on your list. Begin with the least difficult and gradually work your way through to the most difficult. As you gain mastery with resolving the less intense conflicts, you and all parts of yourself become more confident and trusting with each other, and they will be more willing to take the next steps.
- Using an inner safe space, meeting room, or by talking inwardly, determine whether all parts of you might agree that relaxation might be a good thing if it were completely safe and allowed. If so, good: You can take the next step. If not, stop and reflect on why parts of you believe relaxing would not be helpful even if it were safe and allowed.
- Let yourself imagine, all parts of you, a foreign land in which relaxation and free time are encouraged as a natural part of every day. In this land, everyone works hard, but they also play hard. No one is in a hurry. No one is critical of others. No one is punished. Imagine yourself watching people in this foreign land as they relax, rest, laugh, play, and enjoy themselves after work. Notice how this image affects all parts of you.
- You might talk inwardly to remind all parts of you that when you (all of you) feel safe and relaxed in a safe environment, there is less chaos and noise inside. All parts might benefit. Critical or angry parts might

find they have to spend less energy managing young parts of yourself if those parts feel safe and more relaxed, and even have fun.

- Remind all parts that enjoying relaxation and free time does not mean you are lazy or not completing your work. It is well known that people who take time off to relax and rest are more productive and effective when they do work.
- Remind all parts that it is possible to be alert and relaxed at the same time.
- If parts continue to feel unsafe in relaxing, ask whether perhaps one part of you might remain "on guard" while other parts of you rest. Various parts of you could take turns with "guard duty" so that each part of you has rest times.
- Make sure you take time to orient all parts to the present and reassure them that relaxation and free time are allowed and healthy, and you will not get in trouble for taking some time for yourself.
- If traumatic memories or intense emotions are triggered when you have free time, help vulnerable parts to stay in a safe place during that time, assuring them that they will be attended to in the near future. And continue to orient them to the present. Be sure to keep such promises as all parts must learn to trust each other.
- Engage in inner discussions and negotiation about what to do in your free time. If there are conflicts, try taking turns, doing one activity one time, and another activity the next time. Or try finding activities that are enjoyable to all parts of you (or at least acceptable). Negotiate healthy "deals" internally. For example, if a critical part allows you an hour of free time without complaint, agree that you will work on a specific task in return after your free time. Be sure to follow through.
- Take small steps. For example, practice relaxation for 1 minute, if 10 minutes is too much. Or 30 seconds if a minute is too much. Go only as fast as the slowest part of you, while always helping such parts by giving them the resources they need to take a step. Above all, do not be critical of yourself or other parts of you.

Next you will find some tips on relaxing safely and using your free time effectively.

Tips for Managing Free Time

- Schedule some free time for yourself every day. Begin by structuring small amounts of free time, for example, 30 minutes or an hour (less if this amount is not tolerable).

- Become more aware of what activities you, and other parts of you, might like to do or what you would like to learn to do for enjoyment. Do not eliminate ideas with arguments about why you cannot do them. Try to be open to new possibilities and help other parts be open to trying something new as well.
- Make a list of what you might like to do. Setting aside differences, are there any activities that all parts of you might enjoy? Start with one of these activities first.
- If you avoid free time or relaxation, reflect and ask yourself (or other parts that might be involved) of what you are afraid or ashamed.
- If you have too much unstructured free time, be willing to add more activities and use your time toward healing, for instance, by attending to parts of yourself that need your care.
- If you have no idea what you want to do, notice what other people do and see whether something appeals to you. Try taking an art class, volunteering, hiking, or joining a choir. Do not wait until you are sure about an activity. Try it, and if you do not like it, you can always stop. Remember that trying new things is a great way to learn whether you like them and to have fun in the process.
- Try not to worry about failing. The task is to enjoy learning, even if you do not do something well.
- Be persistent and patient with yourself.

Learning to Safely Relax

People who have been traumatized often find it difficult to relax, because they, or at least some parts of themselves, are almost always on high alert. They may feel it is not safe to relax because they would not be able to notice danger. But in reality, relaxation occurs at many levels of awareness and alertness. A person can be extremely relaxed, present, and alert or relaxed in a drowsy kind of way. Being simultaneously alert and relaxed is actually the most adaptive and flexible way to be most of the time. Parts of you can help each other to realize this state of mind. In chapter 8, you learned how to begin to develop an inner sense of safety. That sense of safety is a foundation that will allow you to learn to relax more effectively and easily.

To practice relaxation, try one of the following exercises at a time when you are not pressured to do something or go somewhere, and when your mind is relatively quiet.

Once you become accustomed to practicing an exercise and are able to relax, begin using it when you are tired, stressed, or feeling low. The earlier you intervene with yourself by helping yourself feel calmer, the more effective the exercise. The following imagery exercises are meant to help you and all parts of yourself feel better, stronger, and to regain more emotional balance.

Try making an audio file of one of these exercises so you can listen to it when you choose. You can do it yourself, or perhaps ask your therapist or a friend or partner to make it for you. Play around with the wording first, so that it fits just exactly right for you and all parts of yourself.

Try one or more of the following exercises. Read through them first to see whether one is especially appealing to you. If you wish, you can change the setting (that is, imagine a mountain instead of a safe tree; a forest instead of a healing pool).

RELAXATION EXERCISES

The Tree

Sit or lie down somewhere quiet and pleasant and breathe quietly, closing your eyes safely. Remind all parts of you that you are safe and that you are working to help each part of you feel better. Invite all parts to participate. If some parts do not wish to do so, they may watch from a distance or go to their own safe place. Gradually direct all parts of you that want to participate to an imagined scene. This place is a quiet and safe spot in the open air with beautiful scenery, just the right temperature, in your favorite season of the year. And around you, you see magnificent trees, resplendent in their green finery. Look around slowly for a tree that appeals to you, one that almost seems to invite you to become acquainted. Perhaps it is a tree standing alone, tall and proud, or perhaps a tree in a forest, one of many in a wise and strong community of trees. Your tree may be short or tall, fat or thin, young or old, firm or willowy. Take your time to choose your tree and remember that you can always change to another tree if and when you wish. Some parts of you may want to choose different trees, each having their own, and of course, this is just fine. Once you, all parts of you, have a clear image of your special tree, take your time to examine it carefully. Notice its shape and texture, its warm wood scent and palette of colors. Become aware of the branches spreading out to shelter you, the leafy, soothing green that extends an invitation for you to relax and rest. Take your tree in until it becomes a natural memory, indelible in your mind.

Walk up to your tree and get acquainted. Begin by exploring the trunk and all its nooks and crannies. Run your hand over the bark. Notice any knotholes or hollows. Put your arms around your tree; notice if you can get your arms right round it, or whether it is so thick you cannot encircle it. Lean up against your tree. Feel its strength, solid and unyielding, protective and grounding. If you wish, you can sit under your tree, with your back comfortably against it, with confidence that it will support you no matter how hard you lean. Now notice that your tree is not standing on its own. It has powerful roots that go deep and deeper, and deeper still into the earth, anchoring it to the ground, and drawing sustenance up and up, all through the tree, to the tiptop. Your tree is always grounded and dwells in the present, its rich history inscribed in its rings, and its branches ready for the winds that blow. It fears neither fair weather nor foul, bending with the storm, swaying with the breeze, resting under the heavens when all is quiet and still. In rain and wind, sun and snow, storm and showers: always steady and grounded. Feel this stalwart and faithful presence in your mind, in your body, and in your heart. Let you and all parts of you feel rooted to the earth with your tree. Let you and all parts of you feel the power and strength, the grounding and readiness to meet what is, and what shall come, unwavering and constant. Let yourself feel the power of your tree with its enormous root system, connected to the earth.

Now draw your attention upwards, to the branches and boughs, to the limbs and leaves. Each branch is unique, each weaving with the other to design beautiful foliage that is never exactly the same from day to day and year to year. The leaves take in light and create energy. They provide you with shelter and shade, safety and soothing, their gentle rustle a pleasant sound in your ears. The play of shadow and light as the branches move is pleasant to your eyes, giving you a sense that all is right with the world. You may even want to climb your tree and sit on one of those branches, gleefully swinging your legs or thoughtfully surveying your world from up there. Perhaps you take a nap in the shady haven of your tree. It is a good, grounding, safe feeling, being with your tree.

Your tree is a refuge where birds may safely nest, small animals may shelter from the elements, where a tree house might be built, or a swing hung from its boughs. It is a hideout that no one can see, that is just for you, where you can retreat whenever you wish. The strength and beauty and peacefulness of your magnificent tree give you a feeling of protection and sturdiness. You, and any parts of you, can go there whenever you like; you can picture it in your mind and look at it, lean against it, or hide in it, as you wish or need.

The Healing Pool

Imagine a beautiful pool of water with just the right surroundings. Perhaps you discover it in a quiet forest, or nestled in the mountains, or in the midst of a meadow. The air around it is fresh, clean, and just the right temperature for you. The season of the year is your favorite. Perhaps it is spring, with all living things blooming and growing. Perhaps it is summer, lazy and languid. Or perhaps it is autumn, cool and crisp. Or perhaps it is winter, a soft blanket of white on the ground. The water is beautiful, inviting. Perhaps it is still, gently fed by deep springs, reflecting back to you the sky or trees above. Perhaps it is flowing and bubbling, at the bottom of a waterfall or fed by rivers or streams. It may be shallow or deep, or both at once. It is pleasant to watch, its freshness smells joyful and clean. So pleasant that you feel almost drawn to its safety and soothing. The sounds around you are delightful: rustling trees or meadow grass, the bubble and babble of water, happy little animal sounds, and birds calling out joyfully. Notice what is right for you. Take your time to notice your pool, its shape, its surroundings, its depth, whether there are little fishes or just clean, fresh water. Perhaps it is a shimmering blue or sparkling green, or clear as a crystal. The light dances and skips across the water and back again to you, inviting you to take it all deeply in. This water calls you to relax, to feel utter and complete contentment and safety. It is healing water, the kind that soothes the sorest body and satiates the thirstiest soul. It refreshes the worn-out mind, a balm for wounds of the heart. When you are ready, allow all parts of yourself to explore your pool and take in its healing energy. Perhaps some parts of you would like to sit thoughtfully next to the water, while some might dangle their feet, their toes dabbling in the water. Some might get in and sit or even float. In fact, you become aware that the water in this pool is the most special you have ever encountered. It buoys you up so you cannot sink. It supports you as you sit, as though you were leaning back into loving arms. It nurtures and soothes, calms and restores, filling you with a peace and a lightness so sweet and splendid that you take it deeply within yourself, to each part of you, to every nook and cranny of pain and stress and sorrow. Let your tension and fear, your burdensome shame and worries be drawn from you to the water and carried away. Let the water surround you, flow around you, refreshing, relaxing, restoring every part of you. Let the water surround you, flow around you. Feel it soothing your body, your mind, your heart. You may remain as long as you like, until every part of you can feel its gentle healing power. This is your pool, where all parts of you can come as they please. It is your special place of healing and hope, soothing and safety, relief and release. It is yours and yours alone to have within you, a wellspring of well-being.

If it is hard for you to use imagery for relaxation, try this exercise:

Physical Relaxation

Sit or lie comfortably. Take a deep breath in through your nose to a slow count of three, hold for three counts, and breathe out slowly through pursed lips for three counts. Repeat three times. Now take in a deep breath and tighten every muscle in your body as tight as you can from head to toe, hold to the count of five, and let go, breathing out as deeply as you can and intentionally relaxing your muscles as much as you can. Repeat the three deep breaths from the beginning of the exercise. Then again take in a deep breath and tighten all your muscles for the count of five, let go and relax, repeat the three deep breaths. Continue until you feel physically relaxed.

Progressive Muscle Relaxation Technique

The following exercise is a well-known technique that might help you gradually relax your entire body (Jacobson, 1974). When you are anxious or fearful, your body becomes tense and you may experience symptoms such as pain in your neck, shoulders, or back, tension headaches, tight jaws, tensed muscles in legs or arms, and sometimes your whole body may seize up. To train yourself to progressively relax, you will begin by tensing specific groups of muscles and then releasing the tension; focus on the differences between the feelings of tension and relaxation of each group of muscles. You will practice with one area of your body at a time: head and face, neck, shoulders, back, pelvis, arms and hands, legs and feet. If you have any injuries, skip that area of your body if needed. Parts of you may or may not want to participate. As always, pace yourself and do not force any part of you. Spend some time collaborating internally to reach an agreement that is acceptable for all parts of you.

Sit or lie comfortably in a quiet and safe place where you will not be interrupted. You will tense and relax each muscle group twice, taking a short break of about 30 seconds between each cycle, and then move to the next area. When tensing a muscle group, hold for about 5 seconds, then release and rest for about 10 seconds. If you wish, you can combine this exercise with one of the ones described earlier or with your inner safe space.

- Begin by focusing on your hands. Clench your fists, feel the tension of your muscles for 5 seconds, and then release 10 seconds. Concentrate on the differences between tension and release. Repeat once more.
- Now focus on your arms, draw your forearms toward your shoulder, feel the tension in your biceps (5 seconds), and then let go and relax (10 seconds). Concentrate on the differences between tension and release. Repeat once more.
- Tighten your triceps—muscles on the underside of your upper arms—by stretching your arms out straight and locking your elbows. Feel the tension in your triceps and then let go, relaxing your arms. Concentrate on the differences between tension and release. Repeat this once more. As your arms relax, just let them lie by your side or rest on the chair.
- Next, concentrate on your face. Tense the muscles in your forehead by raising your eyebrows as far as you can, feel the tension in your face and eyebrows, hold and then relax. And again, concentrate on the differences between tension and release. Repeat a second time.
- Tense the muscles around your eyes by squeezing them tightly shut and then relax. Observe the different sensations when you tense and when you relax your eyes. Repeat.
- Tighten your jaws by opening your mouth as wide as possible, hold and then relax. Repeat.

- Focus on the muscles in your neck, bow your head, your chin on your chest, then turn your head slowly to the left, return to the center line and lean your head back as far as it will go, then again return your head to its normal position. Turn your head to the right and then again to the normal position. Repeat this slowly and carefully, since there is often a lot of tension in your neck. And again, concentrate on the differences between tension and release.

- Focus on your shoulders. Raise them as though you were going to touch your ears, hold and feel the tension, and then relax. Focus on the different sensations between tension and relaxation of your shoulders. Repeat.

- Then focus on your shoulder blades; pull your shoulder blades back as though you want them to touch them together. Tense and release. Notice the difference between the tension and release. Repeat.

- Stretch your back by sitting up very straight, tighten and let go, then relax. Repeat and focus on the different sensations between tension and relaxation.

- Tighten your buttocks by squeezing them together, hold, and then relax. Repeat.

- Hold your breath, pull your belly in, tighten it, and relax. Repeat and feel the difference in your stomach and belly.

- Now focus on your legs. Stretch your legs out and feel the tension in the muscles of your thighs, hold on, and then relax your legs. Notice the difference between tension and release. Repeat.

- Now extend your legs and point your toes back towards you. Feel the tension in your calves and feel the relaxation after you let go. Repeat.

- Finally focus on your feet. Point your toes down as far as possible and feel the tension in the muscles of your feet; tighten them and then relax. Observe the different sensations when you tense and when you relax the muscles in your feet.

- Now scan your whole body mentally and look for any residual tension. If a particular muscle group is still tense, return to this area once more.

- Now imagine that relaxation is spreading through your whole body; your body may feel warm, a bit heavy, and very safe and relaxed.

Homework Sheet 11.1
Developing a Relaxation Kit

In the same way that you developed a sleep kit in chapter 9, you may design your own "relaxation kit."

1. Begin by making a list below of activities and exercises, music, or other items or experiences that are enjoyable or fun. List things you imagine would be enjoyable and relaxing, even if you have not tried them yet. Make sure to take into account the different needs and desires of all parts of yourself. Highlight any activities that might be agreeable to all parts of yourself, that is, that you can enjoy as a whole person.

1.

2.

3.

4.

5.

6.

7.

8.

9.

10.

2. Just as you did with your sleep kit, you may make a special box or basket with various items for your relaxation and comfort, for example, music CDs, relaxing videos, special bath salts, pleasant lotions, a comfortable shawl or sweater, a pair of old slippers, warm socks, candles, special teas or coffees, healthy snacks, a good book, favorite photos, or mementos.

3. List one or two new activities you would be willing to try for relaxation or fun.

4. Describe any inner obstacles to trying these activities.

Homework Sheet 11.2
Exploring Inner Obstacles to Leisure Time and Relaxation

You may find it difficult to enjoy your free time or to relax. Below you will find common reasons why this might be so. Check or circle any that apply and then complete the questions at the end.

You (or a part of you):

- Do not feel comfortable with or know how to "play."
- Do not like to move your body, so you avoid leisure activities that require any physical exertion.
- Are afraid or ashamed of the feeling of excitement.
- Are afraid or ashamed of the feeling of enjoyment.
- Believe enjoyment is dangerous or bad.
- Believe you do not deserve to relax or feel good.
- Feel out of control when you are excited or enjoying yourself.
- Are afraid you will fail at any leisure activities.
- Are afraid people will ridicule you.
- Are afraid someone will criticize what you are doing.
- Feel that people will not take you seriously.
- Have a belief that having free time means you are lazy or not working hard enough.
- Fear that you will be punished if you have a good time.
- Fear that something bad will happen if you enjoy yourself.
- Fear that if you relax, you will not be able to notice danger.
- Find that certain words, such as "relax," "enjoy," "pleasure," or "play," are a trigger.
- Experience flashbacks as soon as you start to relax.
- Have panic or serious anxiety as soon as you start to relax.
- Become immediately depressed when you try to relax.
- Feel too much pressure to work and feel guilty or preoccupied if you try to relax.
- Have inner conflict among parts about relaxation and leisure time.
- Have trouble being alone, and thus relaxation is more difficult.
- Other? If so, please describe.

1. Using the list above, and reflecting on other possible reasons, describe two or three fears, concerns, or beliefs that you, or parts of you, have that impede your ability to relax and enjoy free time. You may also refer back to #4 of the previous homework assignment, where you listed obstacles to trying a new leisure activity.

2. Using the section in this chapter, Tips for Resolving Inner Conflicts about Relaxation and Free Time, spend time identifying inner common ground for relaxation and free time. (For example, all parts might agree to practice relaxation exercises for 15 minutes each day this week and see if it is helpful. If so, you can negotiate a next step. If not, parts can discuss what is not agreeable and why, and renegotiate.) Describe your inner communication and negotiation below, as well as what worked and did not work for you.

CHAPTER TWELVE

Physical Self-Care

AGENDA

- Welcome and reflections on previous session
- Homework discussion
- Topic: Physical Self-Care

  - Introduction
  - Factors Affecting Your Body Awareness and Physical Self-Care
  - Managing Alcohol, Illicit Drugs, and Prescribed Medications
  - Regulating Your Physical Energy
  - Tips for Resolving Inner Conflicts About Physical Self-Care
  - Tips for Improving Your Physical Self-Care

- Homework

  - Reread the chapter.
  - Complete Homework Sheet 12.1, Physical Self-Care Questionnaire.
  - Complete Homework Sheet 12.2, Making a Healthy Change in Physical Self-Care.

Introduction

Taking care of your body and maintaining your physical health are important aspects of healing and living well. Your body is not separate from you, even though it may feel like a "thing" with which you do not want to bother sometimes. But your body is you, and you are your body. Your emotions involve physiological changes in your body that produce physical sensations and movements; your beliefs and perceptions are mirrored in your posture, movements, and level of physical arousal. Your physical health affects your mental health, and vice versa. Many people who have experienced childhood abuse and neglect avoid dealing with their bodies or even find them disgusting or terrifying. Healing comes through more compassionate acceptance of mind and body as one together. This acceptance is not always easy or quick to accomplish, but it is an important goal for you and parts of yourself. In this chapter we will discuss some basic ways to care for yourself physically and overcome some of your reluctance about dealing with your body.

Factors Affecting Your Body Awareness and Physical Self-Care

People with a dissociative disorder may have many reasons for avoiding their bodies and neglecting physical self-care. In the following sections we discuss some of the major factors, which you may recognize for yourself.

Basic Physical Self-Care Was Never Learned

Some families neither practice nor teach their children basic physical self-care. Such children may not have ever been taught to care for their bodies, to prevent disease, to eat healthily and exercise, to get routine medical and dental checkups, or to recognize symptoms that require a visit to the doctor. These skills can be acquired with practice, attention, and persistence, and you can find a multitude of readily available resources on physical self-care.

The Body Is Perceived as an Object of Fear, Hatred, Disgust, or Shame

Many people with a dissociative disorder, or at least some parts of them, find their bodies repulsive. There is no enjoyment of their physical being, and their bodies feel alien to them, a burden, and a reason for others to find them undesirable. They tend to avoid certain physical sensations, movements, or postures. They often perceive their bodies as objects, not as an integral part of existence. In addition, control issues can be evoked if people do not feel well and cannot function in the way that they want or find they are physically weaker or less attractive than they wish. The body can seem like an enemy when it is expected to be perfect and function like a machine.

When people are abused by others, they often experience physical pain in their bodies, as well as emotional pain. And of course, emotional pain can be experienced intensely at the physical level of the body. Thus, survivors sometimes condition themselves to avoid their bodies in order to avoid pain and suffering.

Others tend to blame their bodies as the reason they were abused and thus feel terrible shame. For example, people may believe that if only their bodies had been stronger, they could have stopped the abuse. They blame their bodies for what happened, instead of accepting that they were too young to stop what happened. And sometimes, certain parts of the personality may hold this belief, while others may not.

Some people who were sexually abused may have been told that their bodies were beautiful and thus blame themselves for what happened: *"If only I had not been so pretty!"* They may develop shame and hatred for their bodies. For example, some women (or parts of themselves) come to hate anything feminine about their bodies. They have associated being female with being abused: *"Girls get abused; therefore, I hate being a girl. My body is bad because it is female."*

Dissociation Involves Altered Physical Sensations

Dissociation not only involves mental symptoms but also physical ones, some of which are intense and uncomfortable. On the other hand, dissociation may involve physical numbness or diminished pain sensitivity. You may want to review some of these symptoms in chapter 2. Dissociative parts of the personality that are stuck in the past may reexperience in the present some physical sensations related to past trauma, such as pain or cold. Such seemingly "unexplained" intrusive sensations can be frightening and confusing, and thus people may become increasingly avoidant and unaware of their bodies. Some people have difficulty distinguishing between physical pain that is the result of an injury or illness in the present and pain that is a reexperience of the past. If you are not sure whether a certain symptom stems from a traumatic experience or is associated with a current physical problem, do not hesitate to discuss it with your therapist and your primary care physician.

Many people with a dissociative disorder report some degree of physical numbness and thus may not experience normal levels of sensation and pain. They have difficulty, for example, in determining whether bath water is too hot or cold, or they do not notice when they have hurt themselves. They also may tend to ignore fatigue, hunger, thirst, and other bodily needs to the detriment of physical well-being. Thus, their bodies suffer from neglect.

While some parts are too numb, others may be exquisitely sensitive to the slightest of physical changes and find discomfort or pain intolerable. It is as though they experience their bodies as constant irritants, at best. They may become increasingly reactive to and phobic of body sensations.

And of course, every emotion you experience is accompanied by its own set of physical sensations, muscle tension, posture, and tendencies to move. If you are afraid or ashamed of an emotion (or a particular thought), you likely have also learned to avoid the physical experiences of it as well.

In sum, you, or parts of you, may have learned over time that physical pain could be intolerable (during abuse); you may have associated your body with that abuse; subsequent intrusive dissociative experiences in your body were painful or frightening; and the physical experience of emotions (or thoughts) may have felt overwhelming to you. For all these reasons, you have perhaps learned to despise, fear, or be ashamed of your body, making it difficult to take care of yourself.

Failure of Parts to Accept the Body as Their Own

In DID, some dissociative parts that experience themselves as relatively separate from the individual may not experience the body as belonging to them. Such parts may believe they have a different body and may not experience bodily sensations that other parts do, and they may even want to "get rid of" or hurt the body, as though it is a foreign object or belongs to another person. If the individual has a physical problem, such parts may deny that it exists because they do not feel the body. They may even "see" their body as being entirely different than in reality. Occasionally these parts may hurt the body with impunity because they insist it is not theirs, or they may engage in risky behaviors because they do not believe the individual is affected.

Physical Self-Care May Trigger a Phobia of Inner Experiences

Physical self-care involves at least some degree of body awareness. People with a dissociative disorder have often learned to avoid their bodies in order to avoid particular inner experiences such as traumatic memories, disturbing thoughts, or painful emotions. The image of their bodies, or awareness of sensations or movement, can suddenly evoke traumatic memories. For example, some people find that paying attention to their body as they try to practice breathing exercises, or in the normal course of washing, can evoke difficult memories, feelings, and sensations. For some, looking in the mirror may evoke an instant feeling of shame or self-hatred.

Fear of Doctors or Physical Examination

Many people with a dissociative disorder find going to the doctor and getting a physical exam very anxiety producing; thus, they do not seek medical care when they need it. Some parts may be afraid to be touched or find that being "looked at" is a trigger. They may not trust doctors or nurses for various reasons, or they may fear being out of control or trapped. They sometimes are afraid they are exaggerating and will be ridiculed, or will not be taken seriously, or will be told something is wrong and do not feel they can handle "bad news."

Because people with a dissociative disorder often have a lot of physical symptoms that have no obvious cause, they may have been told that their symptoms are "in their head," resulting in feeling ashamed and belittled. Actually, their physical symptoms are in their mind and also in their body, as are all symptoms for everyone. The mind and body are inseparable. Such individuals are not imagining their symptoms; rather, these symptoms may be a combination of physical intrusions from dissociative parts, and the chronic stress response of the body, the latter of which often leads to more serious physical problems over time.

Note: Make sure you find a competent and understanding primary care physician. Make a list of qualities you would like to have in a doctor and interview several to find a best fit for you. Ask friends for recommendations. If you feel it would be helpful, you may ask your therapist and physician to be in contact with each other to ensure that you have an integrated health team.

Managing Alcohol, Illicit Drugs, and Prescribed Medications

Many traumatized people tend to self-medicate with substances because they have chronic inner chaos, depression, anxiety, flashbacks, loneliness, or other emotional pain. They may misuse drugs or alcohol or prescription drugs to relax, numb out, or feel better in the short run. In some cases, particular dissociative parts of a person will misuse substances and there may be inner conflict about using. In a few cases, a person with DID may have little to no awareness (amnesia) that a part is using drugs or alcohol. Self-medication can easily lead to addiction over time.

Although this manual does not address addiction treatment, if you are dependent on substances or are abusing them, it is of the utmost importance to share this problem with your therapist and make it a major focus of your current treatment. Any addiction seriously complicates the effects of being traumatized and interferes with treatment. If you are not sure whether you are self-medicating or addicted, please discuss it with your therapist. Keep a record of what you use, how much, how often, and what prompted you to use. You can draw on the skills in this manual to help yourself learn to handle your problems more effectively than by using substances.

Many psychiatric medications are meant to be taken on a regular basis, every day, unless otherwise prescribed. You should understand what you are taking, why you are taking it, and have a basic understanding of how it works. Perhaps you have inner conflicts among parts about taking medication. Some parts may believe taking medication is a sign of "weakness" or a "crutch." Nothing could be further from the truth. Psychiatric medications often help your brain function more effectively, just as a heart medication might make your heart work better if you have a cardiac problem, or as insulin augments what your pancreas is not able to produce if you have diabetes. Make sure you take your medication as prescribed. Some medications (for example, antidepressants) take days or even weeks to become effective: They cannot be taken only during times when you feel bad. Others that act quickly and have short-term effects should not be taken too often: These are generally prescribed to take "as needed." For instance, you may have been given something for anxiety that you take only when you feel especially anxious. Either before or when you take this type of medication, also use your skills to calm yourself and all parts of you. For example, talk inwardly to orient and calm parts of yourself, listen to what parts may need, step back and reflect on your inner experience, practice relaxation or safe space exercises, go for a walk, or call a friend. Finally, feel free to discuss your medications with your doctor and share inner conflicts about them with your therapist (and your doctor, if applicable).

Regulating Your Physical Energy

Physical self-care involves regulating your energy level. Almost all people with a dissociative disorder have some difficulty regulating their energy. Some push themselves beyond what is reasonable, for instance, by working too much or spending too much time doing for others, and thus are constantly exhausted and depleted. Others are far too inactive, which further contributes to lethargy, depression, and disinterest in life. It is essential for you to learn to pay attention to your body's signals of hunger, thirst, fatigue, and illness. Your body needs replenishment and rest on the one hand, and activity on the other. It is essential to reach a degree of cooperation among parts of yourself to ensure you have the proper amount of rest and activity for your healing (see also chapters 10 and 11).

Tips for Resolving Inner Conflicts About Physical Self-Care

- Take time to reflect on why you might be having difficulties with physical self-care and/or body awareness and make a list of them.
- Do not judge yourself about these conflicts; just notice them.
- Prioritize as best you can from the least to the most difficult conflicts on your list. Begin with the least difficult and gradually work your way through to the most difficult. As you gain mastery with resolving the less intense conflicts, you and all parts of yourself become more confident and trusting with each other, and you will be more willing to take the next steps.
- Using an inner safe space, meeting room, or by talking inwardly, determine whether all parts of you might agree that physical self-care might be a good thing if it was completely safe and allowed. If so, good: You can take the next step. If not, stop and reflect on why parts of you believe taking care of yourself would not be helpful even if it was safe and allowed.
- You might talk inwardly to remind all parts of you that when you (all of you) take care of yourself, you feel better physically, which helps you feel better emotionally. All parts might benefit.
- Remind all parts of you that your body is safe in the present and that body sensations are normal messages to help you care for yourself.
- If parts of you believe you do not deserve to take care of yourself, remind them that self-care has nothing to do with being deserving. Those parts might prefer, for the time being, to think of self-care as similar to maintenance of your car. Your car needs gas to take you where you need to go; it needs repairs to run. You cannot just neglect it. You need rest and replenishment to do what you need to do and health maintenance so you can continue doing what you do.
- Make sure you take time to orient all parts to the present and reassure them that you will not get in trouble for taking care of yourself.
- If traumatic memories or intense emotions are triggered when you become aware of your body, help vulnerable parts to stay in a safe place during that time (for example, when you shower or bathe), assuring them that they will be attended to in the near future. And continue to orient them to the present. Be sure to keep such promises.
- Engage in inner discussions and negotiation about the ways in which you can engage in physical self-care. If there are conflicts, be open to hearing respectfully another point of view and try to find common ground, that is, those self-care activities on which all parts of you can agree.

Tips for Improving Your Physical Self-Care

- Learn to understand the messages your body gives you. Are you able to recognize when you are tired, hungry, thirsty, cold, hot, in pain, or ill?
- Are you able to distinguish—at least some of the time—between a sensation or symptom that is part of a flashback and those that are indications of present-day illness or injury? If you have pain or other physical discomfort, you might check inwardly to see whether any part of you might be able to help you understand better.
- When you get up each morning, check in with yourself not only emotionally but also physically. How do you feel in your body? Tired? Ill? Energetic? Sore muscles? Achy joints? Stomachache or headache? Relaxed? These physical sensations are messages about your physical and emotional needs.
- Practice physical relaxation every day, as noted in earlier chapters. Develop internal agreement about these activities and times you should practice them. Chronic physical tension adds to mental and emotional stress, and it takes a toll on your body.
- Exercise regularly, even if only a little.
- Make sure you are getting enough rest. Most people need 7 to 8 hours of sleep each night; some need a little more or less. People with a dissociative disorder usually sleep much less, but if sleeping is a problem make sure you are at least taking short rests during the day. All parts of you need to agree that a specific time is set aside for sleep (see chapter 9).
- If doctor or dentist appointments are difficult, try taking a supportive person with you, talk with your doctor or dentist about your anxiety, practice relaxation techniques, and imagine parts of you being in a safe place during the appointment, or perhaps sleeping through it (see chapter 8 on inner safe places). If needed, take a prescribed antianxiety medication before you go, if you have one. It also helps to write down your fears, including those of other parts, and challenge them or think about how you could help yourself make the appointments less scary or shameful.
- Imagine caring for young parts of yourself internally, if that is helpful to you. For example, imagine giving them a warm bath, pampering them physically, giving them a sense of being cared about and cared for. Or imagine that all parts of you are experiencing the self-care you are giving yourself. All parts need to be reminded that self-care is a part of daily life and necessary for healing.

Homework Sheet 12.1
Physical Self-Care Questionnaire

The following questions are designed to help you learn more about your areas of strengths and need for growth in physical self-care. This is not a test: There is no pass or fail. Various parts of you may have different answers to the same question. If so, note it so you can understand and help those parts of yourself. Completing this questionnaire will help you chose one or two target areas on which you would like to work as a beginning to better self-care (see Homework Sheet 12.3).

For each question, circle the number that best applies to you at the present time:

    0   Does not apply to me
    1   Rarely applies to me
    2   Sometimes applies to me
    3   Often applies to me
    4   Almost always applies

1. I pay very little attention to my physical health.   0 1 2 3 4
2. My physical health is poor.   0 1 2 3 4
3. I am afraid to see a doctor.   0 1 2 3 4
4. I do not have a primary care doctor.   0 1 2 3 4
5. I never see a doctor even if I have serious symptoms.   0 1 2 3 4
6. I have trouble feeling pain or cold/heat in my body.   0 1 2 3 4
7. I am afraid to go to the dentist.   0 1 2 3 4
8. I never see a dentist.   0 1 2 3 4
9. I do not eat healthy meals.   0 1 2 3 4
10. I often forget to eat.   0 1 2 3 4
11. I eat at irregular times.   0 1 2 3 4
12. I am underweight.   0 1 2 3 4
13. My weight often fluctuates.   0 1 2 3 4
14. I regularly have bouts of binge eating.   0 1 2 3 4
15. I frequently vomit after eating.   0 1 2 3 4
16. I take laxatives regularly.   0 1 2 3 4
17. I am inclined to overeat.   0 1 2 3 4
18. I am overweight.   0 1 2 3 4
19. I exercise more than 2 hours a day.   0 1 2 3 4
20. I exercise regularly.   0 1 2 3 4
21. I do not get enough exercise.   0 1 2 3 4
22. I have physical problems that I am ashamed to discuss.   0 1 2 3 4

23. I do not follow through with medical recommenda-
    tions.   0 1 2 3 4
24. I am afraid to take prescribed medication.   0 1 2 3 4
25. I take medications for all my aches and pains.   0 1 2 3 4
26. I have daily aches and pains that really bother me.   0 1 2 3 4
27. People tell me I drink too much sometimes.   0 1 2 3 4
28. I drink alcohol when I feel upset.   0 1 2 3 4
29. I sometimes drink until I pass out.   0 1 2 3 4
30. I use illicit drugs socially.   0 1 2 3 4
31. I use illicit drugs when I am upset.   0 1 2 3 4
32. I do not recognize hunger or thirst.   0 1 2 3 4
33. I do not recognize when I am tired.   0 1 2 3 4
34. I have physical problems, but a doctor has told me
    there is nothing wrong, or that it is "in my head."   0 1 2 3 4
35. I do not get enough rest.   0 1 2 3 4
36. I stay busy all the time.   0 1 2 3 4
37. I do not have any energy.   0 1 2 3 4
38. I sleep too much.   0 1 2 3 4
39. I have trouble sleeping.   0 1 2 3 4
40. I cannot tell if I am really physically sick or not. 0 1 2 3 4

Homework Sheet 12.2
Making a Healthy Change in Physical Self-Care

Look over the previous questionnaire. Choose one or two target areas on which you would like to work. Complete the section below. Remember to take small steps toward changing your behaviors and habits. It takes a few months for a change to become a habit. Enlist the support of your therapist and others who can help you.

Example
Item number (from the questionnaire): #22 I have physical problems I am ashamed to discuss.

Describe your problems in this area: I feel ashamed to talk about my body. I feel like I have done something wrong, if something is wrong with my body. I hear an angry voice telling me not to say anything. Sometimes I can't tell if I am exaggerating a symptom or if it is real.

My objectives (what I want to do differently about the problem): To tell my therapist about at least one physical problem so I can work with all parts of myself to resolve fear and shame about that problem.

Inner conflicts or concerns about changing my behavior: A part of me thinks I am weak and whining if I mention something physical. If I start telling my doctor all the physical symptoms I have, I am afraid she will think I am a hypochondriac.

Steps to achieve my objectives:

1. I will choose one small physical problem: pain in my back from lifting something heavy that is keeping me awake at night.
2. I will ask internally whether all parts are aware of the pain and how much it interrupts my sleep.
3. I will ask whether any part of myself has some suggestions to help me take care of my back by helping me be more aware of how I am moving and lifting things.
4. I will rest my back for 2 more days. If it is not improved, I will see the doctor.

5. In the meantime, I will discuss with my therapist the shame and fear I feel when something is wrong physically, as well as my reaction of shutting down and suffering in silence.

Following the example above, complete your targeted change in self-care.

Item number (from the questionnaire):
Describe your problem:

Your objectives (what you want to do differently about the problem):

Inner conflicts among parts or concerns about changing your behavior:

Steps to achieve your objectives:

CHAPTER THIRTEEN

Developing Healthy Eating Habits

AGENDA

- Welcome and reflections on previous session
- Homework discussion
- Topic: Developing Healthy Eating Habits

  - Introduction
  - The Many Meanings of Food and Eating
  - Eating Problems in People With a Complex Dissociative Disorder
  - Tips for Resolving Inner Conflicts About Healthy Eating

- Homework

  - Reread the chapter.
  - Complete Homework Sheet 13.1, Record of Your Eating Patterns.
  - Complete Homework Sheet 13.2, A Plan for Improving an Eating Problem.

Introduction

The focus of this chapter is to help you resolve problems with eating related to traumatization and dissociation. Eating is an integral part of healthy living and an often overlooked partner in healing from trauma. Sensible and healthy eating nourishes and helps heal your body, which is under chronic stress when you have a dissociative disorder. When your body feels better, you feel better in general. But if you grew up in a home in which eating was associated with tension and stress at mealtimes, or food was not healthy or readily available, or was used as excessive reward or punishment, various aspects of eating may be difficult for you. We begin with an understanding of the many meanings of food and eating, and then discuss ways in which you might deal with any eating problems that may be related to your dissociative disorder.

The Many Meanings of Food and Eating

Food and eating are often associated with positive thoughts and feelings for most people. Being fed as an infant is one of the very first ways we experience a relationship. Eating is a way we care for ourselves and receive care from others. Thus, it is connected with giving and receiving, with nurturing and care, that is, with people and relationships. At social gatherings, food is often central. We experience food in many ways: through sight, smell, taste, touch, and even sound (the sizzle and pop of some dishes), so that awareness of foods can affect all of our senses. Certain foods also evoke emotions because they have become associated with particular memories.

Eating is also a necessity, providing us with the energy and nutrients we need for living. Poor eating habits can cause both physical and psychological symptoms. Eating too little can lead to becoming seriously underweight, vitamin and mineral deficiencies, brittle bones, dental problems, anemia, poor memory, and difficulties in thinking clearly and rationally. Overeating can result in obesity, an increased risk of heart disease, diabetes, asthma, joint and bone problems, and even of certain types of cancer. In addition to physical symptoms, eating problems can give rise to numerous psychological symptoms, such as shame and self-loathing, depression and anxiety, a disturbed body image, and a tendency to isolate from others.

Attention to and knowledge about healthy eating habits differ from person to person, family to family, and culture to culture. If you need basic nutritional guidance, cooking skills, help with efficient food shopping, or tips for healthy meal planning, there are many Web sites and books readily available on those subjects. If you need more personalized guidance, we suggest that you consult a nutritionist, whom your therapist or primary care physician can help you locate.

Eating Problems in People With a Complex Dissociative Disorder

A majority of people with dissociative disorders have at least some difficulties with eating (for example, Boon & Draijer, 1993; Goodwin & Attias, 1993; Vanderlinden & Vandereycken, 1997). Different parts of yourself may have different eating preferences or problems, resulting in unstable or chaotic eating patterns. Some parts of you may have reasons to avoid food as much as possible, while others may have a tendency to overeat or binge.

If you are not yet very aware of dissociative parts of yourself, it may be difficult for you to understand certain eating problems that occur due to the activity of these parts. For example, perhaps you find evidence that you have been eating during the night without awareness, or find food in the kitchen that you do not like but must have bought, or feel intense urges to binge or purge, or limit your food unreasonably. You may have food preferences or craving that suddenly begin and end without warning. It may be uncomfortable or perhaps even frightening to realize that other parts of you have actually bought, prepared, or eaten food outside of your awareness. But as you become more comfortable with parts of yourself, you will feel less afraid and more able to negotiate and coordinate the essential activity of eating.

Following is a list of eating problems that are often experienced by people who have a dissociative disorder. Check or circle the ones that may apply to you or to other parts of yourself.

- Bingeing (eating excessive amounts of food in one sitting, beyond what is healthy, to the point of feeling bloated and sick)
- Purging (forced vomiting, use of diuretics or laxatives to get rid of food and decrease weight)
- Food restriction (eating too little or a very limited variety of food compared to what the average person consumes)
- Being triggered by particular foods or by eating in general, and associating food with negative feelings and beliefs, or memories
- Lack of knowledge about basic nutrition
- Difficulties shopping for food
- Difficulties making food choices
- Difficulties with food preparation (for example, it feels too complicated or overwhelming to make a meal)
- Sudden loss of knowledge about how to prepare food or sudden lack of familiarity about how to use kitchen appliances
- Problems establishing healthy and regular eating routines
- Forgetting to eat due to problems with time management and/or inattention

- Inability to feel hunger or thirst due to physical numbness and avoidance of physical sensations
- Desire to maintain a body shape that is not within a healthy range because it feels protective (for example, being overweight helps you feel insulated; being underweight helps you feel less like an object of desire, or it gives you the certainty that you cannot get pregnant)
- Conflicts among parts of yourself about whether, what, and when to eat
- Food and eating are associated with shame and self-loathing
- Difficulty being around others when eating
- "Emotional" eating, that is, using food to cope with emotions
- Food restriction or withholding as punishment

Tips for Resolving Inner Conflicts About Healthy Eating

- Learn to recognize and understand your difficulties with food and eating. Reflect on any inner conflicts about aspects of eating (for example, regarding shopping, staying within budget, preparation, types of food). Make a short list of any problems and check the ones with which you want to begin. Remember to begin with easier problems before you work on more complex ones.
- Recognize that some parts of yourself may be stuck in trauma-time and may have found solutions in the past to regulate intense emotions through their eating habits (under- or overeating), and other parts may be triggered by certain foods or mealtimes. Begin by acknowledging the purpose and intention of these eating problems, rather than blaming parts of yourself.
- Eating problems, like many other problems, can take time to resolve. Be patient and empathic with all parts of yourself. Allow yourself to be content with taking small steps at a time.
- Begin by choosing one small problem area about food and eating, for instance, shopping, or cooking, or irregular meal times. These are tasks that are usually accomplished by you or other parts that have a function in daily life. Make a list of small and very specific steps you need to put into action. Spend time communicating internally to get a sense of how various parts of yourself should be involved with a plan.
- If some part of you is triggered by food to the degree that it makes you unable to eat, help this part of yourself be in an inner safe place during food preparation and mealtimes as a temporary containment. Later,

when you are ready, you can help this part overcome what is triggering.

- You might spend a little time considering what foods you appreciate and enjoy, and whether there are different preferences among parts of yourself. If helpful, use a diary or your computer to create a file where all parts may list their food preferences. You can learn to take into account wishes of other parts in a reasonable way, instead of ignoring or criticizing them.

- Notice what happens when you think about your eating problem, for example, shopping or eating irregularly. Of what beliefs are you aware? What emotions and sensations? Are you aware of any parts of yourself that might have a different experience with eating than you do? Be compassionate with yourself as you become more aware.

- Make every effort to eat at least three times a day in order to get into a healthy routine. Reach an inner agreement with other parts to do so. Make a plan to remind yourself to eat by using a timer or alarm, if you need it. Set some dates to go out with friends to eat. Put a list of meals on the refrigerator and cross them off when you have eaten.

- If you have a daily inner struggle about cooking, or if you have little time for cooking due to work or other obligations, make large portions of food at a time, divide them into individual servings, and freeze them or store them in the refrigerator, so that you will have something healthy to pull out and eat quickly when you do not feel like cooking or do not have time.

- If particular parts of you have strong food preferences or aversions, try to allow some flexibility in responding to them. Perhaps you can temporarily avoid a food if it is triggering to a part of you. Or you might provide a food preference in moderation for a part of you.

- It is important to set healthy limits on the food that various parts want to eat. It will not help you to give in to a part that only wants to eat ice cream or cookies, for example. After all, your job is to begin to provide yourself (including all parts) with a healthy lifestyle.

- Eating patterns often have an underlying emotional goal: You may eat when you are tired, bored, angry, depressed, and so forth. When you feel hungry, yet do not need to eat, notice what emotions or thoughts you are having. Are there any feelings or situations that you might want to avoid by eating? Also pay attention to whether a part of you needs something, such as comfort or attention from you.

- When you have eaten well, and some part of you still feels the need to eat, determine whether this part is oriented to the present. If not, try to orient this part to the present so that you can share your physical sensations of being satiated. You may also imagine an inner safe space where food is plentiful for parts of you that may feel chronically deprived.

- Binge eating is usually a way of regulating unbearable feelings. If you suffer from (nocturnal) attacks of binge eating (with amnesia), inner communication and cooperation with parts can help stop this behavior. For example, perhaps parts will agree that nighttime is only for sleeping (see chapter 9 on sleep), and not for eating. A safe inner place with plentiful food may be sufficient to stop parts of you from actually eating during the night. With the help of your therapist you can begin to understand more about the parts of yourself that engage in such behaviors and then try to help them make positive changes, which may include finding suitable alternatives that meet their needs adequately.

- Try to make more social contacts that involve eating. If you have problems with regular meals, make an agreement with friends or colleagues that each person will cook a large meal to share with everyone each week (for instance, a big pot of soup, stew, pasta, chili, etc.), so you do not have to cook as often. This activity and sharing also helps you become more accustomed to socializing while eating.

- If you or parts of you find it hard to eat, pair your eating with something enjoyable about which all parts can agree, for instance, taking a picnic to eat on a pleasant hike; sitting outdoors and enjoying the breeze while you eat; arranging your food nicely on the plate and adding a special garnish; setting the table nicely and adding flowers, candles, and music; and so forth.

- If there is a day that you really cannot eat, use liquid nutritional supplements.

- If you have serious eating problems, be honest with your doctor, dietician, and therapist and let them help you make a stepwise plan that works for you.

Homework Sheet 13.1
Record of Your Eating Patterns

1. List healthy eating habits you and parts of yourself already employ and wish to continue.

2. In the chart below, list your successes and challenges in eating. Successes might include eating at a regular time, eating healthy food, preparing a meal. Challenges might include forgetting to eat, refusing to eat, bingeing, eating junk food, or difficulty in shopping or preparing a meal. Use this chart to keep track of your eating.

	Breakfast	Lunch	Supper	Snacks	Nights
Monday					
Tuesday					
Wednesday					
Thursday					
Friday					
Saturday					
Sunday					

Homework Sheet 13.2
A Plan for Improving an Eating Problem

Based on the example below, list one eating problem, your objectives for what you want to change, any inner conflicts among parts of yourself, and specific steps to help yourself. Objectives should always be measurable, defined, specific, and include simple steps.

Example

Eating Problem	*Describe Your Problem*
Eating unhealthy food	Eat a lot of junk and fast food; not enough vegetables; too many sodas; hate to cook
Eating at irregular times	Forget to eat; eat on the run; snack all day; find evidence that I am eating during the night

My objectives (what I want to do differently):
Eat a healthy meal (including fresh fruits and vegetables or salad) *at least* once a day at a regular time: lunch (between noon–1 p.m.) or dinner (between 6:30 p.m.–7:30 p.m.)

Inner conflicts or concerns about changing my behavior:

1. Parts of me like junk food, and it's a comfort for them and me.
   o Possible solution: Buy one type of junk food and have it, but in limited quantities; that is, eat one serving portion. Chew your food slowly and mindfully, and savor it; this will make you feel more full and satisfied. Be mindful that you have given yourself a treat.
2. I don't like change and I am afraid of additional inner struggles.
   o Possible solution: I will try to communicate (maybe with help of my therapist) with parts of myself so I can understand more about the fear of change. I will find and discuss with all parts of myself. I will start small, changing one thing at a time. I will introduce one healthy food at a time, and I will begin with one regular meal that includes some healthy food.

Steps to achieve my objectives:

1. Take time for inner communication, cooperation, negotiation, and joint decision making about each step of my plan.
2. Gain a better understanding of what foods are and are not healthy.
3. Set specific times to eat each day and set an alarm as a reminder.
4. Choose a couple of healthy and easy recipes or find places where I can buy prepared healthy food that is within my budget.
5. Make a list before going to the grocery store; take into account different preferences of all parts of myself.

6. Ask a friend to shop with me, so I will stick to my list.
7. Go to grocery store only once a week.

Eating problem (describe your problem in detail):

My objectives (what I want to do differently; be specific):

Inner conflicts or concerns about changing my behavior:

Steps to achieve my objectives (begin with small, manageable changes; be specific).

PART THREE
SKILLS REVIEW

You have learned a number of skills in this section of the manual. Below you will find a review of those skills and an opportunity to develop them further. As you review, we encourage you to return to the chapters to read them again and repractice the homework a little at a time. Remember that regular, daily practice is essential to learn new skills.

For each skill set below, answer the following questions:

1. In what situation(s) did you practice this skill?
2. How did this skill help you?
3. What, if any, difficulties have you had in practicing this skill?
4. What additional help or resources might you need to feel more successful in mastering this skill?

Chapter 9, Developing a Bedtime Routine; Developing and Using a "Sleep Kit"

1.

2.

3.

4.

*Chapter 10, Developing a Realistic and Healthy
Daily Structure and Routine*

1.

2.

3.

4.

*Chapter 11, Relaxation Exercises (The Tree, The Healing Pool,
and Muscle Relaxation)*

1.

2.

3.

4.

Chapter 11, Developing a Relaxation Kit

1.

2.

3.

4.

Chapter 12, Making a Healthy Change in Physical Self-Care

1.

2.

3.

4.

Chapter 13, A Plan for Improving an Eating Problem

1.

2.

3.

4.

Coping With Trauma-Related Triggers and Memories

Understanding Traumatic Memories and Triggers

AGENDA

- Welcome and reflections on previous session
- Homework discussion
- Break
- Topic: Understanding Traumatic Memories and Triggers

  - Introduction
  - Autobiographical Memory and Traumatic Memory
  - Understanding Triggers
  - Recognizing Triggers
  - Types of Triggers
  - Triggers for Positive Experiences

- The Store: An Exercise for Support, Strength, and Protection
- Homework

  - Reread the chapter.
  - Practice The Store exercise.
  - Use the Learning to be Present exercise from chapter 1 as needed.
  - Complete Homework Sheet 14.1, Identifying Triggers.
  - Complete Homework Sheet 14.2, Reflecting on Reactions to Triggers.
  - Complete Homework Sheet 14.3, Identifying Positive Triggers.

Introduction

The instability experienced by people with a complex dissociative disorder is often related to the reliving of past traumatizing events, also known as *flashbacks* or *reactivated traumatic memories* (Boon, 2003; Van der Hart et al., 1992). In this chapter you will learn more about traumatic memories and how they are different from everyday, normal memories; why they are so overwhelming; and how they are related to dissociative parts of yourself. Traumatic memories are often evoked or triggered by a stimulus (*trigger*) in the present that is a reminder of some aspect of the original traumatizing event. You will learn more about triggers and how to recognize them. In the next chapter, you will then learn how to reduce and cope with triggers.

Autobiographical Memory and Traumatic Memory

Generally people are able to recall important events they have experienced in the past. They realize the event has happened to them and that it is not happening now. The memory is, so to speak, a part of their "autobiography." But as you may painfully experience at times, this is not the case with traumatic memories. When you, or a dissociative part of you, reexperiences a traumatic memory, you feel as though it (or at least some aspect of it) is happening in the present.

Traumatic memories may include intense or overwhelming feelings, such as panic, rage, shame, loss, guilt, despair; conflicting beliefs and thoughts; physical sensations such as pain; visual images, sounds, and smells; and also behaviors, such as running away, fighting, freezing, or shutting down. Each of these aspects of a traumatic memory can occur simultaneously, in succession, or separately at different times. Typically, these reactions are not appropriate to the current situation, or they are far more intense than the situation warrants. You may want to return to chapter 4 for a review of traumatic memories (flashbacks).

Understanding Triggers

A trigger (or reactivating stimulus) is something that bears a literal or symbolic similarity to an aspect of an unresolved traumatic experience. It may be a present-day situation, an interaction with another person, an object, or even an inner experience such as a particular feeling or sensation, a smell, or a position of your body. Parts of you then may automatically react in similar ways as during the original traumatizing situation, that is, parts of you have conditioned reactions that you cannot consciously control.

Being able to accept traumatic experiences as your own is not easy, and it may take some time and work before you are ready. This manual is meant to offer you opportunities to learn and practice the skills you need to be able to achieve the task of fully realizing what has happened to you. In the meantime, you may find that you continue to have problems from time to time with being triggered, because some dissociative parts of yourself remain stuck in trauma-time and thus are vulnerable to reliving past experiences. Therefore, it will be helpful for you to be able to recognize triggers and your reactions to them in order to change these conditioned responses.

Recognizing Triggers

It may be hard to recognize when you are triggered unless you have an extreme reaction. But it does help to recognize some possibilities that you might be triggered:

- Your reaction to a situation seems more intense than is warranted, or it is significantly different than your usual reactions.
- You are not able to step back and reflect in the situation, but feel stuck in your reaction.
- Inner parts of you become activated to the degree that you are aware of them.
- You have a defense reaction, that is, flight, fight, freeze, or collapse.
- You seem to watch your reaction unfold, not feeling in control of it, as though another part of you is having the reaction.
- You switch to another part of yourself and lose time.
- You have a sudden flashback; these are almost always triggered by something in the present.

Sometimes you may be able to recognize the link between a trigger and the original traumatizing event. For example, a person might be aware that the smell of gasoline evokes fear and panic because of a traumatic past experience involving gasoline. However, at other times, you may not be aware of what has triggered you. Perhaps you have no memory of the event and thus cannot make a connection with a trigger. Or even if you know about it, you may not be (very) aware of the part of yourself that has become triggered, or you may simply not understand the link between them. As we have noted, the parts of you that function in daily life are adept at avoiding parts stuck in trauma-time, as well as the traumatic memories that they hold, so you may find yourself not wanting to know why you are triggered. Unfortunately, this avoidance has serious disadvantages. When you cannot understand and accept your inner experiences, they become confusing and frightening, seemingly arbitrary and out of control. This only increases your fear of inner experiences and you then make your life ever smaller to avoid dealing with yourself (see chapter 5 on the phobia of inner experience). Therefore, you need to learn to reflect on triggers and the reactions they evoke in you and other parts of yourself.

Although it may sometimes seem as though "all of life" is a trigger, it can be of great help to distinguish specific triggers. Then you can notice that not all situations are equally disturbing to you and that you have already learned to cope successfully with certain triggers.

You may be puzzled by the fact that you can be triggered at one time by a stimulus, but not at another time. Your vulnerability to triggers is determined to a large degree by your physical and mental condition in the moment. If you are more tired or spacey, sick or seriously stressed, or faced with new challenges or problems that seem overwhelming, you are more likely to be triggered. If parts of you are in inner chaos and conflict, you are very prone to becoming triggered more easily. And as you work on particular aspects of your history, the triggers related to that time may be more active for a while.

Triggers can involve an infinite variety of experiences or objects, depending on what has become associated with a particular traumatic episode. Although it is important to recognize triggers, you do not necessarily need to know at this point in time the history related to the trigger in order to cope differently. In the early stages of treatment you may not yet be ready to deal with painful memories to which they are related.

For example, if you feel panic in crowded stores, regardless of whether you know why, you can begin to help yourself with practical solutions. Perhaps you might choose to shop during times when stores are less crowded. You might make a list before you go, so that you minimize time in the store. You can help parts of you remain in an inner safe place while you shop. You might take your partner or a friend with you. We will discuss strategies such as these to cope with triggers in the following chapter, but your first task is to be able to recognize that you have become triggered and to notice your conditioned reactions, that is, your thoughts, feelings, impulses, sensations, movements, and so forth. To that end, we describe various types of triggers, which may help you become more aware of your own.

Types of Triggers

Following you will find an explanation of different types of triggers.

Time-related triggers. You may have heard of "anniversary reactions," in which a person has a predictable and involuntary reaction on or around the anniversary of a traumatizing event. This experience is most well known in people who have intense grief reactions each year around the anniversary of the loss of a loved one. But anniversary reactions may be evoked for a wide variety of other events. At first, you may not recognize an anniversary reaction, but you or your therapist may begin to notice that you, for instance, become depressed, or very anxious, or feel suicidal around the same time each year, time after time.

Time-related triggers may also involve a time of day or a particular period of time, such as weekends or holidays (see also chapter 16). For example, some traumatized people may become increasingly fearful and anxious as it becomes dark each evening, related to overwhelming experiences that may have occurred around that time.

Place-related triggers. Many people find it hard to return to places where they were abused or had other highly distressing experiences. This avoidance can generalize to other places that remind them of the original situation, prompting them to evade more places and experiences to prevent triggering. For example, if a person had been robbed or assaulted on a bus, he or she might be inclined to avoid all busses. And eventually, this person may come to avoid any public transportation, including trains, trams, and planes.

Many traumatized people regularly report that they are upset or overwhelmed by crowded spaces, such as shopping malls, long checkout lines, or crowded waiting rooms. Their aversion often has nothing to do with a traumatic memory, but rather they feel overstimulated and trapped, which may be similar to inner experiences they felt during traumatic events in the past.

Even though some parts may be triggered by certain places, other parts may not be; they may even enjoy, for example, riding in the train or flying, or being at the mall. These contradictory experiences may set up internal conflicts, because some parts may dismiss or even be unaware that a trigger is problematic for other parts.

Relational triggers. Relationships themselves are often triggers. Relationships and any perceived threat to them evoke the most powerful feelings in everyone, for better or worse. When you have been mistreated by others, intense feelings of abandonment, rejection, humiliation, shame, panic, yearning, and rage are often easily triggered by the minor ups and downs that are a natural part of even the best of relationships. And when a serious relational disruption occurs, it can feel catastrophic. Some parts of you may always be on guard, looking out for any cues that perhaps you are being rejected or criticized, and thus they may overlook important cues to the contrary. Others may desperately seek out relationships, not attending to whether they are healthy (see chapters 28 and 29 for more about relationships).

Many patients with complex dissociative disorders rightly felt criticized, lonely, and misunderstood as children. Anger or critical remarks by a partner or a friend in the present may quickly give rise to a partial reliving of old experiences, such as intense fear of being abandoned or misunderstood, or fear that you cannot speak your mind without terrible consequences.

Internal triggers. People who have a dissociative disorder have typically learned to avoid much of their inner experience in order to avoid traumatic memories (see chapter 5). Any inner experience may be triggering, such as the sound of another part talking or yelling, certain emotions (anxiety, anger or shame, and so forth), sensations (such as pain, sweating), needs (such as wanting to be comforted), or thoughts (such as *"I wish I was dead"* or *"I am not happy in this relationship"*).

Some parts may even provoke other parts as an internal reenactment of old experiences. For example, a highly critical part might scream that you are stupid when you are trying your best to cope with a difficult problem at work. This inner experience may be quite similar to some you may have had as a child. We will further discuss ways to deal with this type of internal triggering from dissociative parts of yourself in chapter 22 on anger, and chapter 24 on shame and guilt.

Sensory triggers. Body sensations are a particular type of internal trigger. These may resemble similar sensations that occurred around the time of a traumatizing event. Smells are particularly potent triggers. Other sensations include pain, the racing heart and breathlessness of anxiety, feeling too hot or cold, nausea, thirst, hunger, stomachache, the need to eliminate, or even certain body postures. Some women may be triggered by the sensations that accompany menstruation. The sense of being touched by another person may be especially triggering from some individuals.

Triggers for Positive Experiences

Triggers are usually thought of as negative, but some triggers evoke positive feelings and memories. For example, looking at pictures of a nice holiday that you enjoyed, the smell or taste of a specific food, or particular music may all evoke positive memories and feelings of contentment or warmth. Positive triggers are important because they can help you find some enjoyment and calmness in the present. In fact, your personal anchors are positive triggers that help you stay in the present.

THE STORE:
AN EXERCISE FOR SUPPORT, STRENGTH, AND PROTECTION

This imagery exercise is intended to help you cope with triggers by girding yourself with resources that can help when you feel overwhelmed. Practice this exercise often, or a similar one that fits better for you, when you are feeling calm. Once you are familiar with the exercise, you can begin using it when you feel stressed.

Imagine a store in which anything you want or need as a resource for healing can be found and taken for free. This is no ordinary store, with ordinary aisles and ordinary merchandise. This is a magical place, a special place, beautiful and comfortable. Perhaps you see it as a quaint village shop, or an old bookstore with comfortable chairs and steaming pots of tea, or a sleek high-tech store with all the latest gadgets, where espresso and lattes are available as you browse. You can envision it in just the right way for you. It is your store that you create. In your shop you feel completely at ease, wandering up and down the familiar aisles, where the lighting and temperature are just right, where all is well and just as it should be. Perhaps it is quiet, or perhaps your favorite music is playing in the background. Perhaps there is even a little stage where your favorite musicians are performing just for you. This is one store where you really enjoy lingering, choosing just the right items for your strength and protection. And indeed, there is an endless selection: shields; screens; transparent bubbles; magic stones; books of great wisdom; vials of liquid with healing properties; protective spirit or animal guides; magic cloaks of many colors, and some invisible to all but you; form-fitting, lightweight suits of armor; emotional Kevlar, and on and on. Each is an equally strong and effective protection from the slings and arrows of life, from the vulnerability of being triggered. You may choose as many as you like, and exchange them as you wish. And as you wander around, or sit comfortably in a chair, allow all parts of you to have their time in this store, because it is for all of you.

Just to practice, try out one of the special protective suits or cloaks. Just as a raincoat or waterproof suit keeps the water out and allows it to slide off of you, or just as a windbreaker protects you against icy winds, so you can imagine that you have found just the right suit of protection for yourself in your store. And allow each part of yourself that wishes or needs to have their own suits, each suit just right for each part of you. You will be amazed at how flexible and lightweight, yet sturdy and comfortable it is. You can don it in an instant, so quickly that no one notices. You can take it with you wherever you go, and wear it whenever you like. Your suit or cloak is just the right weight, the right material, the right texture and color to help you feel completely protected from head to toe, front to back, up and down, all around, where not a single chink or crack or hole will allow negative forces to gain entry, and where you are comfortably ensconced in safety and calm. You are completely protected in body, mind, and heart. You are protected from other people's emotion that set you on edge, from triggers that might evoke you, from the stresses and strains of life and living. If you wear the suit even when you feel more tranquil and secure, it offers you extra protection, adding even more serenity, calm, and safety.

Now allow a situation to come to mind, one in which you felt uneasy or insecure. Imagine wearing your suit or cloak and walking into that situation with a sense of deep protection, confidence, relaxation. It is as though you cannot be touched by the situation, unaffected by the stress of it, yet still you feel very present because you feel safe and protected. Take your time to imagine yourself in the situation with this protective suit. And be aware that at any moment, you may make adjustments to your suit or return it to your store and find another. When you are ready, you can return to your store. Look around once again, taking all the time that you need to be familiar with every aspect of it. This is your store. You can return whenever you need or want. It is there for each part of you whenever it is needed. And when you are ready you can return to the present, feeling strong and serene, supported and safe.

Homework Sheet 14.1
Identifying Triggers

Choose a time when you were recently triggered. Reflect back on the situation and answer the questions below, as you are able. This reflection will help you become more aware of yourself and what evokes you and other parts of you. *If this exercise evokes too much for you, simply stop and practice a grounding or relaxation exercise. It is essential to pace yourself.* Discuss with your therapist how you might be able to learn more about triggers without becoming overwhelmed.

1. Where were you and what were you doing when you were triggered?

2. Describe the trigger, if you know.

3. What was your inner experience of being triggered (for example, feeling like you were out of body, anxiety or panic, visual or auditory flashbacks, nausea, loss of time)?

4. If you lost time, what is the last thing you can recall (for example, a sound, smell, image, thought, feeling)?

5. Are you aware of any specific parts that may be involved? If so, please describe what you understand about that part of yourself.

6. If you were with someone, what, if anything, might have been stirred up for you in the relationship (for example, you felt hurt, angry, invisible?)

7. Note the date, season, and time of day when you were triggered, if you have a sense that the trigger may be time related.

Homework Sheet 14.2
Reflecting on Reactions to Triggers

In the chart below, choose a time each day this week when you have been triggered (if you have). Do not focus on any traumatic memories at this point, but only your reactions to them. As you reflect on the experience, answer the questions below as best you are able. If you are not being triggered, that is wonderful! You may then use this chart to describe previous examples of being triggered.

	What triggered you, or a part of you?	What did you think and feel?	What was your physical reaction (fight, flight, freeze, collapse?)	What resources or help would you need to respond differently in the future?
Monday				
Tuesday				
Wednesday				
Thursday				
Friday				
Saturday				
Sunday				

Homework Sheet 14.3
Identifying Positive Triggers

Make a list of positive triggers and what they evoke for you. Use these experiences in your daily life to help you feel better and more grounded.

Examples
　1. **Positive trigger**: snowfall
　　 Reaction: a feeling of pleasant excitement and fun memories of playing in the snow
　2. **Positive trigger**: the smell of freshly baked bread
　　 Reaction: a feeling of comfort, of having pleasant and basic things in life
　3. **Positive trigger**: a funny joke or movie
　　 Reaction: laughter, feeling grounded, a feeling of being lighter for a time

　1. **Positive trigger:**
　　 Reaction:

　2. **Positive trigger:**
　　 Reaction:

　3. **Positive trigger:**
　　 Reaction:

CHAPTER FIFTEEN

Coping With Triggers

AGENDA

- Welcome and reflections on previous session
- Homework discussion
- Break
- Topic: Coping With Triggers

  - Introduction
  - Reducing or Eliminating Triggers in Daily Life

- Homework

  - Reread the chapter.
  - Complete Homework Sheet 15.1, Identifying Triggers and Coping Strategies.
  - Complete Homework Sheet 15.2, Skills to Cope With Triggers.

Introduction

In the previous chapter you learned about triggers, and that parts of you stuck in trauma-time are most vulnerable to being triggered, unable to distinguish between the past and present. You may not always be completely aware of these parts. The more you can reflect on your inner world, the more effective you can be in helping all parts of yourself cope with triggers. But of course, managing triggers is difficult. The first steps are usually the hardest. Do not expect yourself to completely control all your triggers immediately. And some triggers are easier to manage than others. Any person can be triggered by completely unexpected situations. Just take your time and learn to be more reflective and tolerant of your experiences.

In this chapter we focus on specific ways to deal with triggers effectively.

Reducing or Eliminating Triggers in Daily Life

Regardless of whether you are ready to directly cope with your traumatic memories, you must still deal with being triggered in ways that interfere with your daily life. In the following sections we describe specific methods to cope with triggers.

Eliminating or Avoiding Triggers

When you become more aware of your triggers, you may temporarily eliminate or avoid certain objects or situations, and thus become triggered less often. *This should be a temporary measure only,* until you are able to resolve what is being triggered. Otherwise you will feel the need to restrict your experiences more and more. But once you are triggered less often, you can begin to work on your skills and resources so you can overcome what is upsetting you. Temporarily stow away, give away, or throw away objects in your home that trigger you, for example, photographs, art, a particular blanket, a knick-knack, a book. It is important to remind yourself and other parts of you that a particular object or situation does not have to overwhelm you the rest of your life. You and other parts can learn to be less reactive in the present as you begin to feel safer and calmer. It might be helpful to remind all parts of you that the object or situation is reminiscent or representative of something painful from your past, but it is not dangerous itself.

When you are not able to eliminate a trigger, you might temporarily avoid it. For instance, if you are triggered by seeing someone drunk, avoid places where such people are likely to be found (parties, bars, pubs, weekend nights in the city). If a part of you is terrified of crowded areas, you can choose to shop at times when stores are likely to be less crowded, while you are working with that part to overcome the fear of crowds. If a part of you is afraid of the dark but you want to see a movie, you can choose to watch a DVD at home instead of going to the theatre. Again, these are only meant to be temporary solutions, until such time that you can approach and handle the cause of being triggered more adaptively. You can also have empathy for these parts of you instead of being angry or frustrated with them, and assure them you are taking their needs into account as well as helping them gradually overcome their fears or concerns.

Anticipating Triggers

If you anticipate that you might be triggered by a certain situation that cannot be avoided, you can plan ahead to cope with it effectively. For example, perhaps you need to make an appointment to receive a flu shot, but some part of you is terrified of shots. You may find the crowded waiting room intolerable, and feel exposed and vulnerable when visiting a doctor. Nevertheless, you need your influenza shot for your health, so this is not a situation to be avoided.

You can prepare yourself by reflecting with all parts of you to discover what you need to cope. You can calm and reassure parts inside that you are getting medication that keeps you healthy: You, as an adult, will make sure nothing bad will happen. You might take time before the appointment to help parts of you go to an inner safe place, or you might imagine allowing them to stay at home, and only adult parts that can distinguish the past from the present of yourself should go to the appointment. Some people may have inner helper parts that can calm and reassure, but it is doubly effective if you can join with these helpful parts in reassuring all parts of you. You can use your own imagination to help vulnerable parts in this way until they are able to heal.

Above all, do not ignore parts of you that are triggered by acting "tough" and belittling these parts of yourself. You run a far greater risk of losing control or switching than when you anticipate what you need.

In addition to inner preparation, you might also ask for the support of others when you are faced with a situation that triggers you. In the aforementioned example, you might ask someone to go with you to the doctor— someone who will keep talking with you to help you stay present. You can ask to make your appointment the beginning or end of the day, or immediately after lunch, so you can be in and out without spending too much time sitting in the waiting room.

Imaginal Rehearsal

All too often, when people imagine an upcoming situation, they imagine themselves failing or being overwhelmed. That is, they imagine a negative outcome. Imaginal rehearsal is the opposite: You imagine yourself being completely successful, walking through the situation step by step (Bandler & Grinder, 1975). Many people find it helpful to imagine successfully negotiating through a challenging situation ahead of time. You may begin by imagining that you are watching yourself. For example, imagine watching yourself walk into the doctor's office feeling calm and adult-like. Imagine being able to reassure yourself if you begin to feel anxious. Imagine being wrapped in your protective suit or your favorite colors, and not even feeling the injection. Imagine that all parts of you feel perfectly safe in the present.

Imagine having all the support you need. Imagine supportive people being with you, encouraging you, cheering you on. After you have successfully "watched" this scenario, imagine it from your own perspective. Imaginal rehearsal is more successful when you share its purpose with all parts of you, and as many parts as possible can participate.

Recognizing Options

Often when people are triggered, they feel trapped and helpless. Recognizing that you have options is essential to feeling more control and choice. You might be surprised at the choices you do not realize that you have. And you are only limited by your own creativity! For example, continuing with the example of the flu shot, if you become too triggered, give yourself the option of leaving if parts of you become too afraid. Or give yourself the option of walking outside to calm down or allowing the nurse to help you calm down. Give yourself the option to either watch or avert your gaze when you get the shot: whichever helps you more. Give yourself the option of being assertive and asking the nurse or doctor to tell you every step of the procedure ahead of time, so you will know what to expect and can be a part of deciding how and when the injection is given.

Neutralizing the Effects of Triggers

You can learn to create distance from the emotional and physical experience of being triggered. Usually this method involves imaginal techniques that you have already learned in this manual. For example, you can use an inner safe place in which parts of you can be protected from the overwhelming experiences of being triggered. Parts of you may voluntarily go to sleep in their safe place if you anticipate a time when you may be triggered, so that only adult parts aware of the present need cope with the situation. You can use The Store exercise in chapter 14 and imagine having on a special suit or cloak, or a shield that triggers cannot penetrate. Or try The Tree or The Healing Pool exercises from chapter 11 to immediately calm all parts of yourself if you become triggered. In chapter 18 you will find suggestions for putting your feelings in a container such as a bank vault or a computer file.

Distinguishing the Past From the Present

It is essential for all parts of you to learn to distinguish between here and now and then and there. For example, a particular knife or fork from the kitchen or the color of the living room wall in the present may remind you of a painful experience in the past, but it is not the same knife or fork or the same living room. Of course, before you can make a distinction between the past and present, you must be aware that you are in the here and now. Continue using your various anchors to the present from chapters 1 and 2.

The more quickly you can ground yourself, the easier it will be to cope with triggers. You may also find it helpful to carry a small object, such as a beautiful small stone, as a tangible reminder of being in the safe present. As soon as you touch it, you can immediately feel yourself become more present.

Once you are present, you will find it helpful to describe the differences between an experience in the past and present in detail, to actually say it out loud to yourself, and to keep reminding all parts of these differences. For example:

The green color on the wall is the same as in the past, but the wall, the room, the house, the city, the year, and even I am not the same as in the past. The only similarity is green, only paint. I am not there, I am here. I can see the pictures on the wall that are different than in the past. The carpet on the floor is different. When I look out the window, I see the scenery of the present, which is different from the past. This green wall reminded me of something that I am not yet ready to handle. I will put that memory in a safe place and contain it until I am ready.

This repetition gradually helps all parts to notice these differences, instead of only focusing on what is similar to the past.

It is particularly important to pay attention to differences when a person in the present reminds you of someone from the past with whom you felt uncomfortable or unsafe. For example, if a friend becomes irritated with you in the present, you or other parts of yourself might automatically react with fear because an angry person was dangerous in the past. However, you notice that your friend's voice is not raised, and he is not screaming or cursing. He is speaking to you respectfully, and you know his intentions toward you are good in general. His body language shows no indication that he might be physically violent. These are cues that tell you this interaction is different from the past. Draw the attention of all parts of you to these cues and bring them back again and again to these cues in the present. In this way all parts of you can learn that although an aspect of the present might be similar to the past (irritation or anger), many other aspects are different enough that you can learn when it is safe. You are teaching parts of yourself the early beginnings of reflection about the motivations and intentions of others in the present.

It is also helpful to notice what is different about *you*, that is, you are an adult, not a child. You are stronger, have more wisdom and experience, and have supports and resources that you did not have as a child.

Inner Orientation, Cooperation, and Support

You have begun to experience times of being able to orient parts of you to the present, help parts cooperate for your well-being as a whole person, and share mutual inner support. These skills are essential in helping you overcome the effects of triggers. When inner parts feel more trusting of each other to attend to, care for, and respect one another, they will feel calmer and less afraid and chaotic. When they are helped to become more oriented to the present, they can reflect more on their inner experiences. And when parts can cooperate, for example, to help other parts remain in an inner safe place without disturbance or to avoid situations in which you may be triggered, all parts of you will feel better. Some degree of inner cooperation is already present when you talk inwardly to all parts of yourself, when you remind them of the safe present, when you create inner safe places, when you practice relaxation exercises, and when all parts of you pay attention not only to what is similar to the past, but more important, to what is different.

This inner cooperation and support can grow exponentially over time, as you will see. People with a dissociative disorder often know at some level, or in some part of themselves, which situations are best avoided or how a triggering situation might best be handled. Inner dialogue and reflection among parts about the best approach to situations is helpful, and it must go beyond merely telling all parts to "just do it." You are a team and must work as a team. Be compassionate with yourself and all parts inside; and help them to engage cooperatively with you as often as you are able. Of course, we are aware that inner cooperation, communication, and support take time to develop and are not always easy to achieve. It may not always seem clear or obvious how you can accomplish these skills. Be patient with yourself and all parts of yourself. In chapter 27 we will return to the subject of inner cooperation, as well as to more advanced work on distinguishing between the past and the present.

Homework Sheet 15.1
Identifying Triggers and Coping Strategies

As in your homework from the last chapter, choose a time when you were recently triggered and reflect back on the situation and answer the questions below, as you are able. This reflection will help you again practice identifying triggers but also to become aware of what coping strategies you might already use. *If this exercise evokes too much for you, simply stop and practice a grounding or relaxation exercise.*

1. Where were you, and what were you doing?

2. Describe what triggered you, if you know.

3. What was your inner experience of being triggered (for example, feeling like you were out of body, anxiety or panic, visual or auditory flashbacks, nausea, loss of time)?

4. If you lost time, what is the last thing you can recall (for example, a sound, smell, image, thought, or feeling)?

5. If you are aware of specific parts of yourself that were triggered, describe their experience as best you can.

6. If you were with someone, what, if anything, might have been stirred up for you in the relationship (for example, you felt hurt, angry, invisible?)

7. Describe what you did to cope with being triggered at the time, and what you did afterwards. You may have used some of the coping skills discussed in this chapter or others. You may even have coped in ways that were not healthy. Do not judge yourself; simply describe what you did.

Homework Sheet 15.2
Skills to Cope With Triggers

Choose a time when you were recently triggered and reflect back on the situation and answer the questions below, as you are able. This reflection will help you become more aware of how you might employ some of the skills you have read about in this chapter. *If this exercise evokes too much for you, simply stop and practice a grounding or relaxation.* Refer back to the chapter as needed. You will be using one or more of the following skills:

- Eliminating or avoiding triggers
- Anticipating triggers
- Imaginal rehearsal
- Recognizing options
- Neutralizing triggers
- Distinguishing the past from the present
- Inner orientation, cooperation, and support

1. Describe an object or situation in the present that triggered you recently.

2. Describe the reactions of you, or other parts of you, to the trigger (for example, feeling like you were out of body, anxiety or panic, visual or auditory flashbacks, nausea, loss of time; being frozen or collapsed).

3. If this trigger can be eliminated or avoided, describe how you could accomplish that for the future (for example, avoiding violent movies, putting away a photograph or book; deciding not to visit a particular place).

4. If you were to anticipate this trigger in the future, how might you prepare for it? For example, helping parts be in an inner safe place, using images of protection, or practicing imaginal rehearsal.

5. Describe in retrospect any options you had but did not realize that you had at the time you were triggered (for example, you could have left the situation, called a friend for support, oriented parts of yourself to the present, or calmed and reassured them, but you did not think of it).

6. Practice protective imagery (for example, from The Store exercise) and containment strategies for the feelings, sensations, and memories that are evoked when you are triggered.

7. Describe the differences between the trigger in the past and its present-day context, for example, the bed is similar, but the room is different; the beard on a man is similar to the past, but it is not the same man.

8. Describe any inner orientation, communication, cooperation, and support you were able to accomplish when you were triggered. If you were not able, describe what stopped you and how you might support your inner parts in the future.

CHAPTER SIXTEEN

Planning for Difficult Times

AGENDA

- Welcome and reflections on previous session
- Homework discussion
- Topic: Planning for Difficult Times

  - Introduction
  - Planning Issues for People With a Complex Dissociative Disorder
  - Difficult Holidays and Other Special Times
  - How to Plan for a Difficult Time
  - Reflections to Help With Planning for Difficult Times
  - Tips for Effective Planning
  - When Obligations to Others Conflict With Your Needs

- Homework

  - Reread the chapter.
  - Complete Homework Sheet 16.1, Preparing for a Difficult Time.

Introduction

People with a complex dissociative disorder often have specific periods of difficulty with depression, anxiety, fear, shame, posttraumatic stress, or other problematic symptoms. Many of these difficult times can be predicted based on how people have reacted in the past to similar situations. These times might include weekends, extended time alone, holidays, times when contact is necessary with people who were abusive in the past, or painful anniversaries of past events (which often are not recognized as such). Planning is always needed for times in which you are likely to encounter an unusual amount of triggers. When you are able to predict that you might have a hard time, you can plan ahead to deal with the situation effectively, instead of being blindsided by it. These important coping skills of forward thinking and planning, the ability to "deal with it before it happens," are essential in daily life and also vital in learning to help dissociative parts of yourself. This chapter will help you learn to plan for difficult times so they are a little easier to manage.

Planning Issues for People With a Complex Dissociative Disorder

Planning ahead may be difficult and can be an enormous challenge for individuals with a dissociative disorder, especially when it involves the need for self-care and boundary setting. Such people, or at least some parts of them, generally avoid dealing with painful or conflicted feelings and situations. As a consequence, they often avoid thinking about or planning ahead to help themselves better manage a potentially difficult time. In the following sections you will find some of the major reasons why planning is difficult when it involves conflicted dissociative parts of yourself. You may also have your own unique reasons that are not listed.

General Feeling of Being Overwhelmed in the Present

When people are already overwhelmed and depleted, thinking about the future can seem like a monumental task, much less planning for it. Thus, it is essential to do your best to care for yourself, manage your time, get sufficient rest, and use your relaxation skills.

Inner Chaos and Confusion

Cognitive confusion and fogginess, blankness, and inner chaos among parts can make it difficult to think through and plan. Often this is due to being overwhelmed in the present and/or conflicts among dissociative parts.

Inner Conflicts Without Sufficient Capacity for Negotiation

Various dissociative parts may have conflicting needs or desires about an upcoming time. These conflicts may make the time more difficult than it needs to be. People may not be aware of these parts, or they may ignore or belittle them. For example, while one part may enjoy a free weekend, another may find it a waste of time, and yet another may find it lonely and overwhelming. One may dread a holiday while another comments on how ridiculous it is to dread just another day. It can take time to learn how to be more aware of inner conflicts among parts and how to negotiate satisfactory outcomes. You can begin by acknowledging the conflicts and taking them seriously, and trying to help those parts of yourself as best you can. Gradually, negotiation will become easier.

Difficulties With Time, Time Management, and Time Loss

Most people with a complex dissociative disorder have some difficulties with time (see chapter 10; Van der Hart & Steele, 1997). Some are forgetful and may not recall making an appointment, or they may engage in the same activity twice, not remembering they have already done it. Some may be so overwhelmed or depressed that they sit and do nothing or sleep away the day, unable to focus either on the present or the future. Some people with DID report recurrent problems with double bookings of appointments made by different parts of themselves or cancellations of appointments by other parts.

Difficulties Setting Priorities

Some people find it hard to prioritize what is most important, and for people with a dissociative disorder this may involve inner conflicts among various parts about what is important (for instance, feeling safe is a priority that may conflict with being in a particular relationship, which is a different priority).

Problems With Executive Functioning

Executive functions are cognitive skills involved in our ability to organize thoughts and activities, prioritize tasks, manage time efficiently, and make decisions. These skills may be limited or lacking in some traumatized people because traumatic stress adversely affects the areas of the brain that are key to using these functions. These problems can be overcome to a large degree, and there are many readily available resources on the Web or in print for coping with problems with executive skills, particularly in material that addresses attention-deficit disorders in adults.

Difficult Holidays and Other Special Times

Specific times of day, time of year, seasons, holidays, weekends, and anniversary dates of significance may trigger painful feelings or traumatic memories (see chapters 14 and 15 on triggers). In addition, free days and times such as weekends, evenings, holidays, and vacations may be hard because they lack sufficient structure for people who do not yet know how to manage their free time (see chapter 11 on relaxation and free time). During such days people may have more time to feel and think about painful issues or memories, which they might prefer to avoid. And if they are avoiding dealing with inner parts, these times are fertile ground for such parts to emerge unbidden. Therefore, empathic internal communication and collaborative planning are invaluable to prepare for these times.

Next we discuss holidays as one example of a stressful time for which it is helpful to plan in advance.

Managing Holidays

Holidays are painful for many people, not just those who have a dissociative disorder. Some degree of depression, anxiety, loneliness, hurt, and general stress are fairly common for people in general. Everyone knows about the "holiday blues," and at some level most of us realize that expectations of ideal holidays rarely match reality. Yet even when people may realize their expectations are unrealistic, they still may be affected emotionally. And there are added complexities for people who must make difficult decisions to be with family who might have been abusive in the past or continue to be abusive in the present; furthermore, some people are faced with the prospect of being alone at an important time. Finally, there may be pressure from those around you, or parts within you, to act like everything is fine, when you feel anything but fine. Such demands compound feelings of loneliness and being misunderstood, and even of shame or despair.

Many people with a dissociative disorder did not have positive experiences of holidays in childhood, and these memories may be triggered, resulting in anxiety, depression, inner conflict and chaos, and flashbacks. Inner reflection, including communication with dissociative parts of yourself, may help you identify triggers and help you make plans to cope with them. You might decide to consciously avoid the trigger for the time being or help parts of yourself cope differently. For example, you might decide to use different holiday decorations, if the usual ones remind you of painful times. Or you might notice the similarities and differences between here and now and then and there, for example, the holiday is the same, but what happens during the holiday now is quite different from then, and you are an adult now. The problem is not the holiday (the trigger) itself, but what it represents for you. You might plan to find ways to contain painful memories so you can enjoy the present holiday, and then deal with these memories at a later time, for instance, storing them in an imagined vault, or box, or on a computer file. It is often helpful to plan how you want to spend a holiday instead of waiting to find out what friends and family will do and whether they will invite you to join them. Learn to be proactive and deal with it before it happens!

Times of Day, Anniversaries, and Seasons

Many people with a dissociative disorder struggle during other kinds of situations that are reminders of painful events in the past. Perhaps nights are hard because that is when they were hurt by someone or when they feel the most lonely. Sometimes the date of an overwhelming experience brings back all the pain. For others, a season may be difficult, for example, summer brings up painful reminders of events that occurred during that time of the year or, conversely, may evoke a sad yearning for wonderful summers spent with loving grandparents when life at home was hard.

Other Difficult Times

There are many times in daily life that may be especially stressful, such as a big meeting at work, an ongoing conflict with someone, a visit to the doctor, a medical or dental procedure, a separation or divorce, being alone when you need the support of others, or having to meet with family members whom you find difficult or even unsafe, and many others. Some of these situations may be challenging in their own right, while others are difficult because they trigger you or some parts of you. We have addressed many of these issues in other chapters, for example, dealing with doctors in chapter 13 on self-care, coping with triggers in chapters 15 and 16, and regulating overwhelming emotions in chapters 17 and 18.

Coping With Being Alone During Difficult Times

There may be important times when you wish to be with others but instead find yourself alone. This happens from time to time for almost all people. Perhaps it is a weekend or holiday, your birthday, or a difficult anniversary for you. The loneliness that is evoked can be profound and painful.

Make efforts to plan for these times. Even though you are alone, you do not have to feel lonely. Use your relaxation kit (chapter 11) and plan healthy activities to occupy yourself. Make a list of activities that you or some parts of you would like to do with and without other people. Try choosing a couple of activities that are agreeable to your whole self. If you cannot be with someone during your difficult time, plan to get together with someone a little later. You can always celebrate holidays or birthdays on a different day if you are flexible. After all, it is the enjoyment of the day, not the date itself that is important. If you are alone during a holiday or other important time, volunteer somewhere or make other active plans instead of sitting at home doing nothing and feeling lonely. You will find more help in dealing with being alone and lonely in chapter 30.

Regardless of the type of situation, if you think you might have a hard time, the planning process is similar, with certain predictable steps, which we discuss next.

How to Plan for a Difficult Time

If you know of an upcoming time that will likely be difficult for you in some way, begin early with inner reflection and communication among parts of yourself. Reflect on what happens for you during those times, noticing what you feel and think, how your body responds to the stress (for instance, freezing or agitated), and how various parts of you react. The awareness you gain from reflection allows you to make different choices instead of feeling hopelessly captive in your experience.

For example, if you are aware a part of you always criticizes you during these times, you might be able to communicate more with this part of yourself to understand why. Perhaps this part believes you will fail and criticizes you in the hopes that you will try harder, or perhaps it uses anger to avoid shame or fear about the situation. If you know you always freeze, you might be able to begin to notice and to change that physical reaction instead of being stuck in it. If you can be aware that you are feeling hopeless, you might be able to provide yourself with comfort, meaningful contact with others, and inner support for parts of yourself.

You may dialogue with parts of yourself, write in a journal or on the computer, or imagine an inner meeting. If you find these tasks difficult, ask your therapist to help you. Do not wait until the day before to communicate internally about upcoming difficult times. Give yourself sufficient space to think it through, to reflect, and to make a plan that will help you, so you can "deal with it before it happens." Even if you do not have "direct" communication with parts, you may already be aware of certain activities, people, foods, and so forth that might trigger you, as well as some ways to help yourself be more comfortable and safe.

In the next section you will find some questions that will help you reflect on how you, including all parts of you, can best plan for difficult times. Find a quiet time at home to reflect on these questions. Try to take into account thoughts and ideas from as many parts as possible, because various parts of you may perceive the situation differently from each other.

Reflections to Help With Planning for Difficult Times

- What times tend to be your most difficult?
- When you have a difficult time, what happens? For example, what do you feel and think, how does your body react?
- How do you usually make a plan? For instance, do you think it through, avoid it, prefer to be completely spontaneous, talk about it with others?
- What obstacles do you encounter while planning? For instance, beginning a plan, identifying the steps needed to complete a plan, getting lost in too many choices or details, inner criticism or conflicts among parts, trouble completing a plan.
- What techniques and skills do you already use to help yourself with planning? You may also check on the Internet, look for books on planning (and executive functioning), or ask for help from your therapist or other supportive people.
- What has helped you in the past with difficult times?
- List any triggers for which you know you need to prepare yourself.
- What are the fears and concerns of various parts of yourself about a particular time?
- How might you ensure your emotional and physical safety during this time?
- What obligations might you have to others during this time? Do these obligations conflict with your own self-care?
- Are there relational limits or boundaries that you need to set? If so, what would help you set them?
- Are particular parts of yourself especially vulnerable during this time? If so, what do they need to feel safe, supported, and cared about by you?
- Notice whether you prefer activities with other people during difficult times or if being alone is more helpful.

Tips for Effective Planning

- Put your plan in perspective. The need to plan is usually not an emergency, so you do not have to do it urgently. Give yourself time to think and to check in with yourself.
- Try to let go of the belief that there is only one single "right" solution or choice. There are almost always many "right" pathways, and if you

make a mistake, you can deal with it. Many plans involve a combination of pros and cons, so often there is not a "perfect" solution, but rather one which likely requires some compromises.

- Most importantly, include all parts of yourself in your planning. Attend to their concerns, needs, and desires without judgment.
- Listen to both your head and your heart, that is, reflect. Sometimes your logic and your emotions (or "gut") tell you something entirely different. Various dissociative parts typically base a choice either on too much feeling or on avoidance of feelings and needs, and they often do not know enough about the present. If all parts of you can work together to learn more about the present, acknowledge feelings, needs, and wants, and offer inner empathy and support, making plans can be a lot easier and clearer.
- Think before you act. Take your time, even if you feel "urgent." Imagine being in your safe space or use a relaxation exercise to get yourself in an alert, calm space. Let all parts of yourself know they will be acknowledged and considered as you make your plans.
- Imagine how your plan will affect *you* and parts of yourself. You are learning how to take care of yourself, which means you need to take yourself into consideration, as well as others. This is not selfish, but rather good self-care. After you anticipate how the plan will affect you and other parts of yourself, then you can take others into consideration.
- Ask trusted others for feedback, but make your own plans, taking their advice into consideration.
- Be willing to modify your plans if they are not working. Making small changes along the way often helps you accomplish your final plan better than rigidly sticking to a plan.

When Obligations to Others Conflict With Your Needs

You may find yourself in conflict during a difficult time between your own needs and those of others. For example, you may have an obligation to attend a family function that you know will be very stressful for you. You prefer not to go, but you must. This may provoke intense inner conflicts among parts inside. Next you will find some suggestions for dealing with these conflicts in such a way that you are able to take care of yourself. You must learn to set healthy boundaries and negotiate compromises that work for you and all parts of you (see chapters 30 and 31 on assertiveness and personal boundaries).

- Negotiate to limit visits with others who are difficult, for example, visit for an hour instead of an entire evening, or a day instead of a weekend. Announce your time limit in advance or at the beginning of the visit. If needed, set the alarm on your watch or phone for the right time so you will not forget, or have a trusted person call you at that time.
- Stay in a hotel rather than in the home of a person with whom you have a difficult time.
- Invite a friend to be with you for support.
- Make plans to leave early if needed.
- Have your own transportation so you do not have to rely on someone else.
- Use imaginary rehearsal, protective suits, and inner safe places.
- Make quiet times for yourself during difficult visits by taking walks, going to your room to read or rest, or going to a movie or other activity.
- Make time for inner reflection and check-ins with all parts of you. Treat their needs seriously and with compassion.

Homework Sheet 16.1
Preparing for a Difficult Time

Choose a difficult time that you predict is likely to occur (not your most difficult, but one that you feel ready to tackle). Record your reflections below regarding this difficult time (you may refer back to the reflections to help you plan). If possible, allow parts of you to participate without making any judgments about them. Try to develop a plan to address your difficult time. It is OK to start with very small steps. If you were able to try the plan after you made it, describe what happened. If you were not able to try the plan (or come up with a plan), please describe what made it difficult.

1. Describe the difficult time on which you have chosen to work in this exercise.

2. Describe what you are most concerned about during this time (for example, having flashbacks, being overwhelmed, being afraid, freezing and going blank).

3. If you are aware of any parts of yourself that are particularly vulnerable during this time, describe what might happen for them (for example, a part may want to engage in self-harm or may feel suicidal; it may want to be with someone who is hurtful to you; or it may be terrified, ashamed, or become enraged).

4. Begin your planning by finding a quiet time, free of distraction and chaos. Use some of the relaxation exercises in chapter 11 to help you be calm and clear headed. Also use your inner safe place(s) to help all parts of you feel safe and secure. It is essential to stay focused on the present, not on the imagined catastrophic future.

5. Next, check in with all parts of yourself to survey your needs and desires for this time and describe them below. It is fine if various parts have conflicts: Do not judge them or worry about the conflict, but rather simply write down what each part of you wants or needs during the difficult time. For example, one part may want to self-harm, while another part wants to hide; yet another part may want to explode in anger, while another part wants to be extra good so that she might be loved by someone.

6. You may be able to find some common ground among parts in these conflicts you have shared in #5 above. For example, if a part wants to self-harm, you likely are feeling overwhelmed with some emotion, and the self-injury may be a way to reduce the sense of being overwhelmed. And certainly all parts could agree that being less overwhelmed might be a common goal each of you could work toward. Likewise, if one part is terrified and another part is furious about this "cry baby," it is possible that both parts need and want safety. The one is expressing fear, while the other is acting "tough" to protect vulnerability: Both are simply different ways to respond to threat. And all parts might agree that feeling safe is a worthy common goal.

Describe one or two inner conflicts (if you have any) about your difficult time, using the examples above as a guide. After you describe the conflict, see if you can determine the underlying common goal among parts. If you need help, make sure you take time in therapy to understand these conflicts and any possible underlying common goals.

7. Describe your plan for being emotionally and physically safe during your difficult time, using inner consultation and, if needed, help from trusted others.

8. Describe the resources you or parts of you may need to cope with your difficult time. For example, parts may need to feel safe or comforted, may need to remain in an inner safe place, may need to know the adult part of you is capable of dealing with the situation, or that a safe person is available to talk, if needed.

9. Finally, describe what you will do if you become overwhelmed. For example, you can leave, take a time-out and go for a walk, call a friend, take time to go to an inner safe space, practice relaxation exercises, or take prescribed medication to calm you.

PART FOUR
SKILLS REVIEW

You have learned a number of skills in this section of the manual. Below you will find a review of those skills and an opportunity to develop them further. As you review, we encourage you to return to the chapters to read them again and repractice the homework a little at a time. Remember that regular, daily practice is essential to learn new skills.

For each skill set below, answer the following questions:

1. In what situation(s) did you practice this skill?
2. How did this skill help you?
3. What, if any, difficulties have you had in practicing this skill?
4. What additional help or resources might you need to feel more successful in mastering this skill?

Chapter 14, The Store Exercise

1.

2.

3.

4.

Chapter 15, Identifying and Coping With Triggers

1.

2.

3.

4.

Chapter 16, Strategies for Effective Planning for Difficult Times

1.

2.

3.

4.

Understanding Emotions and Cognitions

CHAPTER SEVENTEEN

Understanding Emotions

AGENDA

- Welcome and reflections on previous session
- Homework discussion
- Topic: Understanding Emotions

  - Introduction
  - Basic Emotions and Their Functions
  - Problems With Emotions for People With a Complex Dissociative Disorder

- Mindfulness exercise
- Homework

  - Reread the chapter.
  - Practice the Mindfulness exercise at home.
  - Complete Homework Sheet 17.1, Identifying and Understanding Emotions.
  - Complete Homework Sheet 17.2, Sensory Experience of an Emotion.

Introduction

Emotions are part of our basic functioning as humans. They are present in everyone, and they are there to guide us and help us make decisions. Emotions are felt in the body; they involve somatic sensations, specific postures or movements, and tendencies toward certain actions. They are also understood as signals to behave in certain ways during particular circumstances. Generally emotions are not voluntary, that is, you cannot "make" yourself feel a particular emotion. They are a bit like internal weather, coming and going, changing from time to time, flowing from one to the other, sometimes stormy, sometimes calm. This internal weather is as normal and expected as outside weather. And like weather, emotions are influenced by various environmental stimuli, either internal or external effects. Emotions are spontaneous (involuntary) reactions to events outside and inside ourselves. They are primary guides that help us best adapt our behavior to what is happening in the present. For example, love helps us be closer to someone we care about; fear helps us avoid a dangerous situation; joy helps us seek out pleasant experiences.

Because emotions are basic to our functioning, it is essential to understand and learn to "read" them. The first step is being able to name and recognize basic emotions, and then to understand their functions and how to respond to them.

Basic Emotions and Their Functions

There are many lists of basic emotions. We have chosen to describe eight that are based on our evolution from animal emotions and are found universally in people around the world. These emotions are paired in a range from mild to intense.

1. Interest–Excitement
2. Enjoyment–Joy
3. Surprise–Startle
4. Distress–Anguish
5. Anger–Rage
6. Fear–Terror
7. Shame–Humiliation
8. Disgust

Judging Emotions

Although we often tend to view emotions as good or bad, this is not a helpful judgment. Emotions are neither good nor bad; they simply are part of our functioning as humans. It is true that we recognize some emotions as pleasant and others as unpleasant or painful, but you will find it very useful to focus more on the purposes and meanings of an emotion rather than judging them. This is a step toward accepting them as part of you and part of life.

Emotions Help Us Meet Our Needs

One major function of emotion is to motivate and initiate behavior that is directed toward specific goals, that is, behavior that can meet our needs. For example, anger directs us to fight when we are provoked, hopefully keeping us safe; fear prompts us to run away or avoid something that is frightening or threatening; love directs us to behave in ways that draw us closer to the ones we love, because we need safe relationships.

Emotions are not really separate "things"; they are part of bundled experiences that include not only emotions, sensations, thoughts, and physical actions but also our perceptions of what is happening in the present and our predictions of what will happen if we act in a certain way. Emotions are as essential as thinking and behaving to our survival. However, when the ability to regulate and tolerate emotions is disrupted or inadequate, this entire bundled experience becomes difficult to manage.

Two Kinds of Emotional Experiences

Some feelings or emotions are involuntary reactions to events that happen around you (for example, feeling joy because someone is especially nice to you; anger because someone criticizes you or forgets a date you made; fear because something startles you). Other emotions are primarily a reaction to your own thoughts, actions, and feelings (for instance, being ashamed of your body because an inner voice tells you that you are ugly; feeling embarrassed that you feel sad; feeling guilty or afraid because you are mad with someone). These "feelings about feelings," that is, emotions about our inner experience, particularly those that involve variations of shame or pride, are called *self-conscious* emotions (Tracy, Robins, & Tangney, 2007). They can often be problematic, because they are paired with inner negative judgments about what we experience.

Feedback Loops of Perceptions, Thoughts, Feelings, and Behaviors

As noted earlier, our emotions are intimately connected with our thoughts, behaviors, sensations, and the ways in which we perceive the world. These experiences are not actually separate, but rather bundled together, in continuous feedback loops with each other. For example, when people feel afraid, they will tend to view the world through the lens of fear, perceiving many things as threatening, when daily life may not be dangerous in reality. These perceptions are related to fear-related thoughts and beliefs, for example, *"That man is frowning; he must be angry with me; anger is dangerous; I must get away."* These thoughts and beliefs heighten the perception of danger, which heighten the feelings of fear, which heightens thoughts of danger, and so on. And perceptions, emotions, and thoughts induce decisions to act in certain ways. Eventually, people may become so sensitively conditioned to an emotion such as fear that merely having a physical sensation of fear, such as a sinking feeling in the stomach, may prompt them to believe danger is near and to act in a fearful way.

Problems With Emotions for People With a Complex Dissociative Disorder

People with a complex dissociative disorder were often confronted as children with situations that evoked extreme and overwhelming emotions. Generally young children learn from their caregivers how to understand and regulate emotions. People with a dissociative disorder often grew up in families in which it was not acceptable to show or discuss certain emotions. In some cases, it was actually dangerous to express feelings, resulting in punishment, ridicule, or complete disregard. Parents or caregivers of people with a complex dissociative disorder typically had a problem with emotions themselves and were thus unable to teach their children adaptive and healthy skills to deal with emotions. These children learn to avoid or disregard their own feelings. They also have difficulty reflecting, that is, accurately reading other people's emotions and intentions in the present, generally assuming something negative rather than positive.

Intense Emotions Are Often Dissociated

People with a dissociative disorder have compartmentalized, intolerable, intense emotions in various parts of their personality. Sometimes parts that function in daily life do not experience much emotion and have learned to avoid feeling much. They may experience feelings as "all or nothing," that is, far too intense or not at all. Some dissociative parts of the personality, living in trauma-time, may experience the same emotion no matter the situation, such as fear, rage, shame, sadness, yearning, and even some positive ones just as joy. Other parts have a broader range of feelings. Because emotions are often held in certain parts of the personality, different parts can have highly contradictory perceptions, emotions, and reactions to the same situation. As an example, you may be in your therapist's office and hear a door slam in the hallway. You jump and are startled, but the adult part of you is able to think, *"It's OK. It's just a door closing."* Yet a very frightened part of you becomes more and more upset and freezes or wants to run out of the room, because that part is not yet oriented to the present and still feels in great danger as though the past were the present. Intense fear continues to be dissociated in that part of you, while you may not feel it at all. You, or other parts of you, may be highly critical of the scared part of yourself.

You may become so fearful or ashamed of so many emotions, as well as the physical sensations that are a natural part of emotions, that you have learned to avoid (some of) your inner experience at all costs (see chapter 5 on the phobia of inner experience).

Negative Judgments of Emotions Among Dissociative Parts

Dissociative parts of an individual often make negative emotional judgments about each other. For example, one part may feel disgusted because another part feels needy or dependent; or one part feels angry because another part is afraid to try new things. Some parts avoid feeling anything at all and believe emotions are a waste of time. Some people hear these comments in their head or "sense" them in the background. These "feelings about feelings" are often highly problematic, because they generally include harsh, negative judgments about basic emotions, which, in fact, are merely an inevitable part of being human.

Fear of Losing Control

The major parts of you that function in daily life may have little idea of why a given feeling occurs, almost as though it comes "out of the blue." Thus, people with a dissociative disorder may experience anxiety or fear of losing control of their behavior or feelings to other parts of themselves. In addition, emotions can be experienced as so overwhelming that some people describe it as "falling apart," "exploding," "crumbling," or other metaphors for intense loss of control.

Difficulty Attending to Emotional Signals in the Present

We all must attend to the signals that emotions give us. Otherwise the emotion is likely to intensify or evolve into something else even more difficult to manage. Many people find it easy to ignore their feelings. But an ignored minor feeling may escalate to an intense one, for example, irritation at someone who is bothering you may build to outright anger if you do not address it. You might then explode in anger with your friend or partner, and the other person will have no idea why, because you never said anything about being irritated. If you had been able to attend to the signal of irritation, you may have been able to speak up respectfully, set good boundaries, and never come to the point of anger.

Most people with a dissociative disorder have not learned to read their emotional signals, only recognizing that they feel globally overwhelmed, or awful, or bad, or tense. They are not yet able to distinguish the physical and mental signals associated with specific emotions, and how they might differ from the signals of other emotions. They must first learn to read and interpret their emotional signals and match them to particular emotions. Reading emotions may be complicated by the fact that some parts have an emotion, while others may not experience it. The part that does not experience the emotion may only be aware of a vague unease or restlessness. This is one reason why it is vital to develop more internal awareness about your emotions and dissociative parts of yourself.

Triggers May Evoke Overwhelming Emotions

As we noted earlier in the chapters on triggers, they may instantaneously evoke powerful and overwhelming emotions. Various dissociative parts tend to have their own particular set of emotions related to traumatizing events, and thus they will be triggered to experience those emotions, without regard to the present situation. In fact, such parts often do not even experience much of the present. Thus, while one part oriented more in the present may be feeling fine, another part that is stuck in the past might be quite fearful or angry. The emotions of dissociative parts can intrude into present experience so that a person begins to feel fear, anger, or shame that is not related to the here and now. These feelings, stemming from dissociative parts, can be confusing and frightening, leading the person to try to avoid emotions, as well as situations in which these emotions are reactivated.

MINDFULNESS EXERCISE

Emotions can best be understood and dealt with when you are fully engaged in the present moment and able to attend to your inner experience while staying in the here and now. The following exercise is designed to help you practice being present and mindful. It will be most helpful if all parts of you can participate; otherwise your attention is divided rather than concentrated on the present.

You will need a small piece of food that you enjoy, such as a raisin or other piece of fruit, a piece of candy or cookie, cheese or nuts, or a slice of vegetable.

> Take the food and put it in the palm of your hand or between your finger and thumb. Look at it carefully. Give it your full attention and examine it as though you have never seen anything like it before. Roll it gently between your thumb and forefinger. Explore it with your fingers. Look carefully at the parts that might catch the light, and at all the little grooves and ridges or irregularities. Explore every single nook and cranny of it.

And if, while you are doing this exercise, thoughts enter your mind such as "This is stupid!" or "What on earth is the use of this exercise?" or if other thoughts about another topic come, simply acknowledge them and redirect your attention back to your food. Now smell it, holding it right under your nose, and with each breath you take, notice the smell. Slowly move it towards your mouth. You may feel your mouth beginning to water. Put it in your mouth and notice what your mouth feels like, with the food in it. Let it lie on your tongue a little. Then bite down on it deliberately, noticing the taste that is released. Chew on it slowly, notice whether more saliva enters your mouth, and whether the food gradually begins to feel different in your mouth. Chew slowly, savoring each bite. When you are ready to swallow your food, be aware of it going down your throat and into your stomach. Notice that in your mouth the last remnants of the taste of the food may still linger.

Each day this week, practice eating something with complete attention: a piece of cheese, an apple, a piece of candy. Practice with a food that you like.

You can expand this exercise to include other routine actions, such as brushing your teeth, shopping, driving, getting dressed, and so forth. The point is to be completely focused on the present experience, even when there does not seem to be any important meaning to it. Such exercises are meant to help you learn to be present and attentive to yourself and your environment in the moment, a necessary skill for reflecting and keeping yourself grounded.

Homework Sheet 17.1
Identifying and Understanding Emotions

1. Make sure you can identify in yourself or in others the eight basic emotions listed in the beginning of the chapter. Name one or two emotions below with which you feel comfortable.

2. Name one or two emotions that you never or very rarely experience, or of which you are afraid or ashamed.

3. Describe an impulsive urge to act (do something) that you might experience when you are faced with a difficult emotion. For example, when you feel lonely, you feel the need to make the feeling go away by any means possible, even though you know that the behavior is not good for you in the long run, such as drinking, self-harm, (binge) eating.

4. List one or two healthy ways of coping with the feeling you described in #3 above, even if you have not been able to use them yet.

5. Name any emotions you might judge as "bad" in yourself or others and state why you think they are negative.

6. Do you find that pleasant feelings such as happiness, pride, fun, or joy are negative for you? If so, describe what is negative for you about those feelings.

7. Name any emotions that some parts of you might experience and other parts do not. Describe your reaction to those emotions. Describe the reactions of other parts of you to those emotions.

8. Please describe as best you can what you are concerned about or fear if you experience a certain emotion that you now avoid.

Homework Sheet 17.2
Sensory Experience of an Emotion

Choose one emotion and describe how you experience it in as much detail as possible. Feel free to use metaphors, images, and descriptions of sensory experiences. Use the suggestions below as a guide. There are no right or wrong ways to describe your emotion.

- Sensations that accompany emotion: tingly, tense, warm, cold, shivery, sweaty, dizzy, burning
- Colors, such as ice-blue, red-hot, sunny yellow, dreary grey, pitch-black
- Sensations such as bitter, sweet, sour, rough, soft, hard, smooth
- Shapes such as round, square, twisty, ball, triangle, rope, blob
- Metaphors such as "like a storm"; "like a big black hole in my chest"; "like a tornado"
- Creative arts: painting, drawing, doodling, mandalas, collages
- Writing: keep a journal about your feelings or write a story or poetry
- Music: make a collection of music that expresses your emotion
- Movement: explore finding a particular posture or movement that symbolizes your emotion

As you reflect on the sensory experiences above, explore how you might be able to change them to feel better. For example, if you experience an emotion as a hard black ball in the pit of your stomach, ask yourself what the ball wants to do or what it needs. Does it want to be thrown? To change color? Does it want warmth? To be held in your hands? To dissolve into light? Does it have something to say? Does it want to uncurl and stretch out? Does it prompt a movement in your body, a change in posture? Be creative and trust yourself, and get help if you feel stuck in your exploration. Also make sure you are staying within what is tolerable as you explore. If you have trouble doing so, stop and ask for help from your therapist.

CHAPTER EIGHTEEN

The Window of Tolerance: Learning to Regulate Yourself

AGENDA

- Welcome and reflections on previous session
- Homework discussion
- Break
- Topic: The Window of Tolerance: Learning to Regulate Yourself

  - Introduction
  - The Window of Tolerance for Arousal
  - Experiencing Too Much: Hyperarousal
  - Tips for Coping With Experiencing Too Much
  - Experiencing Too Little: Hypoarousal
  - Tips for Coping With Experiencing Too Little

- Homework

  - Reread the chapter.
  - Complete Homework Sheet 18.1, Learning About Your Window of Tolerance.
  - Complete Homework Sheet 18.2, Your Tips for Coping With Feeling Too Much or Too Little.

Introduction

As we noted in the previous chapter, emotion regulation is an essential part of healing. However, many people with a dissociative disorder tend to experience too much or too little in many different areas of life, not only with emotions. They may feel every little ache and pain or change in their body (too much), or they may not feel pain when injured or feel physically numb all over (too little). They may seek out experiences that may be risky (thrill seeking) or avoid new life experiences altogether. They may overthink and be unable to turn off their thoughts, while others may be unable to think much at all and feel blank. Some are highly sensitive to changes in their surroundings, noticing every little thing such that it becomes hard to concentrate, while others are very inattentive to their surroundings. And of course, dissociative parts intrude into the present with unregulated experiences, contributing to feeling too much or too little.

Feeling too much and too little are actually two sides of the same coin: Both indicate difficulties with regulation of physiological arousal. Your arousal level simply indicates how physically and emotionally responsive or even reactive you, or certain parts of you, are to certain stimuli. In particular, you may become dysregulated when you react to stimuli that are especially emotional or stressful for you, such as learning a difficult new skill, having an argument with your partner or friend, driving in traffic, having an unpleasant feeling, or remembering something painful. In order to function at our best, we all need an optimal arousal level—not too high and not too low, depending on the level needed for the current circumstance. In this chapter you will begin to learn how to regulate or modulate your arousal to manageable levels.

The Window of Tolerance for Arousal

A major goal in therapy is to support you, and all parts of yourself, to learn how to experience "enough," rather than too much or too little. This range of optimal arousal is called your *window of tolerance* (Ogden et al., 2006; Siegel, 1999; Van der Hart et al., 2006) (see figure 18.1). It is the range of experiential intensity that is tolerable for each part of you and within which you can learn, have an inner sense of safety, and be engaged with life. You may know from experience that you learn most effectively and feel most comfortable when you are not too agitated or anxious, nor too tired, sleepy, or shut down emotionally. This is true for all parts of you.

When you, or other parts of yourself, are outside your window of tolerance, you experience too much arousal, termed *hyperarousal*, or not enough,

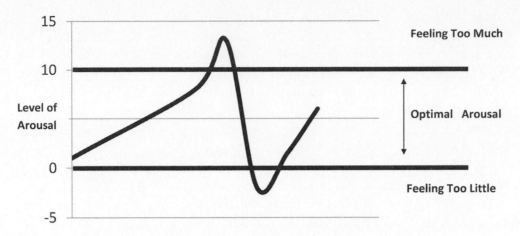

Figure 18.1. Window of Tolerance. Adapted from Ogden et al., 2006; Siegel, 1999; and Van der Hart et al., 2006.

termed *hypoarousal*. Sometimes your window of tolerance might be quite small, like a window that is barely cracked open. Then you, or some parts of yourself, can be overwhelmed quickly and feel out of control or even completely shut down. In that case, your task is to widen your window of tolerance a little bit at a time until it is sufficient for coping with daily life.

Each of us has our rather unique range of what we can tolerate; our window of tolerance is to some degree defined by our inborn temperament and natural level of physiological reactivity. But it is also defined by experiences. When you have been chronically overwhelmed, your ability to regulate your physiological arousal is eventually compromised.

Auto- and Relational Regulation

People regulate themselves by using a combination of relational and self-regulation. The first is referred to as *interactive regulation,* and the second, *auto-regulation* (Schore, 2001). Early caregivers ideally help soothe and regulate an infant or young child by nurturing, encouraging, attending to emotional and physical needs, and comforting. This lays the groundwork for individuals to be able to regulate themselves as they grow and develop. As adults, we call upon others to support us when we are upset, because it can be comforting to have another person present, and he or she helps us view our problems from other helpful perspectives. And at times, others are not available or needed. Then we are able to regulate ourselves by reassuring ourselves, slowing down to reflect, practicing calming exercises, or doing things that help ourselves feel better.

The ability to employ a balance of auto- and relational regulation is important. However, some people find it hard to rely on others for any kind of support, that is, they do not use relational regulation. Others find it hard to rely on themselves, that is, they do not use auto-regulation. Both groups are at a significant disadvantage, since we all encounter situations in which one way of regulating is not sufficient or appropriate. We will discuss more about auto- and relational regulation in chapter 29 on resolving relational conflicts.

Lack of Reflection

A major difficulty in emotional dysregulation is that you are, at times, unable to reflect on what you are feeling, but instead are just "in" the feeling, acting blindly and not able to think clearly. You may find that emotions from dissociative parts of yourself intrude into your awareness. You may not always know where these emotions are coming from, as though they are "out of the blue," and this adds to how overwhelming and frightening they can feel.

Avoidance of Emotion

Most people with complex dissociative disorders are very adept at avoiding emotions. And there are certainly times when it is important to focus on the task at hand and wait to deal with your emotions until a later time. Although avoiding overwhelming or intense feelings may help you function in daily life in the short run, it also leaves you and other parts of you devoid of rich and meaningful connections to yourself, to safe others, and to experiences that make life worth living. And you also have little ability to resolve painful or traumatic experiences.

Perhaps only certain experiences, such as having flashbacks, or the threat of losing a relationship, push you, or some parts of you, out of your optimal level of arousal. But the more afraid or ashamed you are of your inner experiences, the more avoidant of inner parts of yourself, the less ability to reflect, and the more unresolved conflicts or traumatic memories you have, the harder it is to stay within your window of tolerance. Thus, being able to reflect is of prime importance in helping yourself learn to cope with your emotions (review chapter 6 on learning to reflect).

As a first step, you need to find your window of tolerance and learn to stay within it more consistently, and then gradually learn to widen your tolerance level, like fully opening a window that had only been cracked open previously. Each part of you will need to learn to become more regulated. Once your tolerance level as a whole person is wider, you can have a much broader range of experiences that do not overload you. Overwhelmed parts of yourself can feel calmer and more focused, while numb or avoidant parts feel more capable of tolerating emotions and other inner experiences. Thus, all parts of you gradually learn how to regulate emotions and arousal levels, and each part of you can learn to help other parts so that you, as a whole person, learn to deal with emotions and all other experiences in ways that are more constructive and adaptive. And as you learn not to judge your emotions and other inner experiences and are able to reflect on them without so much avoidance, you will find your window of tolerance will increase, that is, you have more tolerance for a wider range of experiential intensity.

A number of exercises in earlier sessions are actually designed to help with emotion regulation and forming a healthy window of tolerance, such as learning to reflect (chapter 6) and creating an inner sense of safety for all parts of yourself (chapter 8). The chapter on sleep (chapter 9) contains methods to soothe yourself when you wake up feeling anxious or scared during the night. The relaxation kit (chapter 11) furnishes you with a list of activities and ways that help you and all parts of you feel more pleasant and relaxed.

Next we explore some of the problems and solutions for experiencing too much and too little.

Experiencing Too Much: Hyperarousal

Typically, some dissociative parts of yourself chronically experience too much, that is, are hyperaroused, because they are stuck in traumatic experiences and feel overwhelmed by fear, pain, shame, and so forth. Or perhaps you, as a whole person, generally feel so sensitive and edgy that it is very easy for you to become overwhelmed and upset in daily life, even when you are not bothered by traumatic memories. You, or some parts of you, might be upset by situations that generally are of little consequence to others, particularly small relational upsets or conflicts, or a last minute change of plans. Once you are upset—agitated, anxious, scared, or angry— it might be hard to calm yourself down (auto-regulation). Time may seem slowed down as though you will be upset forever, and you cannot remember being calm. This makes you even more upset and urgent to stop what you are feeling.

When you are overwhelmed, your judgment is not at its best and you, or another part of you, may impulsively try to stop the intensity of your feelings by acting in ways that may not be in your own best interest in the long run. For instance, people may drink, use drugs, harm themselves physically, get into fights, say things they later regret, or isolate from others. You may find yourself puzzled about why you are so upset and cannot seem to understand what happened: This sometimes occurs when a dissociative part of you has become triggered without your awareness.

Tips for Coping With Experiencing Too Much

There are a number of ways to help yourself when you are feeling overwhelmed. You can temporarily distract yourself and all parts of yourself. You can contain particular feelings or memories or parts of yourself in a safe place. You can express your emotions appropriately. You can reassure and soothe parts of yourself. And you can practice grounding exercises to help keep you in the present.

You will receive the most benefit from the following tips when you are able to reflect on what has evoked your hyperarousal and begin to develop awareness of the struggles of various parts of you that contribute to feeling too much. Empathic understanding of your inner struggles and a willingness to seek out healthy coping strategies to help all parts of yourself are essential to your healing. Without inner awareness and empathy, most coping strategies are not very effective.

Distraction

Temporary distractions help everyone who is feeling overwhelmed from time to time. But it is important for all parts of you to understand that conscious and voluntary distraction as a temporary coping strategy is *not* the same as persistently avoiding the needs of parts of you. Temporary distraction is just a way to slow down your hyperarousal, like using a "reset" button. It gives you some time where you can take a deep breath and rest, so you feel more able and ready to cope with your feelings. An apt analogy is staying busy to take your mind off of a strained muscle while you continue to do the right things to help it heal, since focusing on the pain will not alleviate it and will often make it seem worse. You do not ignore the need to tend to your injury, but once you have done all you can, you may distract yourself as you heal.

Distract yourself with healthy activities and support all parts of yourself to refocus on something other than what you are feeling. However, avoid working too much or engaging in other compulsive distractions that will further stress you. When you distract yourself, always make a promise to yourself that you will return later to what is overwhelming, as soon as you are able.

What works for distraction may vary according to the way in which you are feeling overwhelmed. For example, if you feel overwhelmed with anger you might find a physical activity like walking, running, or gardening helpful. But if you, or parts of you, feel intensely sad, you might chose a soothing activity like watching a nice movie, reading a (children's) book, listening to calm music, or going to your safe inner place. Try choosing activities that match what you are feeling and that are agreeable to all parts of you. Following are additional suggestions for distracting activities.

- Exercise or take a brisk walk; changing your physiology can change how you feel. Encourage all parts of yourself to experience the walk.
- Listen to music while singing the lyrics.
- Do something pleasant or fun that all parts of you can enjoy.
- Call a friend and get together. Talking with another person (not about the problem that is overwhelming you) can take your mind of yourself for a while.
- Engage in an activity that requires concentration, for example, a hobby, a crossword puzzle, or a computer game. Try to encourage all parts of yourself to concentrate on the same thing at the same time.
- Read an interesting or nice book that is not upsetting to any part of you.
- Watch a comedy program or read a funny book. Again, encourage all parts of you to focus on the same activity at the same time. Laughter is a great distracter, and it helps you feel better, too.

Containment

Contain, but do not ignore, feelings and parts of yourself. Containment is entirely different from "getting rid" of your feelings. When you contain a feeling or memory, and thus often a dissociative part of yourself, you are saying to yourself, "*Not now, but I will return to this later*." You are making a promise to all parts of yourself to make the time and energy to deal with it in the right place at the right time. Be sure to take the time to check for internal agreement among parts to contain an experience temporarily.

You can use countless containment images: a bank vault, floating up in a balloon floating high in the air, a submarine, a computer file, a video, and so on. Use your own images that fit for you or parts of you.

A different way to contain is to write or to use art to express what you are experiencing. If this evokes too much for you, there are other ways to contain. But some people find it helps to put their experience on paper or canvas and then leave it there for later. You may allow some parts of you to use this method if it is helpful, while other parts need not be present, for example, by staying in their inner safe place. You can put away these writings or drawings or take them to your therapy appointments to help you move forward in your healing.

Calming and Soothing Yourself

When you soothe and reassure yourself, you are not telling yourself to stop having negative feelings, for example, "*Shut up and don't cry. Put your happy face on.*" This critical approach does not really make any part of you feel better, even though it may be a long-standing habit. Soothing and reassurance are much more effective in calming all parts of you. Soothing includes an empathic acknowledgement of the feeling, for example:

I am feeling sad and angry, and that is a hard combination. I am doing my best to deal with these difficult feelings. It is in the best interest of all parts for me to focus on what I am doing right now and then deal with them when I get to therapy. That way I feel good about how I function in life and also have support to work on these feelings.

This empathic acceptance also includes supporting all parts of yourself, for example:

Since I am feeling so bad, I will do something nice for myself that all parts can enjoy. It is OK for any part of me to have feelings, but I don't want them to overwhelm any part of myself. I will take care of all parts of me.

Following are some tips that help you to calm and soothe all parts of yourself:

- Listen to all parts of yourself and try to reassure and comfort any parts that may be anxious or upset; a little inner communication and empathy go a long way.
- Practice calming, deep breathing exercises. Imagine that all parts of you are breathing together, in perfect synchronization in your safe place.
- Invite upset parts of yourself to go to a quiet, undisturbed safe space where they can be soothed and helped, while promising you will return to what is bothering them as soon as you are able.
- It may also be helpful for you to take a short "time-out" to rest.
- Ask a helpful inner part of yourself to support parts that are anxious or upset.
- Try to slow your thoughts down and each time you notice you are thinking about the problem, shift your thoughts to something else. Help parts of you share thoughts at a reasonable pace.
- Get some rest. Encourage all parts of yourself to rest. If parts are critical, for example, "You are lazy and need to be doing more," try to negotiate with those parts of yourself for a period of rest to see if it actually helps calm you down.
- Listen to soothing music and take into consideration what all parts of you might find calming.

Grounding and Reassurance

- Use all five senses to ground yourself and be aware of the present moment. Say out loud to yourself what you notice with your senses.
- Try just noticing the experience of being overwhelmed, slow your breathing down, and each time you feel the urge to do something about

the experience, allow that feeling or thought to pass through you mind, like a train that does not stop a the train station.

- Remind all parts of you that feelings are normal, a part of life, and that it is safe to feel intensely in the present.
- Remind all parts of you that all experiences, no matter how unpleasant or intense have a beginning, middle, and an end.
- Notice what was happening when you began to feel overwhelmed. This may help you determine what triggered you (see chapters 14 and 15 on triggers). It also reminds you that the feeling had a beginning, and before which you were feeling something else.
- Recall times in the past when the feeling finally passed, that is, remember its ending, as a reminder that this feeling will also end in time.
- Ask your therapist to help you with additional ways to cope.
- Talk to people you know and become curious about how they handle intense emotions and what they do to calm themselves down. You can learn from their experiences.

Experiencing Too Little: Hypoarousal

To avoid feeling the kind of intense hyperarousal described earlier, you, or some parts of yourself, may cope through avoidance and numbing; thus, you experience too little at times. This is called hypoarousal. You, or avoidant parts of you, may evade situations that would evoke too much feeling, which often means you avoid being too close to people, since relationships evoke some of our most intense feelings, positive and negative. Sometimes a part of you may completely shut down for brief periods, going to sleep or being unable to think. Some people may even become unresponsive, unable to hear or respond to someone speaking with them. You might tend to avoid thinking about anything painful or unpleasant, which means you are not able to resolve issues that involve pain and conflict.

Dissociative parts of yourself that feel numb and detached may have little to no empathy for, or even awareness of, other parts of yourself that very much need support and help with feeling too much. It becomes easy for these parts to label certain feelings or experiences as "bad," and thus to be avoided (see chapters 16 and 17). Such avoidance strongly maintains dissociation and prevents healing.

Tips for Coping With Experiencing Too Little

- Because shutting down is often the result of feeling overwhelmed, most of the interventions used for feeling too much are also appropriate.

- You, or a part of you, may tend toward hypoarousal when you are stressed. A major solution is to first become physically and then mentally active. If you, or a part of you, feel sleepy when you are faced with something overwhelming, try to get up and get moving. You must resist the tendency to become more and more still.
- Help inner parts feel safer in the present by reassuring, calming, and orienting.
- Try a brief, vigorous activity to get your heart pumping and your energy level up, for example, jumping jacks, push-ups, or running in place.
- Do not allow your eyes to focus in one place, or you will trance out. Notice your environment. Use all five senses and name the things you notice out loud, in order to ground yourself in the present. If a part of you tends to trance out, you may try putting a little temporary distance between you and that part of yourself, for example, imagining actual physical distance between you or allowing that part of you to go to a safe space.
- Use mental stimulation to get your brain more engaged and active, for example, count backward from 100 by threes or sevens, or go outside and count trees or cars.
- If you have a feeling of being paralyzed, ask inside whether a part of yourself can help you move. You can start with a very small movement, such as moving your little finger just a bit, blinking your eyes, or twitching your nose. Next try to make other small movements in another part of your body. Focus on moving as much as possible. Think of someone whom you may trust—a friend, your therapist, your partner—and imagine that person helping you. Sometimes a particular part of you is immobilized and other parts of you can help by tending respectfully and empathically to that part, giving orienting information, comfort, and safety.
- If you feel cold or freezing (a common experience in hypoarousal), try a warm bath or shower (not too hot). Or wrap yourself in a blanket and place a hot water bottle or heating pad on your stomach to warm your core. Then imagine soothing inner parts as you warm up, using some of the other resources available to you.
- If you, or a part of you, have physical numbness, note where in your body it begins and ends, or whether you are completely numb. Many people have at least small areas of their body where they can feel. If you have such a place (for example, your forearm), touch it gently and intentionally, saying to yourself, *"I am touching my forearm."* Scratch your back with a soft, long brush; rub up against the door frame as a bear rubs up against a tree; or wrap in a blanket to feel your skin.

- If you are emotionally numb, notice whether you can feel just a little bit of emotion, perhaps a 1 or 2 on a scale of 10. Concentrate on the feeling, say it out loud, and draw the attention of all parts of yourself to it. Remind yourself that emotions can be safe; they are merely signals.
- You might ask whether any part of you could "share" a little emotion with you, no more than you think you can tolerate, for example, a teaspoon, a cup, or 5%. Also set a time limit, so you can feel a little of the emotion just for a moment, say to the count of 5, or 10 seconds or 30 seconds. As you feel more able, you can increase both the amount and time you experience an emotion. Notice as much of your inner experience during this time as possible: what you think, feel, sense, what you predict.
- If you are aware of certain parts of yourself that are severely shut down, see if you can become more curious about what they might need in order to be less shut down, and how you might provide for some of those needs. Sometimes merely the reassurance that you are really interested in tending to them is enough to help these parts become more present and alert.

Homework Sheet 18.1
Learning About Your Window of Tolerance

1. Place your current arousal level on a scale of 1 to 10, with 1 being the most extreme hypoarousal (feeling too little) and 10 being the most extreme hyperarousal (feeling too much). On the scale below, mark the range of your optimal level of arousal (not too much or too little), that is, the range that is tolerable and relatively comfortable. This is entirely subjective. There is no "right" answer. For example, you might mark an area between 3 and 7, or 4 and 6. Next, circle the points at which you might begin to work on keeping yourself from going too high or low on the scale. For example, if your range is 3–7, perhaps these points might be 2 and 6. Where on this scale would you need to stop what you were doing to find a way to return to your optimal level of arousal?

Also notice whether any parts of you might have a different window of tolerance.

Too little   Too Much

| 1 | 2 | 3 | 4 | 5 | 6 | 7 | 8 | 9 | 10 |

2. Next, describe how you know you are within your optimal arousal zone. For example, perhaps you feel calm, alert, relaxed, pleasant, or energized. Perhaps you feel warmth or coolness in your body, a sense of competence, a quiet or active mind. Your inner experience when you are within your window of tolerance is like a bookmark. You can memorize that experience, almost as though you were taking a picture of it with your body, and return to it as often as you need.

3. Finally, reflect on what helps you know you are about to, or already have gone outside of your window of tolerance. For example, you feel a whole-body tension, thoughts become disorganized, your mind goes blank, you hyperventilate, parts become noisy or you feel inner chaos, or you become drowsy. If you can recognize these markers as they happen, you can stop what you are doing and get yourself more grounded.

Homework Sheet 18.2
Your Tips for Coping With Feeling Too Much or Too Little

Make your own list of tips for dealing with too little feeling and dealing with too much. Try to include all parts of yourself in this exercise. You might be pleasantly surprised to find that you are already using some skills or that some parts of you might have some helpful ideas.

Helpful Tips for When I Am Feeling Too Much
1.

2.

3.

4.

5.

Helpful Tips for When I Am Feeling Too Little
1.

2.

3.

4.

5.

Understanding Core Beliefs

AGENDA

- Welcome and reflections on previous session
- Homework discussion
- Break
- Topic: Understanding Core Beliefs

  - Introduction
  - The Origins of Core Beliefs
  - Negative Core Beliefs in People With a Complex Dissociative Disorder
  - Realistic and Healthy Core Beliefs

- Homework

  - Reread the chapter.
  - Complete Homework Sheet 19.1, Identifying Negative Core Beliefs.
  - Complete Homework Sheet 19.2, Developing Realistic and Healthy Core Beliefs.

Introduction

In chapter 17 you learned that unduly negative thoughts and beliefs can play an important role in maintaining overwhelming and dysfunctional emotions. Positive thoughts and beliefs that are realistic can reinforce positive self-perception and contentment, satisfaction, happiness, curiosity, and connection with others. Persistent negative thoughts can evoke or reinforce feelings of depression, anxiety, grief, anger, guilt, shame, or fear. And in turn, these feelings reinforce yet more negative thoughts and beliefs. When we are in a bad mood, our thoughts are more negative, and thus we are more likely to see things in a negative light. This interconnection among thoughts, emotions, perceptions, predictions, and related decisions creates a cycle that supports our unique experience of self, others, and the world, whether that is largely negative or positive. Once a negative cycle begins and is reinforced by negative situations, it becomes more difficult to balance our perspective. And for people with a dissociative disorder, various parts will have different perspective and beliefs.

In this chapter you will be working toward gaining a greater understanding of some of your basic thoughts and belief systems that originated in the traumatic past but which are not helpful in your current life. Exploring and challenging these thoughts and beliefs can be an effective point of entry for positive change.

The Origins of Core Beliefs

Our most basic, or *core beliefs*, are those which provide the foundation for our view of self, others, and the world. They often define what we believe about safety, trust, belonging, self-esteem, competence, vulnerability, needs, and risk taking (Janoff-Bulman, 1992). For example, a realistic positive core belief might be: "*Most people are good and well intentioned, though they are not perfect; however, a few people are truly dangerous and should be avoided.*" A negative core belief might be: "*No one can ever be fully trusted because they are looking out only for themselves; I should avoid getting close to anyone for any reason.*"

We all develop certain core beliefs whether they are negative or positive. For those who have a dissociative disorder, various dissociative parts of yourself may have different core beliefs, and these may create much inner conflict (Fine, 1988, 1996). We will discuss more about these conflicts in the next section.

Core beliefs have their origin in childhood and a few can develop later in life based on powerful events. They can be changed, but often people are not consciously aware of them. Instead they might have automatic thoughts that seem true but which they do not closely examine. For example, many traumatized individuals have automatic thoughts such as "*No one loves me. I am worthless and stupid. I always fail at whatever I try. I am so ugly. It is ridiculous that I need help: I am just weak and whiny.*" Positive change requires being able be aware of and reflect on core beliefs.

A number of factors play a role in the development of core beliefs. Your inborn temperament affects the way in which you naturally view the world. A person who is naturally introverted and likes routine is likely to have somewhat different beliefs than one who is extroverted and likes to take a lot of risks. Some people are naturally more sensitive, while others seem less vulnerable to hurts and abrupt changes. Some people naturally feel quite intensely, while others have a more narrow range of feeling. These differences can influence a wide range of core beliefs.

In addition, each family has collective core beliefs that are passed down to the child, whether explicitly or unconsciously. For example, if the implicit message in a family is that one should never make mistakes, a child will develop the conviction that he or she should always be perfect. Gradually such a child will develop fears of making any kind of mistake, will become afraid of trying new things, and will not be easily satisfied with whatever he or she accomplishes. If the family core belief is that children are important, competent, and lovable, a child will grow up with confidence and feel secure in relationships. Core beliefs can also develop based on whether early relationships are secure and enduring. For instance, suddenly losing a parent at a young age may result in feelings of abandonment and the belief that something disastrous can suddenly happen, and that you can lose people you love at any moment. Likewise, being abused by a caregiver at a young age may result in strong beliefs that you cannot trust anyone, ever.

Negative Core Beliefs in People With a Complex Dissociative Disorder

Chronically traumatized people often suffer from persistent negative core beliefs. These are deeply rooted convictions that typically involve all-or-nothing thinking without balance or nuance: "*Things never work out for me,*" "*People always hurt me,*" "*I am completely stupid and unlovable,*" or "*There is no safe place.*" These beliefs often contain words like *always*, *never*, or *none*. Such thoughts and beliefs can profoundly influence, reinforce, and intensify negative emotions. Negative core beliefs are reinforced over time by negative emotions, perceptions, and predictions, and by additional negative life experiences. The same is true for positive core beliefs and attendant perceptions, emotions, and experiences.

People with a dissociative disorder may find that their beliefs, thoughts, and convictions may change suddenly or be in conflict, since various dissociative parts may have different core beliefs (Fine, 1988, 1996). Some thoughts and convictions are so fundamental to the individual's life experience that all dissociative parts share them, for instance, *"I cannot trust anyone"* or *"I will never be safe."*

Individual differences in beliefs among dissociative parts are related to the fact that each part has somewhat different life experiences. Parts of you that deal with tasks and functions in daily life are sometimes better able to observe and interpret the reality of the present moment, without being influenced by too many old thoughts or convictions. These parts have more distance from the past, largely because they avoid it. Most dissociative parts that are stuck in trauma-time suffer from negative, undermining thoughts and convictions, because they view the world only through their past experiences, without considering that the present may be quite different. As a result, the reality of the present moment can easily be distorted and relived in similar ways as the past as parts intrude into daily life: This is what we have called living in trauma-time. Even if there is some factual acknowledgment that the present is different from the past, these core beliefs often seem so compelling that they drown out current reality. Talking inwardly to these parts and helping them by respectfully challenging their deep-rooted convictions is a start, beginning with orienting them to present-day realities. Correcting core beliefs is not easy and will take some persistent work, but you can be successful over time.

Core beliefs affect your ability to reflect on your experiences. For example, suppose you are walking down the street and see a friend on the other side, walking in your direction. You wait for her to say hello, but she just keeps walking without acknowledging you at all. You could consider many different possibilities for what she was thinking, and not just assume that she did not care about or was angry with you. Depending on your core beliefs and your perceptions, you or different parts of you may have some or all of the following thoughts: (a) This person is preoccupied and did not even see me; (b) This person is deliberately ignoring me; (c) This person seems angry (with me); (d) She is walking fast to get away from having to talk with me; (e) She feels hurt that I did not say hello.

It is important for you to consider the possible intentions of others, rather than jumping to the same conclusions based on certain core beliefs, such as *"People never like me."* Do your core beliefs allow you to assume that people generally have no reason to dislike or ignore you, and that most people are well intentioned? Or do you believe that most people do not care about you and are just out to get what they want from you? Perhaps different parts of you might have different beliefs. Regarding the earlier example, some part of you may think, *"See! She ignored me. Nobody likes me. I am worthless and will always be alone."* Yet another part of you has an entirely different perception: *"This isn't about me at all. She probably didn't even see me."* These two very different sets of thoughts, beliefs, and perceptions have different emotional tones: one is highly negative, and one is positive or at least neutral. The first statement reinforces old negative beliefs, whereas the second statement supports a more positive and realistic view of the world.

Realistic and Healthy Core Beliefs

There are a number of generally accepted healthy core beliefs that allow for a more balanced view of self, others, and the world. They are more flexible and realistic. A healthy core belief is based on both the positives and negatives of reality. For example: *"I prefer not to make mistakes, but I know I will, because no one is perfect. When I do, I will work to correct it and not be too hard on myself."* Or *"Everyone needs help from others from time to time. Needing help does not mean I am weak or lazy; it means I am human."* Or *"I can allow myself to relax and have a good time, just as I allow myself to work hard when I need to."*

Of course, not everyone can always live in accordance with all their beliefs or put them into practice every moment. You may be quite convinced that something is healthy and good, but this does not mean that you can always "practice what you preach." But the more you practice, the more healthy beliefs can become part of your life. In Homework Sheet 19.2 you will find a list of some realistic and healthy core beliefs, which might be helpful in formulating your own.

Homework Sheet 19.1
Identifying Negative Core Beliefs

Below you will find lists of negative core beliefs about yourself, about others, and about the world. Read each list and check or circle five beliefs that affect you or parts of you most often.

Negative Core Beliefs About Yourself

- I am a failure; I never succeed in anything.
- I am an outsider and have no place to belong.
- I cannot connect with other people.
- I am utterly worthless.
- I am a bad person, ashamed of who I am.
- I am a weak person, always dependent on others.
- I should have never been born.

Negative Core Beliefs About Others

- Other people will always betray or hurt me.
- People are dangerous.
- Even if someone is nice, he or she is just waiting for the right time to trick me.
- Nobody understands me.
- Nobody will ever love me.
- People will always take advantage of others.
- People will always abandon or reject others.
- People are only out for themselves.

Negative Core Beliefs About the World

- The world is a dangerous place.
- At any moment something terrible can happen.
- The world is always unpredictable.
- There is no place for me in the world.
- The world is full of pain and misery, nothing more.

List any other negative core beliefs not listed above that affect you or other parts of you.

1.

2.

3.

4.

5.

Notice whether all parts of you share the core beliefs that you checked or wrote in above, or whether only some parts do. Choose one of the beliefs and take some time to have an inner dialogue about whether it is always correct in the present. Describe your experience during this inner discussion. If you are not able to have such a dialogue, please describe what stopped you from doing so.

Homework Sheet 19.2
Developing Realistic and Healthy Core Beliefs

Below you will find lists of healthy beliefs about yourself, others, and the world. Please read each list and then complete the homework below.

Healthy Core Beliefs About Self

- Pleasure and relaxation are normal, acceptable, and essential life experiences.
- I accept myself the way I am. I have my stronger and weaker points just like everyone else, and there is room for improvement and growth in my life.
- I can set healthy limits and boundaries with other people.
- I am competent in being able to solve everyday problems by myself most of the time.
- It is OK to ask for help when I need it, and I can manage when help is not available.
- I can be in charge of my own life. I do not always have to give in to what others want if it is not good for me.
- I feel I belong in the world and with others.
- It is OK that I don't know everything.
- I don't have to be perfect, just human.
- I am a decent human being.

Healthy Core Beliefs About Others

- Most people are decent and trustworthy; a few are not.
- Others are willing and available to help if I need support or assistance.
- People care about and understand me for the most part.
- Important relationships can be stable and good, though not perfect. Conflicts can be resolved.
- I can choose to be with safe people and avoid those who are not.

Healthy Core Beliefs About the World

- There is a place for me in this world.
- Unpredictable things can happen in the world, but I have resources and support to cope with most things.
- The world can be relatively stable and predictable much of the time.
- The world can be dangerous, but I am usually safe.
- There is pain and suffering in the world, and there is joy and love as well.

1. Check or circle any of these healthy beliefs you, or at least some parts of you, already have. Describe any inner conflicts or disagreements about those beliefs.

2. Check one belief in each category (self, other, and the world) that you would like to work toward developing. Make sure you share these beliefs with your therapist and the people around you whom you love and trust. It might be helpful to ask others what helped them develop healthy beliefs.

3. Notice any of your negative beliefs that include the words *always, everyone, none,* or *never*. Try to shift the beliefs to a more moderate position using words like *sometimes, some people*, or *occasionally*. For example, if one of your beliefs is "*I never succeed*," challenge yourself and parts of you by naming a few times when you have succeeded at something, even if small. At the least, you have succeeded in staying alive, getting yourself into therapy for help, and are trying your best to become healthier. See if you can change the belief, "*I never succeed*" to "*Sometimes I succeed and sometimes I do not. I am doing my best, and I accept that I cannot be perfect.*"

CHAPTER TWENTY

Identifying Cognitive Errors

AGENDA

- Welcome and reflections on previous session
- Homework discussion
- Break
- Topic: Identifying Cognitive Errors

  ○ Introduction
  ○ Common Cognitive Errors
  ○ Reflections to Identify and Explore Cognitive Distortions

- Exercise: The Necklace of Positive Experiences
- Homework

  ○ Reread the chapter.
  ○ Complete Homework Sheet 20.1, Identifying Your Cognitive Errors.
  ○ Complete Homework Sheet 20.2, Identifying Types of Cognitive Errors.
  ○ Practice the exercise The Necklace of Positive Experiences, or a variation of it.

Introduction

In the previous chapter we discussed negative core beliefs, from which dysfunctional thoughts stem. We noted that when you have a dissociative disorder, you may experience conflicting thoughts from other parts of yourself, which can influence your emotions and actions in the present. Core beliefs are influenced and reinforced by *cognitive errors,* which are exaggerated and irrational patterns of thinking that perpetuate your problems (Beck, 1975; Burns, 1999). These make it even more difficult to challenge and eventually change your dysfunctional core beliefs about yourself, other people, and the world around you. Cognitive errors are based on insufficient and highly selective attention, that is, they do not take into account the whole and complex picture of a given situation and thus lead to inaccurate thoughts. As we have explained, various dissociative parts are often geared to attending only to certain aspects of an experience, for example, whether there is danger, whether people are frowning or otherwise seem angry, whether there is a way to get a certain need met. Such parts exclude from awareness many essential cues that would help you, as a whole person, to respond appropriately. In this chapter we will explain several of the most common cognitive errors, and we will help you learn how to identify these ways of thinking. In the next chapter you will start to learn how to challenge and change rigid thought patterns and cognitive errors.

Common Cognitive Errors

Everyone employs cognitive errors from time to time. This is normal. But when they dominate your thinking and make life difficult, they need particular attention. A major difficulty for people who have a dissociative disorder is that many parts have serious cognitive distortions (Ross, 1989, 1997). Typically parts of you living in trauma-time have severe cognitive errors. These influence your life in confusing ways, because not all parts of you may think in the same way. Following are several commonly identified cognitive errors (Beck, 1975; Burns, 1999).

- *All-or-nothing thinking.* You, or parts of yourself, perceive everything as either black or white, yes or no, either/or. Things are either good or bad; there is no middle ground. Anything that is less than perfect is a disaster. People either like you or hate you; they are kind or cruel; honest or completely dishonest. If they ever say "no" to you, they have permanently rejected you. This pattern leaves no room for balance, nuance, or human frailties.

- *Overgeneralizing.* You, or parts of yourself, assume that one experience generalizes to all others, so that once you have had a bad experience, you believe that every similar situation going forward will also be negative. For instance, you ask someone out to see a movie, but she cannot go at the time you suggest. You decide, or another part influences you, to never to ask this person again, because it will never work out anyway. You do not invite anyone else either, because you have concluded that no one will ever want to be with you.

- *Mental filtering.* You, or parts of yourself, focus on a single negative detail of an event and you can think of nothing else. Positive experiences are rejected because you believe they are not real, do not last, do not count, or are only the result of luck. You lose perspective. For example, you prepared a nice dinner, except the salad dressing was a little too tart. You keep having negative thoughts about the dressing, how people think you are incompetent and a terrible cook, and you are convinced that the whole dinner was a complete failure.

- *Premature (arbitrary) conclusions.* You, or parts of yourself, make a conclusion without sufficient evidence. For example, you conclude that you cannot go back to school or change jobs; you cannot take up a new hobby because it would be too time consuming; you cannot cook because you are bad at it; therapy will not work for you; or your boss will never give you a raise. Such conclusions are not based on facts, but on underlying, often unconscious assumptions.

- *Mind reading.* You, or parts of yourself, assume you know what another person is thinking. You do not check out whether your assumptions are accurate. In other words, you do not use reflective skills. For example, your boss asks you to come into his office for a moment. You immediately assume he is angry with you and is going to fire you because he does not like you.

- *Catastrophic predictions.* You, or parts of yourself, assume that something awful is going to happen, that things are going to end badly no matter what you do. You consider this an unchangeable fact, as though it had already happened. For example, "*Why should I study for this exam? I'll fail anyway.*"

- *Magnification.* You, or parts of yourself, magnify personal failings or mistakes and blow situations out of proportion. For example, you forgot an appointment with your therapist and think: "*I am a terrible, irresponsible person. My therapist will fire me. I am so stupid. This is unforgivable.*" Or perhaps another critical part of you begins to berate you for being so "irresponsible and stupid."

- *Emotional reasoning.* You, or parts of yourself, assume, because your feelings are all powerful, that reality is determined only by what you are feeling, regardless of other facts and experiences to the contrary. For example, *"I feel like a bad person; therefore, I am bad." "I feel anxious and unsafe in the presence of that person; therefore, she is not safe." "I feel like something terrible is about to happen; therefore, I must get away before catastrophe strikes."* All things being equal, you should be able to trust most of your feelings. But if they derive from dissociative parts of yourself that live in trauma-time, that is, are not oriented to the present or are hyperfocused only on specific aspects of an experience to the exclusion of others, these thoughts are more likely to be inaccurate and not fit with current, external reality.

- *"Should /ought to" explanations and statements.* You, or parts of yourself, bombard yourself with statements such as *"I ought to . . . I should . . . I could have. . . ."* Often these statements are experienced as an inner voice that berates you, that is, a critical part of you that continually tries to correct your actions. Examples: *"You ought to be more available after hours for your work: Don't be so lazy"; "You should be able to make therapy work faster; you aren't trying hard enough"; "You should have been able to stop thinking about the past by now."* This constant inner criticism does not lead to healthy change, but rather to more shame, guilt, anger, resentment, and sense of failure.

Reflections to Identify and Explore Cognitive Distortions

To correct cognitive errors, you must be present and use reflective skills (chapter 6). It is also essential to begin to learn to connect, communicate, and collaborate with all parts of yourself over time, so you can understand their thinking. Next you will find a number of questions on which you and all parts of you can reflect to help you identify and explore cognitive errors. When you have an immediate negative thought about a situation, it is a good idea to examine that thought more carefully than usual. Because it is so automatic, it may involve a cognitive distortion. You will need some communication and collaboration with parts of yourself. It is usually quite helpful to check with all parts of yourself to see whether there are conflicting thoughts about an experience. It may be helpful to write answers to these questions and understand that different parts of yourself may have different answers. If this is so, the conflicts are the place to begin with empathic reflection: "I wonder why that part of me has such a different experience than I do? What can I learn about that part of myself, and how can I help that part of me?"

- Is there evidence that a bad experience from that past will always happen in the future?
- Have I taken into account the complete context of the situation? Can parts of me help me to do so?
- Do I have memory loss about a situation and thus have made assumptions that may be incorrect? Do other parts of me have a different perspective on what happened?
- Are there also positive aspects of an experience that I (or other parts) am ignoring or have not noticed?
- Did I check with all parts of myself to see whether there is internal agreement on a certain conclusion, especially if my conclusion seems to fit one of the cognitive error categories (see earlier discussion)?
- If the worst would happen, is it really true that I could not handle the situation? Do I have other choices about how to handle a bad situation?
- Is my decision or conclusion based solely on feelings? If so, what are the feelings?
- Do the feelings make logical sense for the situation?
- Is there any evidence that my feelings are influenced by parts of myself that are stuck in the past?
- Are these thoughts helping me to function better and to feel good about myself and others?
- Do all parts of me agree with these thoughts?
- Can I or other parts of myself offer reasonable counterarguments to these thoughts?

IMAGERY EXERCISE: THE NECKLACE OF POSITIVE EXPERIENCES

The following is an exercise that may help you experience more of the positive aspects of life. This kind of experience is not meant to deny or minimize your painful and difficult times, but rather is one of many ways to soothe, calm, and reassure yourself, so you feel stronger and better able to cope.

This exercise uses the image of a necklace or armband made with various beads. If this image is not suitable for you, try another, such as weaving a tapestry with threads of positive experiences, or imagine a garden of flowers or beautiful mosaic, or a book with beautiful pages. You can find the right image for you. You can make a scrapbook or piece of art as well, if you would like something more tangible.

Imagine that you, and all parts of yourself, are making a beautiful necklace or armband for yourself. It is crafted from lovely beads. Wooden beads, glass beads, ceramic beads, metal beads, beads of light, beads of water, beads of stone—you can use whatever material appeals to you. But in addition, these beads have a very special quality: Each one represents a good, positive, enjoyable experience in the present. These experiences do not have to be big, just simple things that have added a moment of contentment, satisfaction, happiness, or calmness to your life. For example, it could be a nice cup of tea with your feet propped up, a walk in the woods, a good night's sleep, a dinner with a friend, a feeling of being accepted and understood by your therapist, a sense of progress in your healing, satisfaction in finishing a project. Let each part of you add beads. You might add proud beads, poignant beads, hopeful beads, happy beads, silly beads, playful beads, safety beads, loving beads, funny beads, or friendly beads. And also beads of strength and serenity, perseverance and peace, courage and kindness, resilience and rest. You are making your creation just as you want it. You can even turn it into a vest or coat or blanket that covers you! You can look at your creation, wear it, hold it, see the light glint off the various beads. Feel their weight, whether they are light or a little heavy; feel their texture, whether they are smooth or rough. There may even be beads that make sounds like little cheerful tinkling bells or soft clicks and clacks. You are completely free in the design of your creation. And if it helps you, you can also imagine that you have a very special box in which you can keep it. If you have such a box, or choose to make one, you can also keep notes or other mementos of special events or moments in your life. In this way, you can return time and again to experiences that are good and pleasant. After all, our memories are not only of painful experiences but also of good and positive ones.

Homework Sheet 20.1
Identifying Your Cognitive Errors

1. Review the list of cognitive errors in the text above. List below those patterns of thoughts that apply to you, or to other parts of you, on a regular basis. Give examples, if possible.

2. Describe any instances when one part of you does not share the cognitive error(s) of another part of you.

3. Describe a recent situation in which you had to contend with one of these patterns of thought. Describe the thought and name the particular cognitive error(s) involved, and a possible challenge to the thought.

Example

Cognitive error: *People ignored me at a party, and I felt no one cared about me.*

Effects of cognitive error: *During the party I felt ashamed and like I was an alien. A part of me was screaming to go home, and another part was telling me what a jerk I was. Afterwards I felt really lonely and wanted to hurt myself and withdraw from the world.*

Possible challenge: *I am not yet comfortable at parties and made no effort to speak. A few people said hello, but I hardly responded, so they moved on. Perhaps it isn't that they do not like me, but that I am too anxious to make conversation. I wonder whether maybe I give off a message to leave me alone.*

Homework Sheet 20.2
Identifying Types of Cognitive Errors

Below you will find three examples of cognitive errors. Read each one and then read the challenge to each distortion. Below each example write the cognitive error at play. You can refer back to the list of cognitive errors, if needed.

Example 1

"I can see by your face what you are thinking. You are angry with me."

Challenge: Actually, although facial expression may give you a hint about what someone is thinking, you cannot actually know for sure without checking it out; that is, you cannot read someone's mind. And because of negative experiences in the past, you (or certain parts of you) often only pay attention to signs that might indicate threat, and not to those that might indicate safety. So if the person is slightly frowning, you may interpret this as being angry and expect that this person will harm you in some way. In fact, the person may not be angry, but rather may be trying to concentrate on what you are saying, or maybe even has a headache.

What is the cognitive error?

Example 2

You are having dinner at a friend's home and he steps into the kitchen for a moment to finish preparing some food. The phone rings and he hurries toward the phone, which is near where you are sitting. He is still holding the knife he has been using to cut up the vegetables. You see the knife, you or other parts of you are triggered, and you no longer perceive your friend accurately. In a flash you expect he is going to attack you.

Challenge: Although a part of you is triggered, another part knows your friend would never hurt you and is not dangerous. You are able to look around and see where you are. You recall your long and wonderful history with your friend. All is well and the fear is something within you, not outside.

What is the cognitive error?

Example 3

You live next door to a family with small children. Every time you hear one of the children cry, you or some other parts of you believe something terrible has happened to them.

Challenge: In reality, you notice that these children do not cry often or for long periods of time; their parents quickly comfort or help them; they do not scream in anguish; they seem otherwise happy, healthy, energetic, playful, and social. There is no reason to think that their occasional crying is anything but quite ordinary.

What is the cognitive error?

CHAPTER TWENTY-ONE

Challenging Dysfunctional Thoughts and Core Beliefs

AGENDA

- Welcome and reflections on previous session
- Homework discussion
- Break
- Topic: Challenging Dysfunctional Thoughts and Core Beliefs

  - Introduction
  - Feedback Loops
  - Exploring Your Thoughts When You Have a Complex Dissociative Disorder
  - Reflections for Understanding and Challenging Your Core Beliefs and Thoughts

- Homework

  - Reread the chapter.
  - Complete Homework Sheet 21.1, Challenging Inaccurate Thoughts or Core Beliefs.
  - Complete Homework Sheet 21.2, Developing Realistic Positive Thoughts and Beliefs.

Introduction

In the last two chapters, you learned how cognitive errors can influence, reinforce, and maintain negative core beliefs and thoughts. You learned that emotions affect how you perceive situations and the intentions of other people, what you predict will happen in the future, and how you act. It is as though you have on colored glasses and everything you perceive is tinted by that color. And parts of you may have on different colored glasses from each other. In this chapter you will learn more about how emotions, core beliefs, thoughts, and certain cognitive errors are related, and in turn, how these affect your ability to size up a situation accurately, particularly relational situations.

Feedback Loops

As we noted before, emotions, cognitions, perceptions (how you interpret a situation), sensations and movement, predictions (what you expect will happen in the future), and decision making all work together in a seamless feedback loop (Van der Hart et al., 2006). Each gives and receives feedback from the others. In this way, we can develop relatively fixed and closed ways of being in and viewing the world: We are in a negative feedback loop. For instance, negative core beliefs promote and maintain overwhelming emotions, and vice versa.

As an example, let us return to the scenario of the friend who walks past without acknowledging you. If you are not being reflective when you see her walk past, you may have an immediate reaction. This reaction is based on a feedback loop consisting of the following:

- Perceptions (seeing her walk past without greeting you; her eyes straight ahead)
- Thoughts (*"She doesn't like me. I'm such a loser."*)
- Emotions (shame, hurt, anger)
- Sensations (roiling in the pit of your stomach, flushed face)
- Movements (hunched shoulders, downcast eyes, urge to run away and disappear)
- Predictions (*"No one will ever like me; things will always end badly for me."*)
- Decision making (*"From now on I will avoid people. I'd rather be by myself."*)
- Actions (isolation, avoiding phone calls from people, turning down requests to do things with others)

You can see how these experiences are not sequential; that is, one does not precede or cause the other, but each affects the others simultaneously. All are part of one package.

You may only be aware of one of these experiences, such as an emotion. Perhaps as your friend walked past you felt shame. You can identify the shame, but you feel too frozen or collapsed to think consciously. But your perceptions, predictions, emotions, and so forth imply the presence of thought. These cognitions, called *automatic thoughts*, are related to core beliefs, and they can be just beneath the surface of your awareness, so insidious and quick that you do not catch them. They often contain cognitive errors, such as all-or-nothing thinking and overgeneralization ("*Nobody cares about me.*"). As you become more proficient in reflecting—perhaps in retrospect at first—you can begin to identify and explore all the others experiences: perception, prediction, thoughts, sensations, and movements. In this chapter you will be focused on identifying negative thoughts and core beliefs within this feedback loop and learning to explore and challenge them.

The importance of reflection and the ability to adjust your responses to the present carry over into the future, because you base your predictions about what comes next on your current perceptions, thoughts and beliefs, emotions, and so forth. For example, if you or certain dissociative parts of you believe your friend has deliberately ignored you, you may start avoiding that person and remain angry, hurt, or ashamed. If you happen to see her again, you are vigilant in looking for cues that she is rejecting you. Her every movement, every ambiguous sentence, every facial expression is now scrutinized for signs of rejection. And because you predict it, you can easily interpret what you see as rejection. You may completely cut off contact with your friend, reinforcing your beliefs that no one is safe and you are unlovable, and leaving you in a painful state of shame and loneliness. When all parts of you can be more open to the possibilities of more neutral or positive alternative interpretations of a situation, you may not feel so negative about yourself and some of those around you.

You can see from this example why it is vital to learn to recognize thoughts that arise from old negative core beliefs, and then to consider reflectively whether these thoughts are still valid in the present. Are they correct? What proof do you have? Can you think of any experiences that provide evidence to the contrary? Do these beliefs help you achieve your goals of being safe, connected, and self-assured in the world? Using such questions can help you challenge some of your beliefs that may not be adaptive in the present.

Of course, even when you recognize that a situation is not harmful to you, you may still feel strongly that it is, because some part(s) of you may be stuck in the past. This gap between what you know cognitively and what you feel can be bridged with inner reflection with all parts, which will help you begin to understand and resolve inner conflicts and lack of orientation to the present. In the next section we will address how you can explore your thoughts and practice reflecting each day at your own pace. Progress comes, even though it may be in small increments.

Exploring Your Thoughts When You Have a Complex Dissociative Disorder

When you have chronic dissociation, exploring your thoughts can be especially challenging because of inner conflicts and barriers among various parts of yourself. You may not be able to recall specific situations, that is, you may have amnesia, so it may be hard to know what another part of you was thinking at the time. You may have thoughts that seem to pop into your mind out of the blue, and you may have no idea where they came from or what they are about, because they belong to parts of yourself of which you are not very aware. And you may feel muddled and confused if several different thoughts from various parts are swirling around in your head simultaneously. Some of these thoughts may not *seem* to belong to you, but nevertheless they are in your mind and can influence your perceptions, emotions, behaviors, and predictions. As we explained earlier, some parts stuck in trauma-time may have their own feedback loops that are different from yours, so they have difficulty in accurately perceiving the current situation, or even at all. They experience the present as the past and may have never questioned the accuracy of their thoughts and emotions, and their interpretations of the present circumstances.

Even with these inner struggles, you will find it valuable to explore consistently your thoughts and core beliefs and how they affect your emotions, predictions, decisions, and actions. You can begin with thoughts about a situation you clearly remember. As inner communication increases among all parts of yourself, you will become more aware of the thoughts of particular parts and how you can more effectively reflect on and help adjust those thoughts. All parts of you can participate in helping you as a whole person learn to change your beliefs over time. Eventually, parts of you that have more realistic and positive core beliefs and thoughts can help those with more rigid and negative ones.

Reflections for Understanding and Challenging Your Core Beliefs and Thoughts

When you want to explore and challenge upsetting or negative thoughts about a particular situation, you can reflect by using the following questions as a guide. You may not know all the answers. That is fine. But the more you practice, the better you will become at understanding your beliefs and eventually changing them.

- Start with describing the situation. What happened? Do you clearly remember the situation? Have you taken into account the whole context of the situation? If not, can you ask parts inside for help in understanding?
- What thoughts did you, or parts of yourself, have? If more than one thought came into your mind, try to write them down, even if they are contradictory.
- Check the list of cognitive errors in the previous chapter to see whether any apply to your thinking.
- Decide which thought evoked the most negative emotion. Does this thought seem as though it is your own thought, or does it seem to belong to a part of yourself? If to another part of you, can you communicate compassionately with that part?
- What proof do you have that your perception of the situation and thoughts about it are accurate in the present?
- Are there any positive aspects of the situation that you (or other parts) are ignoring or have overlooked?
- Have you or parts of you had any experiences that contradict your perceptions and thoughts about this situation?
- If you were to share your thoughts about your experience with someone whom you trust, what do you imagine that person would say?
- If someone else was involved in the situation, would you be willing to check out your perceptions and thoughts with this person?
- What counterarguments or alternative explanations could you think of that might be different from the way you perceived the situation and the thoughts that you had?
- If thoughts clearly belong to other parts of you, talk inwardly or organize an inner meeting to discuss the possibility that these thoughts might not be completely accurate in the present situation (see also chapter 27 on decision making).

Homework Sheet 21.1
Challenging Inaccurate Thoughts or Core Beliefs

1. Describe below four dysfunctional or inaccurate thoughts and core beliefs of which you were aware this week.

2. Next write down statements or experiences that challenge or refute the thought or core belief (perhaps with the help of other parts of yourself). If needed, reread the list of realistic healthy core beliefs in chapter 20. If some parts disagree with refuting statements, write them down anyway, and put a check or star next to them. You can later establish dialogue with these parts of yourself to reach inner common ground.

3. Describe any inner obstacles to challenging your thoughts and beliefs.

4. Describe, if you are able, options for reducing the inner obstacles.

Example

1. ***Dysfunctional thought or core belief***: *I can never do anything right!*
2. ***Refuting statements and experiences***: *I got out of bed, took a shower, ate a healthy breakfast, and completed my homework. I did all those things right. I can do some things right.*
3. ***Obstacles to changing the belief***: *Part of me kept telling me I couldn't even get out of bed the right way because I just wasn't right as a person. Another kept yelling, "Stupid! Stupid!"*
4. ***Solutions to inner obstacles***: *I need to acknowledge I am a little afraid of being OK, not wrong all the time. I can empathize with parts who berate me with the intention that I won't make more mistakes. I can notice what happens inside when I actually do something right.*

Dysfunctional thought or core belief:

Refuting statements and experiences:

Obstacles to changing the belief:

Solutions to inner obstacles:

Dysfunctional thought or core belief:

Refuting statements and experiences:

Obstacles to changing the belief:

Solutions to inner obstacles:

Dysfunctional thought or core belief:

Refuting statements and experiences:

Obstacles to changing the belief:

Solutions to inner obstacles:

Dysfunctional thought or core belief:

Refuting statements and experiences:

Obstacles to changing the belief:

Solutions to inner obstacles:

Homework Sheet 21.2
Developing Realistic Positive Thoughts and Beliefs

Make a list of your own realistic positive beliefs and thoughts. Include all parts of yourself in this exercise, and write down even those beliefs with which all parts do not agree.

1.

2.

3.

4.

5.

6.

7.

8.

9.

10.

PART FIVE
SKILLS REVIEW

You have learned a number of skills in this section of the manual. Next you will find a review of those skills and an opportunity to develop them further. As you review, we encourage you to return to the chapters to read them again and repractice the homework a little at a time. Remember that regular, daily practice is essential to learn new skills.

For each skill set below, answer the following questions:

1. In what situation(s) did you practice this skill?
2. How did this skill help you?
3. What, if any, difficulties have you had in practicing this skill?
4. What additional help or resources might you need to feel more successful in mastering this skill?

Chapter 17, Mindfulness Exercise

1.

2.

3.

4.

Chapter 17, Identifying Emotions

1.

2.

3.

4.

Chapter 18, Strategies for Coping With Feeling Too Much and Too Little (distraction; containment; calming and soothing; orienting to the present; activity and mental stimulation; taking care of parts of yourself)

1.

2.

3.

4.

Chapter 18, Learning About Your Window of Tolerance

1.

2.

3.

4.

Chapter 19, Identifying Your Negative Core Beliefs

1.

2.

3.

4.

Chapter 19, Developing Realistic and Healthy Core Beliefs

1.

2.

3.

4.

Chapter 20, The Necklace of Positive Experiences Exercise

1.

2.

3.

4.

Chapter 20, Identifying Your Cognitive Errors

1.

2.

3.

4.

Chapter 21, Challenging Your Inaccurate Thoughts or Core Beliefs

1.

2.

3.

4.

Chapter 21, Identifying Realistic and Healthy Beliefs

1.

2.

3.

4.

Advanced Coping Skills

Coping With Anger

AGENDA

- Welcome and reflections on previous session
- Homework discussion
- Break
- Topic: Coping With Anger

    ○ Introduction
    ○ Understanding Anger
    ○ Anger in People With a Complex Dissociative Disorder
    ○ Tips for Coping With Anger
    ○ Working With Parts of Yourself to Cope With and Resolve Anger

- Homework

    ○ Reread the chapter.
    ○ Complete Homework Sheet 22.1, Understanding Your Experience of Anger.
    ○ Complete Homework Sheet 22.2, Understanding and Coping With Angry Dissociative Parts of Yourself.

Introduction

Anger is natural and healthy. However, it can be a powerful and frightening emotion. People who have been seriously traumatized, especially by other human beings, typically have strong feelings of anger, rage, and even hate and revenge. It is completely natural to react with anger as a way of protecting or distancing yourself when someone has hurt you intentionally. However, when anger becomes chronic and unresolved, when it is inhibited over long periods, or is uncontrolled and expressed in destructive ways towards self, other parts of you, or other people, it becomes a hindrance to relationships and to personal healing. In such cases, present-day anger is nearly always intensified by and mixed up with past anger that is unresolved. In this chapter you will learn more about the meanings of anger and how to regulate and manage anger, whether you experience it yourself, or another part of you does.

Understanding Anger

In the sections that follow you will find some facts about anger that will help you change how you view and cope with this emotion.

Common Inaccurate Beliefs About Anger

One of the most difficult aspects of anger is how intense and overwhelming it can feel; a lot of energy is generated in the body, and the physical sensations of anger are very powerful. After all, anger is an inborn tendency designed to support us in threatening situations. Some people believe their anger gives them a sense of strength and makes them feel good; they are afraid if their anger is "taken away," they will lose their power and energy. Of course, it may well give them strength for the moment, but there are many other ways to find energy and a sense of being in control of oneself while still being appropriately angry at the right times.

Many traumatized individuals feel ashamed of their anger, because they believe anger is "bad," or they believe they will be punished and rejected if they express or even feel anger, or because they fear being angry makes them "just like" the people who hurt them. They fear losing control, yet their anger remains intense and easily provoked. Like many intense negative emotions, anger is often disowned and held in various parts of the personality, so that other parts need not experience it but will react in other ways instead.

It is essential to remember than anger is an emotion that guides behavior, not a behavior in itself. Anger as a feeling is not dangerous or bad; it is an inevitable part of life. It is *how* you cope with anger that makes it adaptive or not.

Anger as a Substitute for Other Emotions

Anger can sometimes be a substitute for other emotions that are hard to tolerate. For example, it is not uncommon for people to express anger when they feel ashamed or afraid. They may strike out at others, or toward themselves, or even both, as noted in chapter 24 on shame and guilt. Various dissociative parts may strike out at each other. Anger also inhibits grief: Sometimes it is important to finally grieve over what you have lost and cannot have, rather than continue to be angry that you do not have it. Grieving is an important way of coming to terms with the reality of what is and then being able to move on. Anger can keep people stuck, unable to find other ways to get what they need. When anger is a cover for other emotions, an important part of anger resolution will be to accept and resolve those emotions.

Expression of Anger

Many people are afraid to express anger but also believe the only way to deal with it is to "get it out." Intense physical or verbal expression of anger may be relieving in the moment, but often it does nothing to resolve chronic anger and does not change *how* anger is experienced internally. That is, expression of anger, in itself, does not create positive, healthy shifts in thinking, feeling, and perceiving. There are many ways to express anger, some healthy and some destructive. For example, healthy expressions include respectfully talking about it with someone, writing, drawing, respectful inner dialogue, working toward positive resolution of problems about which you feel angry, dealing with underlying emotions such as shame, or accepting that you cannot change a situation and moving on.

Destructive expressions of anger include persistent revenge fantasies or actions, hurting self or others, "taking it out" on innocent people (or animals), or destruction of property. Some people or parts may feel the need to express anger physically, by hitting a pillow, for example. Although there is nothing wrong with this, it does not solve anger and may actually heighten your emotion. Only when anger is paired with behavioral control and a significant change in core beliefs is it healing. For example, a negative core belief might be, "*I deserve to be angry for all the bad things that have happened to me.*" This could be changed to something like, "*I was hurt and justified in my anger. Now I can let it go and make room for other feelings, since continual anger does not help me function and have a better life. I can accept my own anger and not be afraid of it.*"

The Experience of the Angry Other

Traumatized people often experience the anger of others as dangerous and terrifying: They may associate it with their abuse and thus link it with terrible and out-of-control behavior. However, it is important to realize that feeling angry and acting destructively are two different things, and there are many ways to express anger that are not dangerous. Everyone feels anger from time to time, and most people are able to feel and express it appropriately without being hurtful to others.

Anger in People With a Complex Dissociative Disorder

Next we describe some unique issues regarding anger that need attention in order for you to manage your anger successfully.

- Specific parts of your personality may be angry and are usually easily evoked. Because these parts are dissociated, anger remains an emotion that is not integrated for you as a whole person. Even though individuals with a dissociative disorder are responsible for their behavior, just like everyone else, regardless of which part may be acting, they may feel little control of these raging parts of themselves.
- Some dissociative parts may avoid or even be phobic of anger. They may influence you as a whole person to avoid conflict with others at any cost or to avoid setting healthy boundaries out of fear of someone else's anger; or they may urge you to withdraw from others almost completely.
- Parts of you that are phobic of anger are generally terrified and ashamed of angry dissociative parts. There is often tremendous conflict between anger-avoidant and anger-fixated parts of an individual. Thus, an internal and perpetual cycle of rage-shame-fear creates inner chaos and pain.
- You as a whole person are thus unable to reconcile conflicts about anger and learn to tolerate and express anger in healthy ways. Inner turmoil and dissociation are maintained.

These problems with anger can be resolved with patience and persistence, as you learn to have inner understanding, empathy, communication, and cooperation among all parts of yourself. Next we discuss common types of angry parts.

Dissociative Parts Fixated in Anger

Dissociative parts of a person that are stuck in anger may experience this feeling as vehement and overwhelming, often without words. They may have irresistible urges to act aggressively and have great difficulty thinking and reflecting on their feelings before acting. Angry parts have not learned how to experience or express anger in helpful ways.

There are two types of angry dissociative parts. The first are parts that are stuck in a defensive fight mode, ready to protect you. Their anger at original injustices may be legitimate and naturally accompanies a tendency to strike out or fight, which is an essential survival strategy. However, such parts have become stuck in anger, unable to experience much else. They rigidly perceive threat and ill will everywhere, and they react with anger and aggression as their only option of response. Although these parts of you may not yet realize it, anger is often a protection against vulnerable feelings of shame, fear, hurt, despair, powerlessness, and loss.

The second type of angry part may seem very much like the original perpetrator(s). They imitate those who hurt them in the past, and they can be experienced internally as the actual perpetrator(s). This experience can be particularly frightening, disorienting, and shameful. But be assured this is a very common way of dealing with being traumatized. In fact, although these parts may have some similarities to those who hurt you, they also have significant differences: They are parts of you as a whole person, who is trying to cope with unresolved traumatic experiences. Sometimes these parts may seem more powerful and aggressive internally toward other parts than they are externally, although in some cases, these parts may also act out toward others. And just as fight parts, they also exist to protect you, and they often hold unbearable feelings of rage and powerlessness that you have not yet been able to accept as your own.

Typically the beliefs of angry parts protect them against awareness of any perceived weakness, vulnerability, or incompetence that might lead to rejection, ridicule, or abuse. You may hear voices inside that say things like, *"Therapy is for crazy people; you are crazy and everybody knows it"; "You are such a cry-baby"; "Stop whining"; "Why do you think you would get a raise? Your boss thinks you are an idiot."* These parts make every effort to maintain "safety" by avoiding mistakes and vulnerability, and they do not allow the development of what seems to them to be false hopes that could be dashed. Even in situations where different ways of coping might be more adaptive, they maintain their rigid way of perceiving, thinking, feeling, and acting, because they are still living in trauma-time. For example, no matter how consistent and safe your therapist seems, an inner voice may caution against trust because *"it won't last and she'll just kick you when you're down. She just wants to control you."*

Finally, angry parts are often afraid that they are unwanted. Indeed, until a better understanding of these parts develops, most individuals wish to be rid of them. It is important to realize that angry parts, like all parts, belong to you as a whole person. You may not like their methods, but the underlying intent is to protect you. You can always learn different and more effective ways to protect yourself, and these dissociative parts can participate and actually become your best inner allies. You can learn from them that you indeed are able to protect yourself in the vast majority of situations. The fact is, healthy anger is an innate capacity with survival value and is not only normal but necessary in some circumstances.

Parts that imitate a perpetrator(s) typically reenact aspects of the traumatic past. Often, they parrot what was said to you, or similar messages, in an inner voice that sounds like the perpetrator(s). These statements typically result in your feeling worthless and unloved, ashamed and fearful, just as you did in the past. For example, many people with a dissociative disorder hear angry voices that say things such as, *"You asked for it"*; *"You are so stupid"*; *You don't deserve anything"*; *"If you tell, I'll hurt you, so shut up."* In truth, these parts are not yet able to distinguish between past and present. As we mentioned earlier, they live in trauma-time. Therefore, they often have a lonely position, ostracized from and despised by other dissociative parts, and the objects of inner fear and shame. They are part of an internal reenactment of the traumatic past that endlessly loops and involves all parts of the self.

Dissociative Parts That Avoid Anger

Other dissociative parts avoid anger at almost all costs, as noted earlier. Some may be stuck in the past, believing or merely sensing that anger makes them more vulnerable, that is, invites more pain and suffering. Thus, these parts, just like angry parts, have limited and rigid ways of protecting themselves. Anger-avoidant parts always tend to minimize or deny their needs or desires, work to appease others, and have a propensity to freeze or shut down. Such parts almost never feel anger even when it would be appropriate to do so. They may associate anger with the perpetrator, which is confusing and frightening. They judge the behaviors of angry parts and are afraid or ashamed of them. Parts that avoid anger often associate anger with loss of control, infliction of pain, and being "bad."

The person as a whole thus experiences an impasse: She or he is stuck between the opposing beliefs and defenses of anger-avoidant parts and anger-prone parts. Some parts believe it is dangerous and shameful to be angry, while others believe it is dangerous and shameful to be vulnerable.

Tips for Coping With Anger

- Anger occurs in many gradations, from mild irritation or annoyance, to anger, to rage. The sooner you are able to make these distinctions and can become aware of mild anger, such as irritation, the easier it is to intervene before anger becomes overwhelming.
- You can learn to be aware of your own physical signs of anger. Anger is typically associated with a tight or tense feeling in your body, clenched jaws and/or fists, feeling flushed or shaky, breathing heavily, rapid heart rate, a feeling of heat, or a surge of energy throughout your body. Noticing your body sensations can be a powerful way to know whether you are angry. You may have learned to automatically react to physical sensations that accompany anger as triggers to avoid angry emotions or thoughts.
- Angry parts may seem like internal "enemies" or "troublemakers," but actually they are not, even those parts that act like perpetrators. They are simply one way in which you try to cope. You must learn to empathize with their plight of having very limited coping skills and being shunned by other parts, alone with their hurt and fear and shame, while not accepting their inappropriate behavior, whether internal or external.
- Once you feel some empathy toward these parts, you can begin to communicate with them, listening with more understanding about what is "underneath" the anger. And you can also ask your therapist to help you communicate with angry parts.
- It is important for angry parts to realize that you will not "get rid of" them, that they have protective functions, and are invited to participate in therapy along with all other parts of you.
- Angry parts are strong parts that can be gradually encouraged to use their strength in more positive ways, such as helping you to attain impor-tant goals in your life, and helping you be more assertive when necessary.
- It is not wrong to feel angry. Anger is an inborn, normal, and inevitable human emotion that is universal. It is only important how you express it outwardly or inwardly. Does it help you get what you need without hurting anyone? Is it respectful? Is it within your window of tolerance? Does it lead to positive experiences instead of more negative ones?
- Notice whether the intensity of the anger that you, or some parts of you, feel is appropriate to the situation. It might help to check how other people would respond to the same situation. For example, you might notice whether you are the only person in a meeting that consistently gets angry because people seem so incompetent, and if so, be-

come more curious about why others do not seem to be struggling with anger in those situations.

- Try creative and healthy nonverbal ways of expressing your anger: writing, drawing, painting, making a collage.
- Physical exercise may help as an outlet for the physical energy generated by the physiology of anger.
- Reflect on your anger, that is, try to understand your anger rather than just experience it. You might imagine observing yourself from a distance and being curious about why you are so angry. It is easy to blame circumstances or others for the way you feel, but really, it is your own internal thoughts, perceptions, and predictions that fuel your anger. Noticing them and being able to change them will be enormously helpful, instead of focusing on the external object of your anger.
- Give yourself a time-out, that is, walk away from a situation if you feel you are getting too angry. Count slowly to 10, or even to 100 before you say or do something you will regret later. Practice calming breathing. Distract yourself. Help inner parts calm themselves.
- Of course, what works for one part of you may not work for another part. It is important for each part of you to have ways to calm down that work. While some parts may benefit from distraction or soothing, others might find it more helpful to engage in vigorous physical activity. Listen to yourself, to all parts of you, and take into account the needs of each part of you.
- Have an inner conversation with parts of yourself about anger and how to express it. Allow all parts of you to share their fears and beliefs about anger. Negotiate toward small and safe ways to express anger that are agreeable to all parts of you.
- Anger, like all emotions, has a beginning, middle, and end. Notice when it starts. Notice what intensifies or decreases it. Notice your inner thoughts, sensations, perceptions, and predictions. Notice what various skills and supports are needed by different parts to cope with anger more appropriately.
- Watch safe people in your life and see how they handle their own anger. Do they accept being angry? Are they respectful and appropriate with their anger? Are there particular strategies they use that you could practice for yourself?
- Healthy anger can give positive strength and energy. It can help you be appropriately assertive, set clear boundaries, and confront wrongs in the world. Anger can pave the way to other emotions, leading to the resolution of relational conflicts.
- Learn the most common triggers of your anger. Once you learn these triggers, you can be more aware when they occur and more able to

prevent an automatic reaction of anger. Establish inner communication among parts of yourself to recognize triggers and negotiate possible helpful strategies to cope with them rather than just reacting.

- You can try allowing yourself to experience just a small amount of anger from another part of yourself: a drop, a teaspoon, 1% or 2%. And in exchange, you can share with angry parts feelings of calm and safety.

Working With Parts of Yourself to Cope With and Resolve Anger

As soon as you are aware of feelings of irritation or anger, imagine holding an inner meeting to understand whether this anger is something all parts of you share, or if it is experienced only by certain parts of you. Make an effort to notice what triggered these feelings. It is very important not only to notice external triggers but also internal ones. The most powerful internal triggers for angry parts are any signs of perceived weakness or neediness: crying, yearning, fear, shame. "Child" parts, for instance, may feel terrified or cry internally, which evokes angry parts that typically treat the young parts in the ways similar to how you were treated as a child. Again, they may do so in order to prevent anticipated abuse from others, as they experienced in the past, or as an automatic reenactment. Their goal is to prevent any "weakness" in misguided efforts to keep you safe.

This is why inner safe places for younger parts of yourself are so important (see chapter 8). If they are experienced as being in a safe place they are less activated by triggers. Internal safety for these parts in turn decreases the need for angry parts to feel rage or impotence. Angry parts often learn quickly that it is to their advantage to allow other parts to feel safe and calm; it helps them feel less agitated and exhausted from being angry all the time. In fact, every part of you benefits from every bit of internal safety you can achieve.

Finally, it can be helpful for angry parts to have their own inner safe places and states. This can be an inner space where they do not feel threatened, that is, a quiet place, where they do not have to hear or care for or protect other parts (including younger parts of yourself) and where they cannot do any harm and cannot be heard by other parts. They can thus begin to experience new, more positive feelings simply by temporarily eliminating the vicious internal cycle of vulnerability-shame-rage. *However, it is essential that parts are not "forced" to be locked away in order to "get rid" of them or as punishment.* Safe places and states must be entirely voluntary and for the intent of safety and calm, not avoidance. If you need help, your therapist can help you create these inner safe and calm states.

Challenging Core Beliefs and Using Reflection to Resolve Anger

Anger may arise because situations in the present are interpreted or perceived from the point of view of the past. You can learn how to distinguish whether your anger is a response to the present, to the past, or to both, and whether its intensity is appropriate to the situation. For instance, if someone is late for a meeting with you because he or she was stuck in a traffic jam, a part of you may feel angry in reaction to the feeling of rejection or being ignored. It will be helpful to ensure that all parts of you know what is actually happening in the present so that you can more fully realize that the person's lateness was not intentional nor meant to hurt you. Often parts of you still live in trauma-time and are not fully aware of the present context. They only feel anger and react as they have in the past. They may believe, for instance: "*Others do not think that I am worth anything, so they do not care if they keep an appointment with me. They want to hurt me on purpose.*" If these parts are not aware of present circumstances (for example, a traffic jam prevented the person from being on time), and if they cannot understand that the person may have no bad intentions, they can never correct this belief, and the anger will be perpetuated.

Taking Time Out

If your anger tends to escalate quickly, especially in relation to other people, the best strategy is to leave the situation immediately. If you are in a relationship, you can make a contract with your partner in which each of you has your own particular signal which indicates the need to have a time-out. Once you have left the situation respectfully, it is important for all parts to help each other calm down. The most important skill to use is reflection. Try to stop being in your anger long enough to calm down and recognize your anger. Then you can reflect on the situation, on how overly intense you feel, and what thoughts, perceptions, and predictions you may have that perpetuate your anger. You can use any method to calm yourself that suits you—walking, sports, listening to music, practicing relaxation exercises, or going to your safe place. If you have a partner, it is essential to have an agreed-upon way in which to discuss the situation later in a calm way, when you both are able to empathize with and understand the other's position, just as you are learning to do among parts of yourself.

Homework Sheet 22.1
Understanding Your Experience of Anger

Describe a current situation in which you or some part of you felt anger.

1. Describe the situation.

2. What thoughts did you or other parts have during the situation?

3. Describe any tendency to turn the anger in on yourself (by you or any part of you). What were the thoughts or beliefs about yourself that evoked anger toward yourself?

4. Describe your physical sensations of anger, for example, heartbeat, trembling, sweating, cold, hot, and so forth.

5. Describe any tendency to avoid your anger, for example, spacing out, distracting yourself, feeling depersonalized, or switching to another part.

6. In retrospect, describe any inaccurate or maladaptive perceptions of the situation or of your own anger, for example, some part of you experienced your therapist as "just like" a person from the past who hurt you.

7. Describe any attempts at inner communication during or after the event to better work with and understand the situation. What was helpful (or not) about the communication?

If you were not able to engage in any inner communication, please describe what stopped you. For example, it did not occur to you to do so; you felt it was useless; you did not want to stop being angry; you are too afraid of the angry part(s) of yourself; or some part of you would not "allow" it.

8. What distracting or calming techniques did you or parts of you try to use, if any? Describe how they were or were not effective.

9. List two healthy coping strategies that you and all parts would like to learn to use when you feel angry in the future. Describe the obstacles in the present to using them.

Homework Sheet 22.2
Understanding and Coping With Angry
Dissociative Parts of Yourself

If you are aware of or suspect you may have angry dissociative parts of yourself, please complete the following homework sheet.

1. Describe how you know a part of you is angry (for example, hearing an angry voice, being told you were acting angry but not recalling the episode, feeling anger "out of the blue" that makes no sense to you).

2. Describe your response to angry parts of yourself (for example, you feel ashamed or afraid, or you freeze).

3. Describe reactions of other parts, if any, to angry parts of yourself (for example, they feel afraid, cry, or get busy with other things)

4. Do you know whether angry parts interact in some way with other parts of yourself? If so, in what ways (for example, criticizing or berating)?

5. Could you begin to empathize that angry parts of yourself may be trying to make you function better, although in misguided ways? Describe some possibilities, for example, a part tells you that you are a failure. The intent is to protect you from the painful consequences of failure by convincing you that you cannot succeed anyway.

6. Could you imagine that angry parts of you are trying to keep you away from relationships in order to keep you from getting hurt or disappointed again? If angry parts of you try to convince you that you cannot trust or get close to others, please describe.

7. Even though it might seem strange, try to thank angry parts of you for trying their best to help keep you safe. Could you allow yourself to have a little more empathy for those parts of yourself, even though you should not tolerate any unacceptable behavior? After all, being angry all the time is exhausting and lonely. Perhaps these parts of you would like to learn additional ways to cope that might feel better to you as a whole person.

8. Invite angry parts of you to have their own inner safe space, where they will not be disturbed by inner or outer chaos.

CHAPTER TWENTY-THREE

Coping With Fear

AGENDA

- Welcome and reflections on previous session
- Homework discussion
- Topic: Coping With Fear

    - Introduction
    - Understanding Fear
    - Problems With Fear for People With a Complex Dissociative Disorder
    - Tips for Coping With Fear

- Homework

    - Reread the chapter.
    - Complete Homework Sheet 23.1, Reflecting on Your Experience of Fear.

Introduction

Fear is one of the most pervasive and problematic emotions for traumatized individuals, and it is an essential symptom in trauma-related conditions, such as PTSD and complex dissociative disorders. It is a universal hyper-aroused reaction to perceived threat or danger. From birth, every person has this innate emotion of fear when sufficiently threatened (Panksepp, 1998; Tomkins, 1963; see chapter 17 on emotions). Fear is a "life-preserving" emotion that signals our bodies to initiate survival strategies such as fight, flight, freeze, or collapse. Fear and anxiety become a problem when they are chronically activated in the absence of threat in the present, or when they remain activated for stimuli that are not actually dangerous. Chronic fear is a universal problem for people with a complex dissociative disorder, at least for some parts of the personality, because many parts are stuck in the past in fearful situations, and fear has become a generalized conditioned response.

Understanding Fear

Physiological Reactions to Fear

The physical sensations of fear are very intense and, in themselves, may feel overwhelming. Typical symptoms include shaking, increased heart rate and blood pressure, sweating, nausea, hot and cold flashes, dizziness, racing thoughts or difficulty thinking, and shortness of breath or hyperventilation accompanied by tingling of the hands, feet, and face. When you are afraid, your sympathetic nervous system pumps out adrenaline (among other activating substances) into the body, instantaneously giving you an intense burst of energy for a flight-or-fight reaction. This happens in milliseconds, long before you have a cognitive understanding about what is happening, often before you can even identify the trigger. Your body reacts as though you are in imminent danger before you are consciously able to discern whether there really is actual danger. In fact, you and all parts of you are always anticipating the (near) future: You are forever making instantaneous (and often unconscious) predictions about what will happen, before your conscious thoughts can catch up (Siegel, 1999).

If your relationships and your world have been relatively predictable, safe, and secure, you are more able to predict accurately. But when you have been unsafe, and have lived in an unpredictable and chaotic world, you learn to expect danger, even where there is none. Thus, you have become conditioned to have fear reactions. Normally, once you have evaluated the situation and decided there is no real danger, your body calms down quickly with the help of the parasympathetic nervous system. However, when you have been chronically traumatized it is as though the "alarm bell" in your body is almost always going off, with your fear in overdrive, no matter how much you try to convince yourself that you are safe.

Collapse

When you feel fear, you or a part of you immediately reacts to protect yourself with inborn defense strategies that involve hyperarousal: flight, fight, or freezing. However, if you become too hyperaroused, too terrified, eventually your body may shut down into a collapse mode and become extremely hypoaroused, a state which we discuss further in the next section. This is the last line of defense and is usually related to severe life threat, although it can become a more generalized conditioned response in chronically traumatized individuals.

Fear of Inner Experiences

For most traumatized individuals, fear is not only evoked by external triggers but also can be a strong reaction to inner experiences that may be frightening or sudden, such as an overwhelming emotion, a traumatic memory, or the voice of an angry or crying dissociative part (see chapter 5, on the phobia of inner experience). You may have strong fear reactions to your own inner experiences, for example, avoiding what is fearful in yourself (flight), becoming angry (fight) with another part of yourself, or freezing in fear and being unable to move when you become aware of inner activities of parts of yourself.

Fear Versus Anxiety

Fear can usually be distinguished from anxiety. Fear is a reaction to threat or danger, focused on a specific stimulus, whereas anxiety is more generalized without a specific target and is typically associated with apprehension and dread. Anxiety has a wide range, from mild to severe. Fear is experienced as an intense, even violent emotion, associated with swift and drastic changes in the body. Panic is also intense, but short lived. When people experience anxiety they are often unable to specify the cause of the anxious feelings. Anxious people might generally feel that something bad will happen, but they are unable to know what it is, or perhaps they fear "losing control," having a heart attack, or being unable to function.

Generally, people can distinguish between fear and anxiety. However, for people with a dissociative disorder this recognition is often difficult; although they experience fear, they are often unaware of dissociative parts that have the emotion, or of the reason these parts are so afraid.

Fear and Anxiety Can Be Healthy

There are many situations in which some fear or anxiety is an appropriate reaction. Fear is an important signal of threat, and if you are unable to recognize danger, you may put yourself at risk. Some dissociative parts do not feel fear because they avoid cues of danger, or do not notice potential danger because they are focused on something else. For example, a part intent on being with another person at all costs may ignore, dismiss, minimize, or avoid blatant cues that the other person is seriously dishonest or even violent. Other parts may intentionally seek out danger as a punishment, or because they feel it is their "lot in life" to be hurt, for example, by walking alone at night in an unsafe area.

Problems With Fear for People With a Complex Dissociative Disorder

When you have a dissociative disorder, different parts of yourself are likely stuck in fear responses, while others may avoid fear with distancing or distracting strategies. These reactions have been discussed in a number of previous chapters, including chapter 4 on PTSD, chapter 5 on inner phobias, chapters 14 and 15 on triggers, and chapter 17 on emotions.

Dissociative parts of you that experience chronic fear are almost always hyperalert and easily aroused. Their "alarm bell" never turns off, activating not just the emotion of fear but also the entire response set of thoughts, sensations, predictions, and perception of danger. For example, when you are in session and your therapist gets up to retrieve a calendar or box of tissue, a fearful part of you may be instantaneously afraid, expecting danger or hurt, on the lookout for cues that indicate danger, predicting the therapist is about to hit you, and does not recognize the fact that you are in your therapist's office in the present, and nothing out of the ordinary is happening. Such a part will perhaps have the urge to run out of the room or hide under the desk (flight), or it may be frozen in fear (freeze). These parts are not (adequately) oriented to the present, and thus they do not respond to the present, but rather to the past: They live in trauma-time. An angry part may be evoked that is meant to protect you (fight) and becomes angry with the therapist for being insensitive or even for intentionally scaring you. Occasionally, you, or a part of you, may become so overwhelmed by fear that you collapse and are unable to move and or be verbally responsive. Next we describe some specific problems you may encounter with fear.

Experiencing Fear Without Knowing Why

You may often experience fear but may not have any idea why you have this reaction, because perhaps you avoid your inner experience. Your fear may be so strong that you find yourself reacting without being able to think through what is happening. For instance, you may feel a sudden strong urge to leave a certain situation and find that your legs seem to start walking or even running on their own, or that you cannot sit still and are completely preoccupied with finding a way to leave. Or you find yourself avoiding a common situation at all costs without understanding why, such as going to the dentist, taking a bath, or being in the backseat of a car. You are aware of the urge or behavior, but it does not seem to come from "you." These "unexplained" urges can often be understood as arising from other dissociative parts of yourself.

Sometimes you may not even be aware of the fact that fear is influencing your behavior. For example, suppose you need to go shopping, and you leave your house only to find yourself back in your home some time later, without having done your shopping at all. Or you find that you have been walking around the store in a daze for a while without buying anything. Or you set out to drive to the store but instead drive around town for an hour without thinking very much. You may feel a vague unease but cannot put your finger on it, or perhaps you feel completely numb, nothing at all. You may lose time, or you may consciously decide that you will do something besides shopping without knowing why you have changed your mind, even though you need food.

Perhaps later, you realize these experiences are related to the activation of a scared part of you. A part of you may find shopping terrifying because so many decisions must be made (for example, what foods to choose and how much) that could be judged as "wrong," and then you would be punished. Or a part may be terrified of the crowds in the store. You may not have been aware that these parts of you were activated at the time and you did not feel fear. Or you may have felt afraid without knowing why. You only know that you experienced time loss, were dazed, distracted, or unable to complete your tasks. The more inner communication you have, the more you will be able to deal with situations like this more effectively.

Inappropriate Fear in the Present

You, or some parts of you, may feel fear even though you know it is not appropriate in the present situation. Yet you cannot rationally talk yourself out of the feeling and feel the urge to act on the feeling rather than on what you know. You may even be aware that a part of you is terrified, but no matter how much you try to reassure that part, you feel no less fear.

Failure to Feel Fear in a Threatening Situation

Some people with a dissociative disorder report that they have been in a dangerous situation in the present and felt no fear at all. They were able to act calmly and rationally, sometimes robotically, and managed to come through the situation without harm. This is adaptive on the one hand, but it may leave other parts of you with fear that is unresolved. In this case, a dissociative part of you that does not feel much of anything may be able to cope with a situation, while other parts may hold those feelings of fear and even get stuck in chronic reliving long after the event is over.

Acting Recklessly Without Appropriate Fear

In other cases, the inability to feel fear may not be adaptive at all. Some dissociative parts are so oblivious to danger and fear that they do not register it. This is a major disadvantage of having dissociative parts that are rigid and limited in their emotions, perceptions, predictions, actions, and so forth. Such parts do not attend to real threat cues and emotions, but rather only (or mostly) to cues that fit with their own tendencies, for example, going to work or doing tasks around the house. Some dissociative parts may become "counter-phobic," that is, act the opposite of being afraid of something, even though some parts may indeed be afraid. This may have been an original survival strategy, but the actions of these parts may put you in dangerous situations, such as being in unsafe places or with unsafe people, driving fast and dangerously, or provoking fights with other people without paying heed to the consequences.

Sometimes people with a dissociative disorder may have amnesia for what they have done and only hear reports from other people about these reckless behaviors; others may be aware but unable to influence their actions. These behaviors may create inner critical judgments and conflicts, resulting in more polarization among parts and thus more dissociation. For example, reckless parts often feel disgust and disdain for fearful parts, while fearful parts, of course, are terrified of destructive parts. And parts that conform to social rules are shocked and outraged, wanting to punish or "get rid" of reckless parts of the self.

Although it may be difficult to understand the behavior and motives of parts that engage in endangering behaviors, it is important to realize these may be attempts to overcome fear, however maladaptive, or prove to yourself that you can be tough or that no one can control you. Commonly, these parts engage in high-adrenaline activities to avoid inner pain and to gain a sense of mastery over fear. They seem unaware that they need to reflect on their inner experience rather than focus on external activities that support their avoidance. Thus, internally there remains a vicious cycle of fear that provokes feelings of extreme powerlessness, which provokes disgust and disdain, which provokes shame, which provokes anger, which provokes fear, which provokes more reckless behavior.

Tips for Coping With Fear

In previous chapters we have described many tips and techniques to help you cope with intense emotions: Virtually all of them can be used to cope with fear. In the list that follows, you will find some of the most essential steps toward reducing fear in yourself, and in all parts of you.

- Take some time to reflect inwardly and check with parts of you about whether they feel fear.
- Try to identify the trigger(s) that evokes fear in you or other parts of you, that is, notice what you are reacting to internally or externally that makes you afraid.
- Try to gauge your level of fear and determine whether it is appropriate to the situation. Is your fear based on an inaccurate perception of the present situation, perhaps a perception based in trauma-time? If so, support all parts of you to accurately perceive and become more oriented to the present.
- After reorientation to the safe present, calm yourself or parts inside, using any techniques that are helpful for you or different parts inside. Remember that all parts may not be helped by the same technique. Be flexible with yourself.
- Practice some of the exercises you have learned in this manual (or any others that you know) to regulate yourself.
- If you feel frozen (hypoaroused without being able to move), you may begin by making small movements, perhaps first by blinking your eyes, moving your fingers and toes, and gradually moving your arms and legs. If you feel cold, warm yourself by wrapping in a blanket or having a hot drink or bath, or putting a heating pad or hot water bottle on your chest and stomach. Use safe space and relaxation exercises to help solidify a sense of calmness and safety for all parts of you.
- If you know in advance that a certain situation is likely to evoke fear, you can make a plan to deal with it ahead of time (see chapter 16, on planning ahead for difficult times). Help parts of you go to your inner safe space, so they do not have to endure a potentially frightening experience, such as having an uncomfortable medical procedure, until they can be more oriented to the present. In other situations it is helpful to gather all parts in an inner meeting place and explain the situation ahead of time and make plans for safety. Once parts are able to reflect, they will be able to change their habitual patterns of response, including fear reactions.
- Dissociative parts that do not feel fear may be helpful in many situations, for instance, being able to visit a doctor or dentist, or cope with

other potentially triggering situations without undue fear. While some parts of you may still be stuck in trauma-time and are not yet oriented to the present sufficiently, such parts can be of great help in these situations.

• If parts engage in reckless behaviors, you will need to begin communication with these parts to decrease their risky actions. If needed, you can enlist the help of your therapist to deal with these parts of yourself.

**Homework Sheet 23.1
Reflecting on Your Experience of Fear**

1. Describe a current situation in which you or some part of you felt fear. Choose an example that is not likely to overwhelm you.

2. Describe thoughts or beliefs you or other parts of you had during the situation.

3. Describe what triggered your fear, if you know.

4. Describe your physical sensations of fear (for example, rapid heartbeat, trembling, sweating, cold, hot).

5. In retrospect, do you think your fear was based on an inaccurate perception of the situation, that is, based on trauma-time? If so, describe the perceptions.

6. Describe any attempt at inner communication during or after the event. Describe how it did or did not help you. If you were not able to have any inner communication, describe what prevented you from reflecting.

7. Describe any techniques that were helpful to you, or in retrospect, might have been helpful if you had been able to use them.

8. List two healthy coping strategies that you and all parts of you would like to learn to use when you feel afraid in the future. Describe the obstacles to using these strategies in the present.

CHAPTER TWENTY-FOUR

Coping With Shame and Guilt

AGENDA

- Welcome and reflections on previous session
- Homework discussion
- Break
- Topic: Coping With Shame and Guilt

  - Introduction
  - Understanding Shame and Guilt
  - Shame Scripts
  - Understanding Guilt
  - Tips for Coping With Shame and Guilt

- Homework

  - Reread the chapter.
  - Complete Homework Sheet 24.1, Coping With Shame.
  - Complete Homework Sheet 24.2, Coping With Guilt.

Introduction

Chronically traumatized individuals almost always experience a devastating sense of shame about who they are, in addition to being ashamed of what has happened to them. In addition, people with a dissociative disorder typically feel ashamed of some parts of themselves, and perhaps even of the fact that they have a dissociative problem. Because interpersonal trauma affects sense of identity and self so profoundly, your very essence and existence can feel shameful to you.

Many experts consider guilt as a particular type of shame that is focused on being ashamed of one's actions (behaviors), even though it may feel different than shame. Some describe guilt as about what you do, involving a fear of punishment or retribution, whereas shame is about who you are. In any case, guilt about our behavior can easily lead to shame about ourselves in a broader way. In this chapter we will discuss both emotions, as they are so linked together, with the major focus on shame. Both emotions involve awareness and evaluation (judgment) of ourselves and of how others may perceive us. And both emotions are nearly universal in trauma survivors.

Understanding Shame and Guilt

Shame is one of the innate emotions that all of us experience (Dorrepaal et al., 2008; Nathanson, 1992; Tomkins, 1963; see chapter 17), and yet it can be one of the most destructive emotions for traumatized individuals. Shame involves a sense of failure, incompetence, and defeat.

When children grow up in loving families, they are praised for each developmental step, helping them achieve a healthy sense of pride. But for children who grow up in neglectful, critical, or abusive homes, these achievements may be ignored, disapproved, ridiculed, or even punished. These children feel shame that may become pervasive and destructive over time.

Feelings of shame and guilt can be induced or reinforced by other people. Many perpetrators tell a child the abuse is his or her fault. Such messages have a major effect when the relationship is one of unequal power and authority (for example, a parent blaming a child). Sometimes a perpetrator threatens terrible punishments if a child tells, so his or her sense of guilt and shame, coupled with fear, becomes almost consuming. And certain religious or cultural beliefs may also induce a chronic sense of shame and guilt.

Shame has intense physical manifestations: head down, eyes lowered and averted, flushing, changes in breathing, confusion or inability to think, and a sense of collapse or freezing. In this condition people seem only able to recall examples that prove how bad or worthless they are: the test that they failed, the deadline they missed, how ridiculous they must have sounded in a conversation with someone, how people must sense or know how dirty and disgusting they are on the inside. They have intense flashbacks of shameful moments, relived over and over. When people feel this over-whelming kind of shame, they want to be invisible or even die, and they find it horrifying that anyone might get to know who they really are. In fact, they do not even want to know themselves.

Shame and guilt in small and time-limited doses serve useful purposes, helping us conform to the norms of our social and cultural groups, support-ing development of conscience and morality, promoting good behavior, and even influencing our identity. A little appropriate shame or guilt might prod us to try harder to accomplish a reasonable task well, or be a better friend, parent, or coworker.

But the kind of shame and guilt we are discussing in this chapter goes far beyond those healthy bounds. It is a chronic, pervasive, and sustained expe-rience of yourself as an utter failure, a flawed and defective human being, unworthy of love or life. These unresolved emotions can be paralyzing, and they can profoundly affect your self-esteem and your relationships with others. Shame is often directed towards your body, an extension of how you see yourself as a person: how unattractive or ugly you must seem to others, how ungainly or clumsy, how weak or useless.

When you feel chronic shame, you believe that no amount of punish-ment or corrective actions would be sufficient, and you are unable to for-give yourself or have any empathy for the terrible suffering shame brings to you. It is as though chronically ashamed people have received a life sen-tence of shame with no hope of parole, even when they are unsure of ex-actly why they are bad. In fact, some people will say there is no particular reason they are bad and unworthy: The mere fact that they exist and take up space on the earth is shameful enough. They believe they are not wor-thy of living and do not deserve anything good. In such cases, shame is an emotion of hiding: The last thing an ashamed person wants is to be open, vulnerable, and seen by others. Thus, it is an emotion that often is not ad-dressed sufficiently in therapy, even though it is a major impediment to healing.

As noted earlier, when people feel ashamed, they are reacting to per-ceived failure or inadequacy. Thus, they always view themselves from the perspective of others. In other words, shame is always based on predictions that others will view them as bad, incompetent, or stupid. Shame does not require the actual presence of another person, but merely an inner imagin-ing of how another person might judge and find them incompetent or bad. Often people are unaware of this inner prediction of being judged, but only of a profound sense of worthlessness, unfocused fear, and sometimes of paranoia.

Extreme and pervasive shame and guilt no longer serve as helpful signals

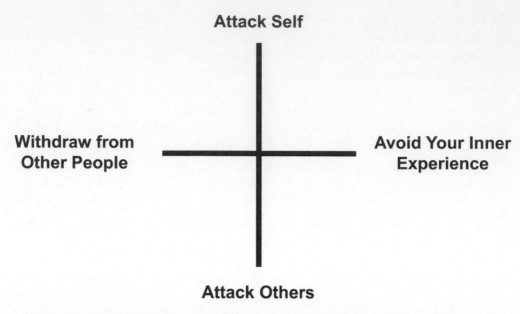

Attack Self

Withdraw from Other People

Avoid Your Inner Experience

Attack Others

Figure 24.1. The Compass of Shame. Adapted from Nathanson, 1987.

that help guide our behavior and the development of our morals and ethics, but rather have become a way of being, a core identity that brings misery to nearly every aspect of a person's life. And quite naturally, people will try to avoid the extreme suffering of shame. To this end, there are four patterns of reactions (or scripts; Nathanson, 1992) that people employ to prevent experiencing the emotion of shame, illustrated in Figure 24.1.

Shame Scripts

Unresolved shame is a major barrier to resolving dissociation (Kluft, 2007). As Lynd (1958) noted, "Shame is the outcome not only of exposing oneself to another person but of the exposure to oneself of parts of the self that one has not recognized" (p. 31). There are four basic maladaptive scripts that perpetuate unresolved shame and that are quite typical for people to employ (Nathanson, 1992). In fact, various dissociative parts of yourself may employ different of these responses. The more you learn how to recognize and intervene to change these automatic reactions in yourself and all parts of you, the more you will be able to resolve shame. These reactions include (1) attack self, (2) attack others, (3) avoid inner experience, and (4) withdraw from others (isolation). Each of these reactions involves a particular set of strategies that attempt to avoid shame, and each is associated with different perceptions, predictions, feelings, thoughts, decisions, and behaviors.

Attack Self

In this strategy, you, or a part of you, accept the beliefs of shame, such as being inadequate, stupid, or incompetent, as true without reflecting on those beliefs. Thus, you turn anger and disgust inward. For example, a person who feels ashamed while working on this chapter might feel self-directed rage for being "stupid," for not already knowing enough to stop being ashamed, for having to deal with shame in the first place, even for thinking about shame. The entire experience is negative, and the more negative, the more self-directed anger, contempt, or disgust is evoked, which only magnifies the effect of shame. Thoughts involve a heightened awareness of all the things you have done wrong, your faults, and negative characteristics. The behavior is to criticize yourself (or one part criticizes another part) in order to prevent reoccurrence of the shameful situation by forcing yourself through criticism to be "better" or even "perfect."

You may be aware of the negative experience of shame (for instance, *I feel so bad that I can't do anything right.*) and the message of shame is accepted as true (for instance, *I'm worthless*), but shame may not be identified as the root of these inner experiences. You simply believe you are worthless, rather than being able to say, *I am feeling ashamed.* Particular dissociative parts that are stuck in this pattern (attack self) are often one side of a coin. The other side is comprised of inner parts that engage in inner criticism, belittlement, and threats.

Attack Other

In this script, you, or a dissociative part of yourself, typically do not feel negative toward yourself, but toward other people. You are not the problem: They are. For example, a person who felt ashamed in therapy might make an intentional comment that could be hurtful or shameful to the therapist. Or a dissociative part may be viciously critical of other parts internally. The experience is negative, and the feeling is one of anger or contempt of the other person (or other parts). Anger is directed away from the self, perhaps toward the source of the shaming event. Thoughts include an awareness of someone else's (perhaps another part's) actions or faults, and they may or may not involve awareness of shame. The motivation is to improve your own self-image by externalizing the shame and perhaps projecting it onto someone else (or some other part). The behavior is a verbal or physical attack to make the other person feel inferior and yourself superior and stronger. Very angry parts may engage in this kind of strategy, always blaming and shaming other parts, or people in the world, unaware of their own shame.

Withdrawal From Others (Isolation)

In this script, you or a dissociative part of you accepts the message of shame as real ("*I am such a loser*") and feels badly about it. You feel so bad that you isolate yourself from others so you do not expose yourself to further shaming experiences. For example, a person who feels ashamed while working on the skills in this manual might consider dropping out of group or individual therapy to avoid the shameful feelings. A strong feeling of anger and anxiety may accompany the shameful withdrawal and isolation. Thoughts include a hyperawareness of discomfort with others, imagining other people's negative reactions ("*Now, she is really a loser!*"), and a heightened awareness of shameful actions, faults, or characteristics. Nevertheless, as in the *attack self* script, negative feelings and cognitions may not be identified consciously as shame based. The motivation is to limit shameful exposure by avoiding other people or situations in which shame might be evoked. Some dissociative parts may have strong urges to avoid social situations or new experiences for this reason, and you might be filled with dread each time you must be with others, or whenever you must try something new at which there is potential for failure.

Avoidance of Inner Experience

A person (or dissociative part) may avoid being aware of inner experiences such as feelings or thoughts that might evoke shame. Thus, he or she is not aware of the experience of shame, typically does not acknowledge the negative experience of self, engages in denial, and attempts to distract self and others away from the painful feeling. For example, a person who felt ashamed in therapy might start making jokes or flippantly comment that the session is boring or useless, or he or she might try to change the subject entirely or even switch to another part that has a different agenda. The experience becomes neutral or positive; shame may be disowned or denied, or overridden with joy or excitement in distracting activities (joking around, talking about something else). There is little to no awareness of shame or one's shameful actions, faults, or characteristics. The motivation is to minimize the conscious experience of shame or to prove that one does not feel shame. *Avoidance* strategies are most likely to operate outside of conscious awareness. Particular dissociative parts may be especially adept at distracting from shame by changing the subject or by being willing only to talk about silly, mundane topics.

Shame and guilt are pervasive in those who have been traumatized. They are painful and difficult emotions to experience and resolve. It will take time for you to deal with them more constructively. In this manual, in your individual therapy, and in your daily life, you will need to pay regular attention to shame-related issues, gradually shifting perceptions, beliefs, and feelings associated with guilt and shame.

Understanding Guilt

As with shame, it is important for you to distinguish between adaptive guilt and guilt that is pervasive and unreasonable. In the case of adaptive guilt, you have done something that society or your own conscience judges as wrong, that is, you have a "guilty conscience." This kind of guilt is remedied when you recognize and take responsibility for your behavior and change it going forward. Guilt often implies that you had a choice about your actions. Yet traumatized individuals have not done anything wrong to cause abuse and were in no position to make choices about what happened to them or what they did as children. And even when they have engaged in unacceptable behavior and did have a choice, they seem unable to eventually learn from it and let it go. Thus, feelings of guilt are often unrealistic or inappropriate in people who were abused as children. Even though they may believe the abuse was their fault, they have no idea of what could have been different, just that traumatizing events would not have occurred if only they had been different in some undefined way. This appraisal is not based on realistic facts or on what would be expected from other people in the same situation. It does, however, provide the helpless child with an internal sense of control to believe that *I could have changed it, if only I fought harder, or ran faster, or stood up to him."*

Tips for Coping With Shame and Guilt

To resolve pervasive shame and guilt, you will find it helpful to learn more adaptive ways of coping instead of using the shame scripts described in the previous section.

- Recognize shame and guilt reactions, and name them. Learn your typical thoughts and feelings that are shame based. For example, you, or some part of you, might often say, *"I could never do that; I would fail, so I won't even try."* That fear of failure is shame based. Or you often compare yourself with others and always come out "less than." If you believe that other people are always smarter, kinder, work harder, are more efficient, and are better at relationships than you are, then you likely are shame based. And the reverse is also true: If you always view yourself as superior to others, you are also likely to have a lot of shame.

- Learn your patterns of coping with shame, that is, how you use shame scripts. Do you mentally attack yourself, or do you tend to attack others? Do you avoid situations, thoughts, feelings, and memories that might evoke shame? Do you isolate and withdraw from others? Each part of you may have used a different shame script to cope with shame.
- Recall how often you tend to feel shame on a scale of 1–5, with 1 being *never or rarely*, and 5 being *every day or almost all the time*. This scale will help you determine how much and what sort of work to focus on to cope with your shame.
- Notice what body sensations you have when you feel ashamed or guilty. Are they different for shame and guilt?
- Once you notice your patterns, try to interrupt or shift them. You may find you need to practice this in small steps. For example, wait a short while to engage in attacking yourself or someone else instead of immediately doing it. Then try changing small aspects, for example, remind yourself that you are experiencing shame and that criticizing yourself will only make it worse.
- Ascertain which cognitions you might need to correct, for example, *"I am worthless. I don't deserve to have good things. People find me disgusting."* Find possible counterarguments, such as, *"No one is completely worthless; each person has some merit." "Having good things is not about deserving them. It is part of life to have good things." "There are people in my life that do not find me disgusting."*
- Notice specific beliefs related to shame and guilt that may be held in particular dissociative parts of yourself.
- Recognize and begin to work with the strategies employed by other parts of yourself. Try creating dialogues about shame and about what all parts want to accomplish with those strategies. For example, respond to critical parts of yourself by saying, *"I know you have my best interests at heart, that you want me to be competent, successful, and well liked. I want that too. Shouting at me or ridiculing me only makes me lose what little confidence I can muster. Let's work together to find a different way that is more effective."* And to a very shameful part, you might say, *"I know that shame is an awful feeling and I am going to help you with it. I*

know you feel ashamed about what happened to you, and I want you to know that it wasn't your fault and that there is a way we can deal with this together. I am glad to listen to what you have to say, whenever you feel ready. I'd like to point out what is different in the present from the past, so you can feel more at ease."

- Be willing to talk about shame in therapy. You can begin by just talking about what it is and how it affects you, rather than talking about particular shameful events. Practice talking about it until you become more comfortable with the topic and know your therapist can talk about it, too. Help all parts of yourself learn to talk about it in therapy.

- Notice your present experience, and whenever shame or guilt is evoked, ground yourself in the present, remind yourself that much of what you believe about yourself when you feel shameful or guilty is greatly exaggerated and not valid.

- Work with your body to shift your physical experience of shame. For example, if you feel frozen, try to move around a little bit, take in some breaths, and squeeze your toes in your shoes.

- Gradually share with yourself, among all parts of yourself, and with your therapist the events in your life that bring so much shame to you. When shame is shared in the presence of an accepting other, it is most likely to resolve. You may not be ready to do this yet: That is fine. This is just a reminder to do so when you *are* ready. The timing should be discussed with your therapist.

- Shame is typically alleviated when you can develop a positive or joyful experience to pair with the shameful one. For example, if you feel "unworthy," recall or imagine a moment when you felt cared for by another person. Or if you feel like a failure, recall or imagine a time when you felt good or proud of something you had done, for example, when you made a good grade in school, learned how to use a computer program, finished a project that was difficult to complete, or were able to make a change in therapy.

- Chronic guilt is best managed by developing increasing empathy for yourself and all parts of you. It is also helpful to begin to realize (with help from your therapist and others) that some of your guilt may not be realistic. The more empathy you develop, and the more you can fully realize the true circumstances about which you experience chronic guilt, the less you will feel.

- Realistic guilt is best managed by (1) accepting that you are fallible and make mistakes and do not always behave perfectly just like everyone else; (2) making a realistic appraisal of what you have actually done (or not done) (this may require the help of a safe other); (3) helping all parts inside come to an inner acceptance in which the offending behavior can be fairly judged but also the human being that you are can be understood and accepted; (4) making amends or restitution if possible; and (5) learning from your behavior so you can do things differently in the future.

Homework Sheet 24.1
Coping With Shame

1. *Event:* Describe an event or situation in the present in which you felt shame (ask for all parts to cooperate as much as possible in this exercise to select a situation that will not feel too overwhelming to you.)

2. List the thought(s) or beliefs you or other parts had during the event that indicated that you were feeling ashamed.

3. Describe the physical sensations that you or other parts of you experienced when you were feeling ashamed (cold, shaking, frozen, collapsed, holding your breath, feeling shut down, tingly, rigid, butterflies in your stomach, etc.).

4. If you are aware of them, list specific triggers that evoke your shame.

5. As best you can, list which of the four shame scripts that you or other parts of yourself tend to use and how they manifested in the situation you described above (attack self, attack other, withdrawal/isolation, and avoidance of inner experience).

6. Can you recall or imagine having a sense of pride, achievement, or accomplishment in a similar situation to the one you describe above? (For example, if you described a situation in which you felt ashamed because you made a mistake, can you recall or imagine a time when you did something well and felt good about it, or someone told you that you did a great job?). If so, take the time to help all parts of you remember or imagine that experience. Notice your thoughts, feelings, and body sensations.

7. Now, make a list of some experiences in which you felt a healthy sense of pride, achievement, or accomplishment. Help all parts reflect on this list often.

Homework Sheet 24.2
Coping With Guilt

1. *Event:* Describe an event or situation in which you felt guilty (again, be careful to choose a situation that is not overwhelming to you or any part of you).

2. List the thought(s) or beliefs you or other parts had during the event that indicated that you were feeling guilty.

3. Describe the physical sensations that you or other parts of you experienced when you were feeling guilty (cold, shaking, frozen, collapsed, holding your breath, feeling shut down, tingly, rigid, butterflies in your stomach, etc.).

4. If you are aware, list specific triggers that evoke guilt.

5. How do you or other parts of you tend to cope with feeling guilty? For example, do you withdraw from others, berate yourself or other parts internally, avoid thinking about it, cannot stop thinking about it, or want to hurt yourself?

6. Describe some ways in which you could approach chronic guilt more constructively. For example, instead of being in it, you could reflect on your experience of guilt and challenge some of your core beliefs.

CHAPTER TWENTY-FIVE

Coping With the Needs of Inner Child Parts

AGENDA

- Welcome and reflections on previous session
- Homework discussion
- Break
- Topic: Coping With the Needs of Inner Child Parts

  - Introduction
  - Understanding Young Parts of Yourself
  - Goals of Working With Young Parts
  - Working With Young Parts
  - Blending: An Advanced Technique

- Homework

  - Reread the chapter.
  - Complete Homework Sheet 25.1, Working With Inner Child Parts of Yourself.
  - Complete Homework Sheet 25.2, Practice Review: Using Inner Cooperation to Solve Problems in Daily Life.
  - If appropriate, practice various forms of blending. Consult with your therapist first.

Introduction

Almost all people with a complex dissociative disorder experience at least one dissociative part of themselves that seems young or childlike. This is natural, given that people with this type of disorder usually were traumatized at an early age: These parts represent the developmental steps they missed or did not completely achieve. Of course, these parts are not actual children, and they must be dealt with in the context of a person's adult life in a responsible manner. In this chapter you will learn specific ways to increase your acceptance of and cooperation with these "young" parts of yourself.

Understanding Young Parts of Yourself

Some parts of you may experience themselves as adolescents, children, or even toddlers or infants. These parts are stuck in various early developmental time periods of the past, having been banished from your awareness or avoided because you may have lacked empathy and a willingness to deal with them. The ages of dissociative child parts often seem to correlate with particularly traumatizing times in your childhood.

Dissociative parts that experience themselves as children often perceive, think, feel, speak, and behave more or less in the ways in which a child might. To a great extent, their behaviors, thoughts, feelings, needs, and wishes are your strivings to achieve the normal developmental experiences from your childhood that you missed, particularly regarding attachment with a caring person.

The Experience of Child Parts

Your experiences of these parts may include hearing voices crying or screaming, begging for help, or asking for activities or objects that a child might enjoy or find comforting (but an adult might not). You may feel intense urges that a child might naturally have, such as wanting to buy a doll in a store, eating dessert instead of dinner, or wishing your therapist could adopt you. At times, a young part might influence or even control your behavior. For example, you might find yourself hiding in the closet or a corner, whimpering like a child; talking in a young voice; or even suddenly being unable to understand a more "adult" vocabulary. These experiences might frighten, shame, or disgust you and other parts of yourself.

Child parts typically hold traumatic memories, especially of fear, shame, anger, loneliness, and yearning for love, a major reason why you might have avoided them. But occasionally they may have positive memories, either real or fantasized, as though they have kept good memories safe for you, or they long ago retreated into a wonderful fantasy world to escape the pain of real life.

Phobic Avoidance of Child Parts

You may have developed a strong phobic avoidance of most of these parts of yourself and the experiences they contain. You, or other parts of you, may find the needs and desires of young parts shameful or disgusting, or exhausting and overwhelming. Perhaps aggressive parts of you criticize these parts as being ridiculous, silly, stupid, childish, and so forth, and try to convince you to ignore or even "get rid of" them. However, avoiding or ignoring these parts of you will only perpetuate their inner experiences of loneliness, yearning, need, shame, and fear. As Marilyn Van Derbur (2004) wrote about a young part of herself:

> Instead of gratitude for sacrificing herself, I loathed, despised, and blamed her . . . she was profoundly vulnerable, completely alone, trapped and scared. (p. 191) . . . Only when I could begin to understand how I really was as a child, could I ever begin to have compassion for the one I hated most, the night child. My perception of her had to change or I would never be able to find a resolution. (p. 242)

When you, and other parts of you, can actively acknowledge, accept, and empathize with young parts of yourself, you will begin to feel more inner relief. You can find ways to help these parts of you that are stuck in the painful wounds of childhood to begin to have more positive experiences. You can take their needs and wishes into account respectfully, even if you cannot always meet those needs in exactly the way that is wished. The point is to take these parts of yourself seriously and take the time to know more about them without judging them as bad or negative.

Problems Related to Switching to Young Parts in Daily Life

Spontaneously switching to a child part in daily life typically occurs when an adult is unable or too afraid or ashamed to cope with a certain situation. Some individuals may switch to a child part as an unconscious avoidance strategy, for example, to avoid a conflict, such as a disagreement with an angry partner, or to deflect attention away from a significant but painful issue in therapy. Other times, switching to a child part is a maladaptive needs-meeting strategy, for example, to gain support or comfort for which the adult is unable or unwilling to ask another person. In these cases, work to help an adult part(s) learn to be assertive and less avoidant is essential.

In the same way that it is not appropriate for real children to be responsible for adult functions in life, young parts should not be in charge of your behavior or be left to cope on their own with daily life without adult parts of you in charge. They should, when possible and appropriate, be present by looking through the eyes of the adult or a temporary blending (see later discussion) (Fine & Comstock, 1989; Kluft, 2003), because it is essential that all parts of you learn to be present. The limited ways of coping and fixation in trauma-time of young parts can result in poor decision making (see chapter 27 on decision making) and problems in relationships with others. It is thus important to learn to prevent switching to younger parts, particularly when you are around other people, because they may not understand or, worse, may take advantage of you when you are too vulnerable. You may choose to allow some time for these younger parts to be out in private for specific activities that have healing goals. But such experiences should be guided by an adult part of you in order to help these parts continue with their growth and development toward adulthood as parts of you as a whole person.

Goals of Working With Young Parts

Every person with a dissociative disorder is different and finds his or her own ways of healing. When you are reflecting on ways to help young parts of you, as with all parts of you, it is helpful to be clear about the goals of what you are trying to accomplish. For instance, if a child part wants to color in a coloring book or call your therapist, it is important to consider the goal(s) of that activity for you as a whole person, as well as how appropriate it may be given relational boundaries or social acceptableness.

For example, does a particular activity help parts of you know that you are allowed to have fun or that you can give yourself a simple pleasure or comfort? Does it help young parts feel more accepted by you and willing to grow and develop, knowing you can meet your needs as a whole person, or does it reinforce their desire to remain childlike and never grow up? Does it help critical parts learn that treating child parts more supportively and empathically is helpful, or does it increase their shame and rage at "childish needs?" Does it support further avoidance of necessary but painful inner grief work by child parts (and you), or does it offer a greater sense of your adult presence to help them tackle difficult issues? Does it soothe and calm parts so that they do not disrupt your daily living, or does it encourage parts of you to become more demanding of "special" separate attention and time? These are some of the important considerations for you and your therapist to take into account when deciding how best to help young parts of yourself.

One reason some child parts remain separate from you is the strong wish to ignore what has happened and to create a loving, wonderful childhood in the present, as though nothing bad had happened. Therefore, a major goal is to find an appropriate balance between the necessary acceptance of and grieving for what you did not get as a child and discovering ways to fill some of those needs in the present. It is not possible to undo what has already been done. It is possible to grieve and move forward to rewarding experiences in the present and the future.

In addition to working toward healing goals for young parts of you, you need to simultaneously balance what is helpful for you as an adult and as a whole person. For example, if a young part wants to take a stuffed animal in hand while you shop at the grocery store, even though that may help that part of you feel more secure, it is not appropriate for you as an adult to do so, and it may not help other parts at all. Moreover, it supports the young part in continuing to be unaware of present-day reality, namely, that you are an adult and that the grocery store is a safe place. In such cases, you might compromise, for instance, by putting a small object in your purse or pocket that represents safety and comfort for that young part. Or perhaps that part might feel safer by looking through the eyes of an adult part who will ensure their well-being or stay in an inner safe place.

Do not be afraid to be creative. As with every interaction with parts of yourself, you must weigh the benefits and risks for all parts of yourself, finding a balance that is acceptable for all parts of you in the context of being an adult in the present. We suggest that you discuss with your therapist the ways that are most effective for you in accomplishing progress toward healing.

As we have noted, young parts of you are not literal children. However, you may use much of what you know about children's growth and development in planning to help these parts of you. Next we will discuss several strategies to do so.

Working With Young Parts

Before you begin specific work with child parts, it is essential to examine your attitude toward these parts with your therapist. Child parts most often remain separate because the adult part(s) of you is avoidant of what they represent. As you work with child parts, it is equally important to help adult parts of you to be more empathic and accepting of the needs, wishes, and feelings of young parts.

Already, in using this manual and in your therapy, you have had opportunities to practice skills that will help you cope with young parts of yourself:

- Reflecting, including paying attention to and listening respectfully to parts of yourself, as well as becoming more aware of and more ac-cepting all of your inner experiences that you previously ignored or avoid-ed
- Communicating with parts of yourself through inner dialogue or journ-aling
- Talking inwardly to other parts to reassure, comfort, and soothe
- Developing a safe inner place for all parts of yourself
- Using imagery and other relaxation techniques to help all parts of you
- Orienting to the present those dissociative parts that are stuck in trau-ma-time
- Understanding and challenging dysfunctional core beliefs of dissocia-tive parts
- Creating an inner meeting place and having inner deliberations about daily life

As with any parts of yourself, you may work with child parts using four different strategies: (1) imagery-based inner experiences, such as safe plac-es and imagined activities; (2) inner cooperation among parts to care for each other; (3) actual experiences that meet a specific young developmen-tal need, such as having a nightlight on during the night; and (4) actual present-day experiences that simultaneously meet the needs of all parts, such as going to the zoo or taking a pleasant walk for enjoyment.

Many people find imagery helpful in working with young (as well as oth-er) parts. You might imagine caring for young parts inside in the same way as you might a literal child. For example, perhaps you might imagine hold-ing or rocking an upset part; teaching a part what it needs to know to grow and develop; or creating an inner space where a part can play freely and feel safe. There are no limits on how you can use your creativity and em-pathic intentions to help parts of yourself heal by using imagery. You may find many additional helpful suggestions from a method called *Developmen-tal Needs Meeting Strategy* (Schmidt, 2009). Of course, you should always check with your therapist before you try any suggestions you may find on your own to make sure they are right for you.

As an extension of imagery work, various parts of yourself can partici-pate internally in caring for child parts. Some people already have parts that are helping internally, perhaps including some mutually trusting rela-tionships between "younger" and "older" parts. Other people may need the help of their therapist to accomplish this step, especially if they are strongly avoidant of dealing with parts of themselves. For example, a part may "babysit" while you tend to adult responsibilities, or various parts can com-fort and orient young parts.

Some people find it useful to allow young parts of themselves private time in which they can engage in actual child's play, for example, coloring in a coloring book or reading a children's book, allowing themselves simple pleasures they did not have previously. Others find it more helpful to imagine offering these activities internally, without the need to actually do them. Still others may find ways in adult daily life to include child parts in adult activities, for example, going on a special excursion that is fun for you as a whole person. Perhaps it might be helpful to establish a comforting bedtime routine for young parts, for example, reading a nice story or having a stuffed animal or other comfort object or music available.

And of course, some people might not find these interventions helpful at all. The point is not to revert back to childhood or to treat these parts as literal children. Rather, the goal is to learn how to give yourself what you need to develop and heal and, most important, to create a greater degree of empathy and connection between you and these young parts of yourself.

Working With Nonverbal Parts

Young parts, and perhaps some other parts as well, are often not very verbal, and thus may have a hard time expressing themselves in therapy. You might allow other nonverbal communications from young parts, such as drawings, to be brought to therapy. Some parts even seem like infants who cannot speak. Fortunately, most people are able to discern what infants need without language. You can help by making an effort to understand the nonverbal behaviors of young parts of yourself, for example, responding to their crying by comforting them. You may also learn to speak for young parts, much as a parent speaks on behalf of a young child to support language development, for example, "*You need comfort. Let me hold you*"; "*You are cold. Let me warm you up*"; or "*You are so hungry! I will feed you.*" A more advanced imagery technique is to help the young part "grow up" to an age at which language is possible. Your therapist can likely help you with these interventions.

Blending: An Advanced Technique

As you develop more empathy and care for young parts (or any parts), you may find it helpful to experience a greater closeness among particular parts of yourself. *Blending* is a temporary coming together of parts for the purposes of enriching the experience of one or more parts (Fine & Comstock, 1989; Kluft, 1982, 2003). Several cautions are important to understand before you try any form of blending. First, be sure to consult with your therapist to determine whether this technique is right for you at this time. Second, blending should be voluntary for all parts involved, not forced, and an agreement made that it will immediately end at the request of any part of you involved. Finally, during the period of blending, as we describe it here, traumatic memories, feelings, or sensations are *not* to be shared. There may be times when blending can support work on traumatic memories, but that is not what you are learning at this time. The focus should only be on present-day experience. If you are unable to practice blending without the intrusion of traumatic material, you should refrain from using this technique for the time being and consult your therapist for further help.

Blending can occur in small steps, according to your own pace. The parts that you may want to blend together should not have major conflicts between them, and be focused on the present not the past.

For example, you can invite a child part (or again, any part) to "come closer" to you so that part can have a more complete sensory experience of the present. First, you might simply allow both of you just to become accustomed to being closer. If this does not yet feel sufficiently safe, you could invite parts to keep a safe distance, but look through special glasses or binoculars, or through a protective window to be able to see the present more clearly. As they begin to experience a current situation "through your eyes," that is, from your adult perspective, their anxious feelings based on the past can be reduced.

If your level of inner closeness feels safe and even positive, you can take another small step to become even closer. Perhaps it involves reaching out and touching together the tips of each other's index fingers, as in the movie *E.T.: The Extra-Terrestrial*, or holding hands, or inviting the child part to sit in your lap, or wrapping up together in a comfortable and safe quilt. Take your time to find the right image for you, and then determine whether this level of inner closeness is acceptable to all parts. If so, you may continue to the next step.

As you and a young part are safely close, encourage her to look out of your eyes, listen through your ears, and feel with your hands. For a short while, you and the child part of yourself are sharing the same experience in the present instead of having different experiences. During this sharing, you can point out the differences of the present that exist alongside some similarities to the past.

A more complete blending occurs when you and another part come completely together for a short period of time. This type of blending is not only for orienting parts to the present, but to help you complete tasks more effectively. For example, several parts of you may merge to function better at work, or to make a plan for safety, or to help other parts internally.

Blending is a precursor to all parts becoming you as one whole person—a major goal of therapy. Many people with a complex dissociative disorder are afraid of having all parts of themselves come together (that is, to integrate), fearing parts will die, disappear, or "be killed off." Blending can offer positive temporary experiences within your control that help you understand more about what integration is like, reducing the fear of all parts of you over time.

To blend completely, you might use an image that works best for you. Perhaps you might imagine one part stepping in the shoes of another, or hugging until you are merged, or standing in a beam of warm light that helps you merge, or blending in a healing pool of water. You may also try to imagine one part standing in front of the other, both facing forward. The part in front steps back just as the other part steps forward. They meet in the middle and merge. There are infinite images you can use for yourself: Choose the one(s) that is right for you.

If you would like, you can try blending for just a moment to see what it is like, and then move away from each other and discuss your experience. Some people have strange physical sensations at first; for example, when blending with a child they feel very short or very tall (depending on which part has the perspective). Some feel wiser, stronger, or just different in a way they cannot explain. Some (but not all) find they have temporary changes in visual or auditory acuity. These are expected sensations and will pass after a brief time. In the beginning, you and other parts may find it helpful to know you can blend and unblend at will, so you will not fear a forced integration. You may set a time frame for blending, for example, 1, 2, or 5 minutes at first during a therapy session, and if that goes well, you can practice at home each day. As you are ready, blending can occur as you need it. You may even find that blending is such a positive experience that you prefer to remain blended together. Just make sure you are going at your own pace, taking into account the needs and concerns of all parts of you.

Homework Sheet 25.1
Working With Inner Child Parts of Yourself

1. Describe your attitude and the attitude of other parts (if any) toward an inner child part; for example, do you feel protective, angry, ashamed, critical, loving, disgusted, exhausted, or helpful?

2. Describe a young part's attitude toward you and other parts of yourself, if you are aware. For example, perhaps this part feels afraid, needy, angry, distrustful, loving, or helpful.

3. Given the attitudes you described in #1 and #2 above, describe any inner conflicts about accepting and working empathically with child parts of yourself.

4. Imagine that your attitudes and reactions to young part(s) of yourself were the same as those you might have to an actual child. What might be different in your approach to your inner child part(s)? For example, would you be more patient, more interested, more caring, or offer more nurturing limits?

5. Describe any difficulties you experience from child parts, for example, hearing inner crying, having flashbacks, feeling a desperate need for attention and comfort, or interference with daily life.

6. Either during a therapy session or during a private time, practice helping a child part of yourself to experience the present more fully by looking out of your eyes, hearing with your ears, feeling with your hands. Explore your surroundings with this child part, talking inwardly to reassure, comfort, and orient. Describe your experience of this exercise below, or if you were unable to complete the exercise, describe what stopped you.

7. List up to five ways you can meet the needs of your child part(s) in ways upon which all parts can agree and which are appropriate in the present. Refer back to the chapter for suggestions, if needed.

1.

2.

3.

4.

5.

Homework Sheet 25.2
Practice Review: Using Inner Cooperation to Solve Problems in Daily Life

This exercise is not specifically about young parts of yourself, but rather is a skills review for inner cooperation.

1. Describe areas of daily life in which you and your parts have achieved (a degree of) cooperation.

2. In which areas would you and other parts like to achieve more cooperation?

3. Which methods of inner communication seem to be most helpful for you?

- Inner dialogue among parts
- Writing/journaling
- Inner meetings with parts
- Blending
- Other (please describe)

Give an example of using one of these methods of inner communication.

4. What do you or parts of yourself do to calm, comfort, and orient parts stuck in trauma-time, including child parts?

5. If you have continued difficulties with inner communication and cooperation, describe the reasons (for example, you feel too much fear; you avoid taking time to do it; parts refuse to cooperate; you do not feel empathy for other parts; or a part of you is highly critical, so you stop trying). Make sure you discuss these difficulties with your therapist.

CHAPTER TWENTY-SIX

Coping With Self-Harm

AGENDA

- Welcome and reflections on previous session
- Homework discussion
- Break
- Topic: Coping With Self-Harm

  - Introduction
  - Understanding Self-Harm
  - Motivations for Self-Harm
  - Helping Dissociative Parts Involved With Self-Harm
  - Tips for Alleviating Self-Harm

- Homework

  - Reread the chapter.
  - Complete Homework Sheet 26.1, Understanding More About Your Self-Harm.
  - Homework Sheet 26.2, Working With a Dissociative Part That Engages in Self-Harm.

Introduction

Self-harm behaviors are coping strategies involving injury to the body that people employ when they do not have sufficient skills to cope in more adaptive ways. Many traumatized people use self-harm as a way of coping with overwhelming inner experiences; thus, the behavior is often related to the phobia of inner experience. In this chapter you will learn more about self-harm, how it affects all parts of you, and new ways to manage it more effectively.

Understanding Self-Harm

Self-harm is deliberate injury to your body in order to cope with stress and inner conflict and pain. It can be understood as a *substitute* action for more adaptive coping that attempts to deal with a variety of overwhelming problems, many involving too much feeling (for example, loneliness, abandonment, panic, inner conflicts, traumatic memories) or too little feeling (numbness, depersonalization, emptiness, feeling dead). Self-harm is thus often related to the need for regulation skills, that is, finding ways to modulate and tolerate unbearable inner experiences, such as painful emotions, or traumatic memories (Gratz & Walsh, 2009; Miller, 1994). Some people harm themselves in secret and carefully hide the inflicted wounds from others. Other people harm their bodies in places that are visible to people around them. For these latter individuals self-harm may be, in part, a way to communicate and express their pain to others because they are unable to say it with words. Some people hurt themselves because they hear inner voice(s) that command them to do so.

Generally, most people feel quite ashamed of self-harm behaviors and find the experience difficult to discuss. They may not mention it in therapy unless they are specifically asked in a nonjudgmental manner. People who self-harm do not intend to kill themselves, and in fact, self-harm may relieve extreme suicidal thoughts for some individuals. Self-harm is a strong signal that you are suffering greatly and that you need help to cope more effectively. Even though self-harm may be temporarily relieving, it inevitably results in an ongoing need to hurt yourself until you are better able to reflect on what is driving this behavior. Then you can make attempts to regulate your emotions and impulses and help parts of you become more grounded in the present.

Self-harming behavior may originate with certain parts of the personality that may or may not yet be very accessible to you. Amnesia is quite common before, during, or after self-harm, so people may find they are injured yet not be aware they have done it to themselves; or perhaps they watch themselves from a distance and cannot seem to control what they are doing (Coons & Milstein, 1990). Parts that self-harm are often reviled and avoided by other parts of self. Inner conflicts among dissociative parts often evoke a tendency to self-harm as a solution to ease the tension of the conflict without resolving it.

Types of Self-Harm

There are different ways to self-injure, ranging from the inflicting mild discomfort or pain with no physical evidence of harm, to severe injury resulting in the need for emergency medical care. Some people feel pain during or after self-harm, while others feel none because they are numb. One may inflict injury intentionally to one's body, for example, by cutting or head banging. A more indirect way to self-harm is to neglect one's body or endanger one's health through severe substance abuse, eating problems, failure to see a doctor when necessary, and inattention that causes frequent accidents, such as falls, kitchen burns, or auto accidents. Also, many people harm themselves by engaging in risky behaviors that could lead to serious physical harm, for example, reckless driving, unprotected sex, going to unsafe places alone or at night, or choosing to be with unsafe people. Some self-harm is very impulsive, while other times it is planned, calculated, and involves a specific routine.

Motivations for Self-Harm

Each person has his or her own unique reasons for engaging in self-destructive behaviors. And various dissociative parts of a person may have different reasons for self-harm. Once you understand your own motivations to engage in self-harm, you are a step closer to learning how to relieve your pain or conflict in a more helpful manner. Following are some common reasons why traumatized individuals might engage in self-harming behaviors.

- To feel real or alive when one is depersonalized or extremely numb
- To evoke emotional numbness in order to stop feeling too much
- To relieve overwhelming emotions, tension, or traumatic memories
- To make the "outside" (body) more congruent with the "inside" (emotional) pain
- To refocus inner emotional pain to the outside, to localize it
- To express anger or aggression toward self (self-hatred)
- As a substitute for expressing anger or aggression toward others
- To cope with abandonment, rejection, or loneliness
- To reduce shame or guilt
- To diminish feelings of emptiness, confusion, or inner chaos
- In response to internal command voices (from other dissociative parts of self)

- To have control over inflicted pain ("I will hurt myself before someone else can hurt me")
- To garner attention from others
- To tell what has happened—as a traumatic reenactment (some part of the body is injured in a similar way as it was during a traumatizing event)
- One dissociative part may be punishing or attempting to kill another
- Punishment for "telling secrets" (one part punishes another part through self-harm for talking about traumatizing events)
- To prevent suicide, that is, an inner bargain for a lesser injury instead of death
- To precipitate a switch from one part to another, or to prevent a switch
- For some people, self-harm becomes addictive, because it may release endorphins, which make them feel euphoric or high.

Helping Dissociative Parts Involved With Self-Harm

People who have dissociative parts that engage in self-harm are often very afraid and ashamed of the behaviors of those parts of themselves. They may have little or no communication with these parts. Thus, these parts are often isolated and feel criticized, feared, and shamed. Often angry parts hurt or command other parts to hurt themselves in reaction to specific internal or external triggers, for example, telling the therapist about a traumatizing event that needed to be kept secret, or a child part desperately seeking contact with another person.

In fact, self-harm often results from an inner cycle of intense conflicts that perpetuate dysregulated emotions. Needy, afraid, vulnerable parts that are in pain evoke anger, fear, and disgust in critical parts. These critical parts strike out internally, causing fearful parts to become increasingly distressed; they also create further inner avoidance of the critical parts, which become increasingly feared, reviled, and isolated. Such dynamics lead to increasingly overwhelming emotions, shame, and self-hatred, which only intensify the risk of self-harm. This cycle is depicted in Figure 26.1.

Tips for Alleviating Self-Harm

- If you have not shared with your therapist that you engage in self-harm, it is imperative that you do so. The more support and help you get, the more you will be able to learn adaptive strategies to cope.

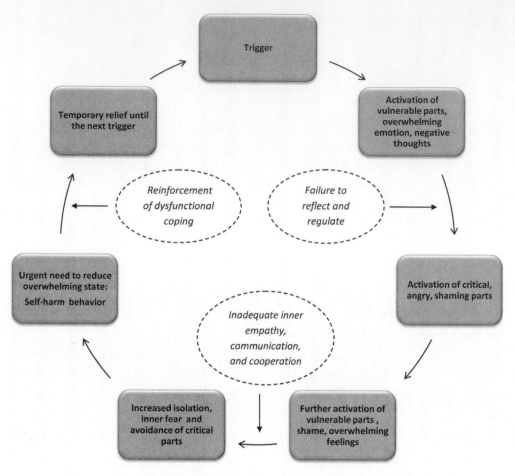

Figure 26.1. Cycle of Self-Harm

- Use your reflective skills (see chapter 6) to try to understand which parts of yourself engage in self-harm and what their motivations are. If you are hesitant or afraid, perhaps some parts of yourself can help you with this task. Your therapist can also help you.
- Try to develop some empathy for yourself and your parts by realizing that self-harm is a way to deal with unbearable experiences, and those parts of you that are engaging in this behavior are in great emotional pain and need help.
- Take yourself and your body seriously. If you need to take care of wounds from self-injury, please do so, and get medical treatment if necessary. This may not be easy, because some medical professionals do not understand why people self-harm, and when the harm is severe, they may mistake it for suicidal behavior. You may need to take special care to find health professionals who will help rather than judge you.

- Realize that each part of you that engages in self-harm may potentially have different reasons for doing so. You may need to help one part at a time with different ways of coping.

- Usually parts inside want contact with you and your therapist; they want to break out of their isolation and self-harm behaviors. However, they are afraid of judgment and need to be assured that you are really willing to help. So there is a double phobia to overcome: You must overcome your fear and shame toward parts of you that self-harm, and they must do the same toward you. Often, self-harm diminishes already as you are more willing to accept and understand these inner parts of yourself.

- Notice what triggers parts of you to engage in self-harm (for example, memories, relationship conflicts, feeling alone, overwhelming anger, shame, or sadness). Once you become more aware, you can use some of the tools in chapter 15 to minimize and manage triggers.

- Use the skills you learn in this manual to soothe or calm you and all parts of you that have the urge to self-harm.

- Develop a plan to use constructive alternatives to self-harm that fit for each part of you. For instance, if a part engages in self-harm in reaction to a flashback, it is important to help this part become more grounded and oriented to the present, and to increasingly realize that those events are over. You may need to communicate with this part to continue to help with grounding and orienting to the present in potentially triggering situations. By staying in contact through inner communication and empathy, you can help this part to stay present, feel more safe and comfortable, and thus feel fewer urges to self-harm. If a part of you engages in self-harm when you experience a perceived threat of abandonment or rejection, you can help by exploring the core beliefs that evoke overwhelming feelings, for example, "I am unlovable"; "Everyone always leaves me"; "People don't really care about me"; "I will always be alone."

- Finally, be patient: It is not always easy to find more constructive ways to cope. Change and healing come one small step at a time.

Homework Sheet 26.1
Understanding More About Your Self-Harm

The more you know about your self-harm, the more you will be able to eliminate it. Use the set of questions below to help you discover more about your need to self-harm. If any of these questions are triggering, you should stop and use grounding and relaxation exercises. Remember to go at your own pace.

1. How do you know when you need to self-harm? For example, *"I feel alone and hopeless"*; *"I have a fight with my partner"*; *"I feel ashamed."*

2. About how long do your episodes of self-harm last? Seconds? Minutes? Hours? How frequent are they? Daily? Weekly? Monthly? Only occasionally?

3. How do know when you can stop an episode of self-harm? For example, *"I start feeling real again"*; *"I feel a release of tension"*; *"I come to and realize I have been hurting myself"*; *"When I make five cuts."*

4. Describe the circumstances in which you would most likely self-harm. For example, when alone; at night; on the weekend, after a fight with someone; when you are very stressed; or when you have flashbacks.

5. Where are you most likely to engage in self-harm (for example, at home, in the bathroom or bedroom, in the car)? Does this location have any special meaning to you?

6. Do you experience amnesia, physical numbness, watching yourself, or other evidence of dissociation? Please describe any symptoms of dissociation and whether these happened before, during, or after self-harm episodes.

7. What do you typically do after you self-harm? For example, do you sleep, eat, go out, watch TV, or cry?

8. What were your thoughts and core beliefs before, during, and after the episode?

9. What were your emotions before, during, and after the episode?

10. What were your physical sensations before, during, and after the episode?

Homework Sheet 26.2
Working With a Dissociative Part That Engages in Self-Harm

1. Using the method of inner communication that works best for you, try to establish a dialogue with a part of you that engages in self-harm. Listen with empathy as that part describes the motivations for self-harm, even if you do not agree. Describe your experience of the inner communication, as well as anything new that you learned about yourself and the tendency to self-harm.

2. List reasons why a part of you might engage in self-harm (review the list of reasons for self-harm if needed).

3. Is it possible that this part of you is not very oriented to the present, that is, lives in trauma-time? If so, use your skills to help this part of you become more oriented and grounded in the present. What was helpful in your attempts to orient this part, and why? What was not helpful, and why?

4. Describe any triggers that might be activating you or a part of you to think about or engage in self-harm.

5. Given what you understand about the reasons for self-harm and its triggers, describe a coping skill that this part of you might use instead of self-harm, for example, avoiding certain triggers, talking to your therapist, providing for the needs of a part, or listening with empathy to a part. Practice these coping skills several times a week and describe your experience of using this skill.

CHAPTER TWENTY-SEVEN

Improving Decision Making Through Inner Cooperation

AGENDA

- Welcome and reflections on previous session
- Homework discussion
- Break
- Topic: Improving Decision Making Through Inner Cooperation

  - Introduction
  - Understanding Decision Making
  - Problems With Decision Making for People With a Complex Dissociative Disorder
  - Improving Decision Making
  - Techniques for Making Effective Decisions

- Exercise: Creating an Inner Meeting Space for Decision Making
- Homework

  - Reread the chapter.
  - Complete Homework Sheet 27.1, Developing an Inner Meeting Space.
  - Complete Homework Sheet 27.2, Using Decision-Making Techniques.

Introduction

Decision making is fundamental to all of our actions. We make decisions both implicitly and consciously. For most people, the many small decisions of day-to-day living take little energy or effort, such as what clothes to wear, what to eat for a meal, what time to go to bed, or when to stop work and relax. These choices are made on a kind of automatic, "subconscious" level and happen (relatively) easily. Particularly difficult decisions tend to involve complex and less than ideal choices, conflicting emotions or goals, sacrifices and compromises, and sustained energy and focus. However, some people, particularly many traumatized individuals, find even the smallest decisions troublesome, much less the more complex and important ones. The ability to make small decisions quickly and easily, and the capacity to reflect and decide on more complex decisions are both necessary skills for your healing. In this chapter you will learn more about how to cooperate and resolve inner conflicts with all parts of yourself toward the end of more effective decision making in your daily life.

Understanding Decision Making

For our decisions to be adaptive, we must not only take into account our immediate needs—which may or may not be completely clear to us in the moment—we also have to consider the potential consequences of our actions in the future. Thus, we tend to base our decision making to a large degree on how we perceive our choices in the moment, and on how we predict the possible outcomes of the actions we decide to take. It is essential to plan for the near and distant future by making good decisions in the present, such as taking time to study now for an exam that is coming up in a few weeks, or saving money now for retirement.

Imagine that you are tired but are reading a very interesting book. You can decide to put the book down at a decent hour and get enough sleep, which meets a longer term need for sufficient rest; or you can continue reading the book into the wee hours, which gives you immediate pleasure but leaves you exhausted the next day. You may decide that finishing the book is a priority over sleep and accept the consequence of being tired, as long as you can still function. Or you may decide that a regular amount of sleep is more important, because you feel irritable and unable to focus when you are tired. What is most adaptive for you depends on how often you skip sleep and how well you can function after not sleeping enough. Staying up too late once in a while is usually not a problem, whereas staying up late most nights is likely to disrupt your sleep patterns and functioning in the day.

Now imagine another scenario: You have bills that are due immediately and you are tired in the evening. You can opt to go to bed early or watch TV, or you can push yourself a little to pay the bills first and then rest. In this case, the most adaptive decision might be to override your fatigue temporarily and pay the bills, because the consequences of not paying them might be painful to you, more so than missing an hour of sleep or relaxation. Even better, instead of postponing such tasks until the last minute, it is helpful to build in time to get them done so they are not left to the last minute.

Some choices require us to think through and analyze the options, while others are best made based on what we feel or need in the moment (Lehrer, 2009), which is different from being impulsive in our decision making. Decisions that involve novel situations that we have never encountered require more reflection, careful deliberation, and creativity. Familiar situations require less reflection, because we often already know what to do. Unfortunately, certain dissociative parts of a person often reflexively make the same decisions in almost all situations, influencing or controlling the decisions of the person. Such parts often do not learn from experience; they act as though their decisions are right without thinking and do not attend to cues that contradict their conclusions.

Decision-making styles can sometimes be problematic. Some people tend to make impulsive decisions based only on how they feel in the moment, rarely stopping to think things through. Others might dither and obsess, overthinking and not using their feelings sufficiently. A flexible and moderate style is most helpful: using your intuition when the situation is familiar and you have successfully made decisions that helped in similar circumstances, and using reflection and consideration of many options when the situation is complex and novel (Lehrer, 2009).

Sometimes it may be hard to know whether to base our decision making on our short- or long-term needs. Thinking through is especially important for these kind of decisions. And even when we make a quick decision in the moment, we need to be able to predict with some accuracy the long-term effects of our actions. However, wise decisions are often made by consciously learning much about the various choices we face and then letting it sink in. Using our intuition, so to speak, we let our subconscious mind work with it, and we subsequently make a decision.

It is important to consider both your thoughts and your emotions when making most decisions. Some people ignore their feelings and act only on rational thoughts, while others might ignore their thinking and decide based on what they feel. People with dissociative disorders are especially prone to either avoiding their emotions when making decisions, because they are too overwhelming, or avoiding their thoughts and being very impulsive, based on the emotion and desires of the moment.

Problems With Decision Making for People
With a Complex Dissociative Disorder

Individuals with a dissociative disorder typically have difficulties making certain decisions due to inner conflicts among dissociative parts of themselves (Van der Hart, 2009). Because various dissociative parts have not yet learned to accept and consider the needs of the person as a whole in a collaborative and empathic manner, even simple choices of daily life can be fraught with conflict, uncertainty, and confusion. Each part may want to make a different decision than do other parts.

In fact, decision making is part of maintaining or resolving your dissociative disorder. Whenever you decide to avoid or to communicate with a dissociative part of yourself, you have made a decision for which there are consequences. Whenever you decide to skip or complete a difficult homework assignment, you have made a decision that will affect all parts of yourself. In every chapter you have learned about new choices, which require new decisions. For example, in chapter 11 you learned more about making decisions about how to manage your free time. In chapter 16 you learned ways to make more effective decisions that help you get through difficult times.

Decisions, especially major ones, most often need to involve all parts of you, just as any person needs to make a decision based on his or her whole self. But when you have dissociative parts of yourself, you may have a greater tendency to avoid hard decisions, find it more difficult to resolve inner conflicts about decisions, and experience impulsive decisions from parts of yourself. You may have experienced how difficult it is to take into account the perspectives, judgments, preferences, needs, or goals of all parts of yourself in making decisions in an area of your life, for example, about what you eat, how you plan and organize your daily life, how you manage relationships, or what you work on in your therapy.

In fact, regardless of whether you are aware, every dissociative part of yourself influences your decisions in some manner, whether through collaboration, fear, shame, anxiety, excitement, criticism, or sabotage.

Dissociative Parts as "Decision-Making Centers"

Each dissociative part is a "decision-making center" that often may involve different perceptions, wishes, needs, and goals than another part of yourself. Many parts fulfill specific functions for you as a whole person, and thus they view certain decisions from a limited or rigid perspective or even find some decisions completely irrelevant, outside the realm of their own area of interests. These competing perspectives and goals can create inner chaos and confusion. For example, in deciding whether to go out to eat with a friend, a fearful part of yourself may not want to leave the house, another wants to be with your friend, another does not trust people in general, one dreads eating in public, and one is completely disinterested, wanting to continue working on a project.

When parts of you are stuck in a rigid perspective, they typically have trouble empathizing with the perspectives and goals of other parts. For example, if a dissociative part is stuck in fear and distrust, it may be hard to convince this part that trusting a person would be helpful. And if child parts are crying and asking for someone to comfort them, while other parts believe that dependency is bad and dangerous, these latter parts will berate the child parts and try to avoid or push the comforting person away. The result is a painful and confusing approach-avoidance to the same person.

Furthermore, even though many important decisions require compromise with other people, many dissociative parts may not have yet learned how to listen to, and deliberate and compromise with, others. Reflecting and overcoming the phobia of inner experience are essential to adaptive decision making, so it is crucial for you to continue to work on those skills. And you may have already been able to come to workable solutions in some areas of your life, for example, some decisions are made by you as a whole person, or you may have delegated certain decisions to particular parts of yourself, which eliminates conflicts about decisions.

Time Pressure and Decision Making

Having to make decisions under time pressure is a stressful challenge for most people, especially when the choices are difficult (Mann & Tan, 1993). The need to choose quickly evokes anxiety or panic, which results in a narrowed perception of options and an insufficient, rather haphazard exploration of the information needed for an adequate decision. The risk for harassed decision makers, as people in such situations have been called (Wright, 1974), is that an impulsive choice may be made that may not be in the individual's best interest.

People with a dissociative disorder are even more vulnerable to time pressures. Some parts of you may feel a chronic sense of urgency, so that even when decisions do not have to be made immediately, they feel the need to do so. The stress of this inner time pressure may urge them to make choices that have not been thought through, and hurried courses of action are not always the most adaptive. For example, a part that always feels harried and overworked may impulsively cancel a therapy session in order to get more work done, instead of working to resolve that extreme feeling of pressure during a session.

Of course, there will always be situations in which you have to decide immediately what to do. For example, while driving in traffic, you make countless decisions to slow down or not, to stay behind another car or pass it, to take one way or another to your destination. In these kind of situations that demand immediate decisions, you need an implicit (if not explicit) inner understanding and agreement that only those parts of self that have the necessary skills and sense of responsibility are to make such decisions.

Harried, pressured decisions often create a vicious cycle, leading to an ever more harried lifestyle, with all parts becoming overwhelmed by the consequences of poor decisions, and thus prone to even more emotion-driven, impulsive decisions that take the least effort.

Effects of Fear and Anxiety on Perception and Judgment

Fear and anxiety affect decision making in the direction of more caution and risk aversion (Loewenstein, Weber, Hsee, & Welch 2001). Traumatized individuals pay more attention to cues of threat than other experiences, and they interpret ambiguous stimuli and situations as threatening (Eysenck, 1992), leading to more fear-driven decisions. In people with a dissociative disorder, certain parts are compelled to focus on the perception of danger. Living in trauma-time, these dissociative parts immediately perceive the present as being "just like" the past, and "emergency" emotions such as fear, rage, or terror are immediately evoked, which compel impulsive decisions to engage in defensive behaviors (freeze, flight, fight, or collapse). When parts of you are triggered, more rational and grounded parts may be overwhelmed and unable to make effective decisions.

Improving Decision Making

One of the most effective ways to improve your decision-making ability is to follow the guideline of "deal with it before it happens." In other words, try to imagine accurately the outcomes of making (or not making) important decisions. For example, in chapter 12 you were asked to develop plans well ahead of time to deal with difficult times or situations. Reflection on what you and all parts of you need, and on the effect of your choices on each part of you and on others, requires that you find adequate quiet time to think through far in advance of the situation. This methodical approach prevents the highly charged and maladaptive decision making that can occur at the last minute when you are feeling anxious and pressured.

Of course, inner communication, empathy, and cooperation are the foundations for improved decision making. To become more effective in decision making about the future (for example, deciding on when and where you will take your vacation, or how you will prepare for an upcoming doctor's appointment, or for your therapist's temporary absence), you need to understand the ways in which parts of you either work together or hamper your decisions. You might consider the ways in which the limited and rigid perceptions and beliefs of certain parts affect your choice of options. You can explore how you can foster further inner communication, cooperation, and negotiation in general, and specifically regarding a given decision.

A basic attitude of mutual empathy for and understanding of other parts' positions, including needs and related goals, is essential in resolving conflicts that make decisions difficult. Decision making is often difficult because it is sometimes impossible to satisfy all parts inside at the same time. Thus, it is essential to learn to make inner compromises, for parts to tolerate a delay in getting what they want, or to grieve for what they cannot have. In your adult daily life you often have to make responsible decisions for actions that some parts might experience as "boring" (for example, paying bills instead of spending money of something fun), threatening (such as going for a job interview where parts might feel they are being judged), or otherwise unsatisfactory.

Once dissociative parts of yourself feel respected and heard by you, they become more amenable to considering different perspectives and compromises. And while the perspective of each dissociative part needs to be taken into account, the responsibility for decision making should be on the shoulders of those parts that have the necessary experience and skills. For instance, a young, impulsive part of yourself should not bear the responsibility for deciding where you will live or what job you will take. Thus, it may be helpful for you to develop an inner "team" that makes joint decisions about important life situations and takes into account the needs of all parts of yourself. Next we describe some specific techniques that help with making decisions.

Techniques for Making Effective Decisions

Examine Pros and Cons
Make a list of options for a particular decision, taking into account the needs and desires of all parts. Of course, no one can always have what he or she wants, but for you to take seriously the desires of all parts helps you to determine what is necessary, and perhaps how parts may be able to get at least some of what they want or need, if not now, then later. Write down the pros and cons (advantages and disadvantages) of each choice and how it might affect different parts of yourself. For example, you need to decide on where to cut your expenses. You cannot cut your rent or mortgage or other essentials, so you must cut those things which are not essential to daily life. Write down the advantages and disadvantages for each of several budget items that you are considering reducing. Take note of how various parts of

you react to each item. Try to encourage all parts together to weigh the pros and cons of each item.

Use a Rating System

Prioritize criteria you, in collaboration with other parts, want your decision or plan to meet on a scale of 1–5. For example, if you are making a decision about a vacation, your criteria might be for the holiday to be safe, fun, comfortable, easy, and meaningful. Which of these is most important? Perhaps you choose this order: 5–Safe; 4–Comfortable; 3–Meaningful; 2–Easy; 1–Fun. If you stay home by yourself, would you meet these five criteria? If you go to a family gathering, would you meet these criteria? If safety is a priority, then any choice must include it. If easy and fun are less important, then a choice may not need to include it.

Make Conscious Decisions: Not Deciding Is Deciding

It is easy to avoid making any decisions when the choices are equally appealing or equally negative, or when you are afraid that no matter what you decide, it will be wrong or stupid. However, if you make no decisions, life always decides for you, in ways over which you have no control and you may not like. In such cases, you might consider whether the timing of a decision is best, whether it is likely that you will have another chance to make a decision at a later time, or whether there is a third option. And these hard decisions are best made by consulting with people you can trust. Most important, such decisions should not be made impulsively, but thoughtfully.

EXERCISE
CREATING AN INNER MEETING SPACE FOR DECISION MAKING

In chapter 8 you learned how to create an inner safe place for yourself and all parts of you. This may be useful for you when you are trying to make decisions that require input from all parts of yourself. In the exercise that follows, you will learn how to create your own inner meeting space, originally called the *dissociative table technique* (Fraser, 1991, 2003; Krakauer, 2001). You may find it helpful to enlist the support of your therapist to practice this exercise, if needed.

> Imagine a place where you and all parts of yourself feel safe and where you can gather to make important decisions. This may be your usual safe space, or it might be a special room, a place in nature, or any other place that feels comfortable. Once you have imagined this place—its sounds, sensations, smells, and sights, its dimensions and shape, and all that it contains—allow yourself to imagine a table in this space that has room for all

parts of you to sit, should you choose. This table is specially made just for you. Perhaps it is of beautiful wood with intricate inlays, a magnificent slab of marble or granite, or sleek glass and chrome. Imagine it just the way you want: a solid table to support solid decisions.

Parts are not required to sit at the table: Perhaps some may feel more comfortable hiding under the table, in a special niche or corner, or other safe spots that are not too close and not too far from the table. Still, you may invite all parts, as they are able, to be seated in the comfortable chairs around the table. Each part of you has just the right chair: the right height, the right color and texture, the right support. Some might swivel, some might rock, some might recline, some might be sturdy executive chairs, some might be tiny chairs for children on special platforms that adjust for their height.

Some parts of you may be willing to listen in but not (yet) participate in the discussions around the table, or they may designate a particular part of you to speak on their behalf. When you can image that all parts of you who are able to join are seated at the table, choose a part of yourself to be the moderator of the discussion. This part of you will structure the meeting, allowing each part to have a fair turn and be heard respectfully. This part of you is able to reflect on what is discussed, is able to take the various perspectives of parts into consideration, and is dedicated to helping all parts of you reach inner agreements that serve the best interests of you as a whole person. If you desire, you may write down the discussion, assign a "secretary" who can take minutes of the meeting, or simply write down the discussion as you are able. If you choose, you can imagine that helpful people come to join you at your table, such as your therapist, a loving partner, a good friend, or someone from the past who may be no longer with you but whom you trusted to have your best interests at heart.

Begin with a relatively small issue in order to practice your inner meeting skills as a team. For example, you might want to discuss how to spend the evening or the weekend, using some of the decision-making strategies mentioned in this chapter. If at all possible, allow time for inner follow-up meetings in which the results of your decisions are evaluated. The more parts of you are assured that you take them seriously and do not ignore or judge their needs and wishes, the more they will be willing to cooperate.

Initially, these inner meetings might have the character of business meetings, such as those that take place in work teams and organizations. Eventually, they may also be used constructively for more personal, emotional encounters, such as inner sharing of joyful or healing experiences, and even sharing of painful memories as all parts of you become ready for that aspect of your work.

Homework Sheet 27.1
Developing an Inner Meeting Space

Practice creating and using your inner meeting space for decision making by performing the following tasks:

- Decide on the room or space in which you want to meet (if you do not have one already).
- If needed, decide which parts of yourself want to participate in the meeting. If you have never practiced this technique, it may be easiest to start with parts of yourself with which you have some awareness, and parts that function in daily life.
- If parts of you remain stuck in the past, perhaps you might assign them a "spokesperson" who can speak on their behalf, while these parts listen in from a safe distance.
- Choose an inner "chairperson." This may be you or another part of you.
- Start with focusing your decision-making process on an easy topic, perhaps something that you suspect all parts of you will agree with.
- Describe your inner meeting, including the decision you were able to make.
- Describe what worked well for you during your meeting.
- Describe any difficulties you encountered during your inner meeting.

Homework Sheet 27.2
Using Decision-Making Techniques

You may use your inner meeting space for this exercise. Review and choose one of the techniques for making decisions discussed in the chapter: (1) examine pros and cons, taking all parts into consideration; (2) use a rating system or another technique that you find more suitable for yourself; (3) use intuition and past experience; and (4) use reflection and creative solutions. By virtue of choosing one of these techniques, you automatically choose to make a conscious decision instead of avoiding a decision. Next, choose a particular decision that you need to make (begin with one that is not too difficult) and apply at least one of the techniques. You may combine several, such as examining pros and cons, and reflection and novel solutions. Write out your decision-making process below.

PART SIX
SKILLS REVIEW

You have learned a number of skills in this section of the manual. Below you will find a review of those skills and an opportunity to develop them further. As you review, we encourage you to return to the chapters to read them again and repractice the homework a little at a time. Remember that regular, daily practice is essential to learn new skills.

For each skill set below, answer the following questions:

1. In what situation(s) did you practice this skill?
2. How did this skill help you?
3. What, if any, difficulties have you had in practicing this skill?
4. What additional help or resources might you need to feel more successful in mastering this skill?

Chapter 22, Understanding and Coping With Angry Dissociative Parts of Yourself

1.

2.

3.

4.

Chapter 23, Reflecting on Your Inner Experience of Fear

1.

2.

3.

4.

Chapter 24, Coping With Shame

1.

2.

3.

4.

Chapter 24, Coping With Guilt

1.

2.

3.

4.

Chapter 25, Working With Inner Child Parts of Yourself

1.

2.

3.

4.

Chapter 25, Blending

1.

2.

3.

4.

Chapter 26, Understanding More About Your Self-Harm

1.

2.

3.

4.

Chapter 26, Working With a Dissociative Part That Engages in Self-Harm

1.

2.

3.

4.

Chapter 27, Developing an Inner Meeting Space

1.

2.

3.

4.

Chapter 27, Using Decision-Making Techniques

1.

2.

3.

4.

Improving Relationships With Others

CHAPTER TWENTY-EIGHT

The Phobias of Attachment and Attachment Loss

AGENDA

- Welcome and reflections on previous session
- Homework discussion
- Break
- Topic: The Phobias of Attachment and Attachment Loss

  - Introduction
  - The Importance of Healthy Relationships
  - What Is a Healthy Relationship?
  - The Effects of Interpersonal Trauma on Relationships
  - The Phobia of Attachment and Difficulties With Regulation
  - The Phobia of Attachment Loss and Difficulties With Regulation

- Exercise: Finding Inner Common Ground About Relationships
- Homework

  - Practice the exercise Finding Inner Common Ground About Relationships.
  - Complete Homework Sheet 28.1, Finding Inner Common Ground About Relationships.
  - Complete Homework Sheet 28.2, Your Experience of Secure and Insecure Relationships.
  - Complete Homework Sheet 28.3, Balancing Self- and Relational Regulation.

Introduction

As humans, we have a lifelong, biologically driven need to connect with others: We are made to be social beings. Healthy relationships can provide safety, protection, emotional regulation and soothing, physical contact, companionship, communication, support, and a sense of belonging. As John Bowlby, an eminent psychiatric pioneer who studied attachment, noted,

> Human beings of all ages are found to be at their happiest and to be able to deploy their talents to best advantage when they are confident that . . . there are one or more trusted persons who will come to their aid should difficulties arise. (1973, p. 359)

However, our most intense emotions are evoked in relationships, for better or worse. This makes relationships more difficult to manage and maintain in a relatively stable manner. Everyone has difficulties in a close relationship from time to time: People are not perfect and their individual needs and wants do not always coincide with those of others. We all misunderstand and misperceive sometimes because we cannot read each other's minds. We occasionally say and do things that are hurtful to others, even though it may be quite unintentional. The experience of being betrayed, abandoned, rejected, or humiliated can evoke some of the most intolerable feelings of hatred, rage, shame, loneliness, fear, and despair. In this chapter we will discuss models for healthy relationships and the difficulties that you may encounter in relationships that are related to traumatization and dissociation.

The Importance of Healthy Relationships

We all base our adult models for interpersonal relations on our early attachments. At that point in development, we learn how relationships work, for better or worse, from our limited experience in interactions with primary caregivers. Ever after, we respond in relatively similar ways in close relationships and expect others to respond similarly. We have thus developed a template or model in which we try to fit all of our relationship to some degree, whether they actually do or not. Relational models include certain persistent core beliefs, for example, *"I can trust others and am lovable," "No one really cares about me,"* or *"People are dangerous."* And various dissociative parts of yourself may have their own relational models that potentially conflict with one another, as we will discuss later in this chapter. Fortunately, dysfunctional models can be changed with mindful reflection and work on your ways of perceiving relationships and other people.

Safe relationships that are nurturing, containing, and predictable are essential to our healthy development from the cradle to the grave. In fact, secure early primary relationships help regulate a young infant's immature physiological systems (including distressed states and emotions), the first necessary step in the infant learning to employ his or her own regulatory skills. Slade (1999) noted that such relationships "predispose a child toward more differentiated, coherent, and flexible functioning" (p. 584), conditions necessary to healthy development across our entire life span. In the next section you will find a partial list of guiding principles for healthy personal relationships. Notice what you have already incorporated into your relational model, as well as those on which you wish to continue to work. And remember, these principles are ideals: Because we are all human, no one is able to live up to them perfectly all the time.

What Is a Healthy Personal Relationship?

- It is based on mutual respect, empathy, and equality.
- You both are able to set clear boundaries with each other and be assertive without being aggressive.
- You both have a relatively healthy balance of autonomy, dependence, and interdependence.
- You both feel secure in the relationship, but this feeling of security *does not depend on whether the person can be available to you at all times.*
- You both have a sense of the other person, even when they are not with you, that is, you can hold him or her in your mind and heart.
- You both can regulate your emotions that are evoked in relationships.
- You both are able to negotiate and resolve most relational conflicts and are willing to ask for outside help if needed to get resolution because the relationship is valuable to both of you.
- You both have a relatively secure and stable sense of self.
- You both have a basic trust that most people do not intend you harm, and you can recognize those that do intend harm.
- You both are able to recognize and respect that the other person has needs and desires, thoughts and feelings, and goals and aspirations that may be different from yours.
- You can both generally accurately understand and reflect on the motivations and intentions of the other person.
- The relationship is based on negotiations about what is best for both of you, not on power and control, or dominance and submission, or winning and losing.
- You can both talk about your inner feelings and experiences without fear of rejection or humiliation.

Perhaps one of the most important aspects of a healthy relationship is that room is made for mistakes, because we all make them. In fact, healthy relationships follow a natural and inevitable *cycle of connection, disconnection, and reconnection*, over and over across time. Your ability to learn to flow along with this cycle and not become stuck in disconnection is a key to making relationships work. We will describe more about this later. But first, we will discuss how being traumatized affects your relationships.

The Effects of Interpersonal Trauma on Relationships

Those who have been significantly hurt or betrayed in major relationships, especially when they were young, generally develop their relational model based on these highly unstable and destructive bonds. Relationships themselves and various relational events have been traumatizing and thus may be major triggers in the present. Therefore, being in close relationship with another may be one of the most challenging and triggering experiences for individuals who have experienced interpersonal trauma.

People who have a dissociative disorder generally expect rejection, hurt, betrayal, or abandonment; therefore, they have major trust problems. They may develop a *phobia of attachment,* an intense aversion to becoming too emotionally or physically close to another person (Steele, Van der Hart, & Nijenhuis, 2001; Steele & Van der Hart, 2009; Van der Hart et al., 2006). On the other hand, traumatized people are in desperate need of stable and caring interpersonal relationships. They may also develop a *phobia of attachment loss,* an intense fear and panic about losing important relationships. The need of the individual to simultaneously seek and avoid relationships leads to severe inner conflict and confusion among various parts of the personality, and it sends mixed messages to the other person, who may also become confused and frustrated. These relational phobias—of attachment and loss—are two sides of the same coin and are the major focus of this chapter.

The Phobia of Attachment and Difficulties With Regulation

In chapter 18, we discussed the importance of being able to regulate yourself both by yourself (self- or auto-regulation) and with the support of others (relational regulation). Individuals, or certain parts of themselves, who avoid relationships generally prefer to find ways to deal with problems by themselves rather than reaching out to others for support and help. They have learned to become self-sufficient and are mortified by their own dependency needs. In fact, they often find that relationships are dysregulating rather than helpful because they are so worried about being hurt.

Some people, however, may have little ability to regulate themselves. They are thus more likely to engage in destructive strategies to cope with relationships, for example, using self-harm, drugs or alcohol, or excessive work. And, of course, some parts may want to avoid relationships but other parts simply do not have the skills to manage much regulation on their own, setting you up to resort to self-destructive coping strategies.

You will likely have one or more parts of yourself that have some degree of avoidance of becoming close to another person. Perhaps you fear betrayal, hurt, indifference, or ridicule and thus hold back. It is important to already begin to become more aware of what you and all parts of you believe about, and expect and predict, in relationships, because you can change dysfunctional beliefs with some help. In addition, some parts of you may fear the intense feelings, needs, and yearning that inevitably arise in a close relationship, and by avoiding relationships, you avoid these strong inner experiences (see chapter 5 on the phobia of inner experience). Because there is so much conflict, fear, shame, and confusion about relationships, you likely have trouble keeping yourself regulated in your window of tolerance.

Most people with a dissociative disorder do not avoid relationships completely but struggle significantly in the relationships that they do have. Parts of you that are phobic of attachment typically have several major innate ways to cope when they feel threatened in relationships. We discussed these reflexive strategies more generally earlier in chapter 4 on understanding dissociative parts of yourself. They include *flight, freeze, fight*, and *collapse*. Perhaps you recognize one or more of these defenses in yourself in the context of a relationship. For example, during a conflict, you or a part of you just wants to leave and get away, or avoid talking about it (*flight*). Or you or a part of you feels so afraid that you are frozen and cannot move or think of what you would like to say (*freeze*). Perhaps you or a part of you becomes angry and gets into heated arguments (*fight*). Or you or a part of you even shuts down so thoroughly that you curl up in a ball and are not responsive, not feeling or thinking anything (*collapse* or *shutdown*). Each of these is an example of how you might avoid or even sabotage relationships with others. Each involves a high degree of dysregulation: you are either hyperaroused or hypoaroused.

At times, some parts of you may be highly critical of other people, warning you that they are not to be trusted, are dangerous or useless, or only out to get something from you. They predict catastrophe because they are so stuck in past traumatic experiences where they were indeed hurt and betrayed. This inner experience only serves to make you more dysregulated and upset. These parts are unfortunately bound by their own limited perceptions to a world where every relationship will repeat the hurts of the past. Inner voices may also attack you internally, criticizing and ridiculing you: *"How could anyone love you? You are so stupid and needy, no one can stand to be around you!"* In this way, they help you avoid relationship by convincing you that no one could tolerate you. Of course, this evokes the shame and despair that you must have felt at times as a child, and these inner voices are re-creating what it felt like in the past, which keeps you from taking any risk in relationships in the present.

Based on understandable reasons, these parts of you that are phobic of attachment often have intense reactions to the parts of you that want to have relationships and feel a desperate need to be with another person. Because they realize that having needs in the past was hurtful to you, they may viciously attack these parts, humiliating and despising them. Although this misguided behavior is hurtful to you as a whole person, the original intent was one of protection, since rigidly suppressing your needs might have been the only protection possible in the past. For example, they may call these parts "crybabies," tell them they are disgusting or ridiculous, that they are just trying to get you hurt all over again, that they should be punished and locked away. Of course, as we have discussed earlier, this provokes the other parts to become every more fearful and needy and ashamed, so the inner cycle of chaos and turmoil continues. Yet it is essential for you to understand and develop empathy for these parts who really only want to protect you from further harm: They just need to learn more healthy ways of doing so.

The Phobia of Attachment Loss and Difficulties With Regulation

Now we turn to the parts of you that may be desperate for connection. Perhaps you or parts of you experience panic when you are alone, feeling that you will be alone forever. Or when you predict that someone might abandon or reject you, intense fear and rage are evoked. Such desperation and need for connection can be profoundly dysregulating and overwhelming. And perhaps you are deeply ashamed of these needs and of the parts of you that have them. However, we all have need for connection and care, to feel special and loved in the eyes of another. These are not bad needs and desires: They are normal. It is important to understand and accept this fact and be empathic toward all your needs and desires as a whole person.

Of course, parts of you may be stuck in trauma-time, reexperiencing periods when you so desperately needed care and support and did not receive it. Thus, they may be in a constant state of frantic seeking and clinging. It is important to understand that this desperate experience is a normal and natural defense in itself: Young animals and humans naturally become panicked when their mother is out of sight, and they cry out for her and cling to her when she returns, because she is their protection against the dangers of the world. This innate seeking and urgent crying is designed to bring the mother back to provide safety, nurturance, and relationship: That is its protective function (McLean, 1985).

Most young dissociative parts have unmet attachment needs. Other parts may attack or be disgusted by them because they continue to reexperience betrayal and hurt by early caregivers. However, this serves only to increase their frantic seeking of help and support, sustaining your inner conflict between approaching and avoiding relationships.

Dissociative parts of a person who have a phobia of attachment loss generally prefer to be soothed and regulated by other people, and they often have serious difficulties with self-regulation. They have learned many different strategies to seek out people and avoid being alone. This comes at a cost, however: They tend to exhaust others, who then pull away, creating the very scenario these parts fear, which further reinforces the beliefs of attachment-phobic parts that relationships are hurtful.

On the other hand, some parts may seek out others by being "people pleasers." Such parts may be rather submissive, avoid being aware of or expressing their own needs and feelings, and try to keep people close by doing whatever they want. But they do not get their needs met, because there is no true emotional intimacy in this type of relational dynamic. This strategy eventually exhausts the person as a whole, and other parts inevitably become resentful and angry. Strategies to be more assertive and realize your own needs are discussed in chapter 32 on boundaries.

In summary, people with a dissociative disorder experience a confusing and conflicting set of relational phobias: Some parts of themselves fear being too close, while others fear losing relationships. This conundrum plays itself out as various parts of yourself simultaneously or alternately seeking and rejecting closeness with others. This fear-based (and often shame-based) dilemma makes it difficult to cope with relational disruptions. Next you will find ways to cope with such disturbances.

EXERCISE
FINDING INNER COMMON GROUND ABOUT RELATIONSHIPS

This exercise will help you learn to empathize with all parts regarding their position on relationships. Use the meeting place technique from chapter 27 (or some other method) to gather all parts together. You may ask for help from your therapist for this inner meeting if you need or want it.

Begin by getting yourself comfortable and calm. In your mind's eye, imagine your meeting space, the one just for you, and allow all parts that are able to attend. Some may sit closer and some farther away. Some may prefer to be outside the room, listening in. Each part of you can find a comfortable place. Begin the meeting with a statement that all parts are welcome and are invited to be heard. Also emphasize that all parts will be respected, and that no criticism is allowed during this meeting. Then begin to find some common ground upon which you could all agree about relationships. For example, you can surely understand that when you have been hurt, no part of you would want to be hurt again in a relationship, and some parts might thus avoid them. You can begin to understand their worldview, their core beliefs, their feelings of fear and anger and isolation, not an easy inner world to experience. Walk in their shoes for just a moment and feel empathy for how difficult it is.

And you can surely agree that all parts of you have been alone and lacked much necessary care and support from others, and thus some parts would quite naturally want to seek out the comfort, support, and enjoyments of what they have missed. You can begin to understand their worldview, their core beliefs, their feelings of loneliness and need and desperation, not an easy inner world to experience. Walk in their shoes for moment and feel empathy for how difficult it is.

Be aware that you are all struggling so hard, each in your own way, and have your own suffering and needs. Perhaps all parts of you could agree that you do not want to be hurt and that you would like to feel better. See if that is so. And perhaps all parts of you could agree that if you could know for sure that a relationship was trustworthy, it would be worth having. See if that is so. Now you are beginning to find some common ground. Just stay with what you are able to agree on, no matter how small, and leave the rest for another time. Experience what it feels like to be in agreement, all together. Savor this moment for awhile.

Now, in the same way that parts need to feel safe, secure, and supported in relationships, free from hurt, free from criticism, free from rejection, each part needs to feel the same with other parts inside. The more all parts of you practice treating each other as you would want to be treated by other people, the more safe and calm and ready to cope with relationships you will be. This meeting is a good start. Come back often to this place and reexperience the common ground upon which you can all agree. Work together, respect each other, take your time, and you will begin to feel better, safer, more stable and strong.

Homework Sheet 28.1
Finding Inner Common Ground About Relationships

1. Reflect back on the exercise, Finding Inner Common Ground About Relationships, and describe your experience of your inner meeting with parts of yourself. For example, what did you feel? What did you expect? Were you able to find some common ground? Did you find that some parts had a more difficult time with the exercise than others? What were the obstacles to agreement; for example, were parts too critical or too scared?

2. Practice this exercise each day at home. If you have difficulties, discuss them with your therapist and practice during your therapy session so you can learn to find common ground.

Homework Sheet 28.2
Your Experience of Secure and Insecure Relationships

1. Describe an experience in which you felt secure in a relationship. For example, what were your emotions, thoughts, sensations, and actions?

2. Using the same experience in #1 above, describe how various parts of you felt, if it was different from what you experienced.

3. Describe any conflicts among parts. For example, were some parts afraid, angry, or mistrustful? Did you feel an urge to withdraw from the relationship? Did any parts criticize you or other parts of you for being in the relationship or for what you felt?

4. Describe an experience during which you felt a little unsure or insecure in a relationship. Choose a minor incident, not a major one. For example, what were your emotions, thoughts, sensations, and actions?

5. Using the same experience in #4 above, describe how various parts of you felt, if it was different from what you experienced.

6. Using the same experience in #4 above, describe any conflicts among parts. For example, did some parts want to continue to be with the person, while other parts wanted to get away? Did some parts want to start a fight, while others wanted to run and hide? Did any part criticize you or other parts of you, or blame you for what went wrong?

Homework Sheet 28.3
Balancing Self- and Relational Regulation

1. Describe times when regulating yourself is preferable to being with someone else to calm yourself down. For example, if you feel stressed or anxious, you prefer to withdraw and think it through and deal with your feelings on your own.

2. Describe how you calm, comfort, or reassure yourself when you are alone.

3. Describe why soothing yourself is preferable to receiving soothing from others in these incidences.

4. Describe times when you find that being regulated in a relationship is preferable to soothing yourself alone. For example, if you feel stressed or anxious, you prefer to call a friend or talk to your therapist in a session, rather than deal with it on your own.

5. Describe what about a supportive relationship helps calm you.

6. Most people have at least some balance between self- and relational regulation. Please describe what (approximate) percent of the time you self-soothe versus what (approximate) percent of the time you seek out

relational reassurance and support. Various parts of you may prefer different ways, and, if so, notice which parts desire self- or relational soothing and support. If you want those percentages to change, please describe what you would ideally prefer, and notice whether there is any inner conflict about changing.

7. Spend some time thinking about and discussing with your therapist how you might achieve a better balance between self-soothing and relational support, if you need to change your balance. For example, you might write below some of the core beliefs that support self- or relational support ("*People should take care of themselves and not ask for help*" or "*I can't do anything by myself, certainly not support myself!*")

CHAPTER TWENTY-NINE

Resolving Relational Conflict

AGENDA

- Welcome and reflections on previous session
- Homework discussion
- Break
- Topic: Resolving Relational Conflict

    ○ Introduction
    ○ Basic Skills for Resolving Relational Conflicts
    ○ Resovling Relational Conflicts for People With a Complex Dissociative Disorder

- Homework

    ○ Complete Homework Sheet 29.1, Using Conflict Management Skills.
    ○ Continue to practice inner safe space, empathy and cooperation among parts of yourself, and relaxation exercises if you feel stressed when managing conflicts.

Introduction

Conflict in relationships is inevitable. Although coping with conflict is not always easy, you can learn skills that will help you resolve disagreements and disruptions with others. We will briefly discuss some of these essential capacities in the next section. But we recognize that merely learning skills does not resolve your own inner conflicts among parts of yourself and the tendency of various parts to react based on the painful past before you can think and respond mindfully. Thus, we will also address ways for you to help all parts of yourself cope more effectively with conflict in relationships.

Basic Skills for Resolving Relational Conflicts

As we noted in the previous chapter, the emotions evoked in our relationships with others are some of the most powerful we experience, for better or worse. And because each of us has at least some different needs and goals from the other, and because we can misunderstand and be misunderstood despite good intentions, conflicts will occur, evoking intense feelings. Thus, staying within a window of tolerance can sometimes be a struggle during disagreements or quarrels, particularly when we feel shamed, threatened, or seriously misunderstood.

We each have our own template or model of dealing with these conflicts, based on our early experiences and on what we have learned since. Some people avoid conflict at all cost and give in to the needs of others; some seem almost eager to argue, ever ready to fight for what they need and want. Others seem to avoid conflict, while quietly making an end run around the other person to get what they want. Some treat relationships almost like a chess game, always thinking ahead to anticipate the other person's moves and their own moves in response. And some people understand that conflict is merely a part of being in relationship. They neither seek nor avoid it, but meet it with equanimity and reflection, searching for solutions that take into account the best interests of both people. Time and experience have shown this last approach works best.

People are able to cope most effectively with relational conflicts when they possess the following abilities:

- They can be present and focused on the here and now. They are not focused on hurts of the past or possible negative outcomes in the future.
- They attend to the verbal and nonverbal communications of the other person.
- They deal with conflicts as they occur, and they do not avoid conflicts.
- They are able to reflect accurately on their own inner experience and that of the other person, and they pay equal attention to the needs and wants of themselves and those of the other (see chapter 6).

- They stay within their window of tolerance (see chapter 18). They are able to regulate thoughts, feelings, and expectations. When people are relatively calm, they can more accurately read and interpret verbal and nonverbal communications. And they can better communicate their own needs assertively without threatening, punishing, or shaming others.
- They are aware and respectful of different viewpoints, needs, and desires. They speak and act in a respectful manner because they are able to reflect and remain within their window of tolerance.
- They are willing to compromise in ways that take into account the needs of self and others.

Of course, these skills are not easy to employ when your relational model of conflict is based on expectations that others will hurt, ignore, exploit, or betray you, and when parts of you react with defensive freezing, flight, fight, or collapse or adapting to every wish and need of the other person. Next we will discuss some ways to address your inner struggles with relationship difficulties.

Resolving Relational Conflicts for People With a Complex Dissociative Disorder

Conflicts in relationships can be one of the most serious triggers for people with a dissociative disorder. Even when minor conflicts occur, you or parts of you may have an intense or overwhelming reaction (for example, terror, rage, shame, panic, collapse). Generally these triggered reactions occur because parts of you are living in trauma-time, and because you have developed core beliefs and a relational model in which disruptions are always interpreted as dangerous or catastrophic. When a conflict occurs, the phobias of attachment or attachment loss, or both, activate various parts of you that already have inner disagreements about relationships (see chapter 28). This only serves to increase your intense and instantaneous reactions, making you feel more out of control. It is important to at least cognitively recognize that relational problems are on a continuum from very minor to, indeed, devastating. Not all are cataclysmic; in fact, most are not. Next we offer some ways to cope with relational conflicts and disruptions.

Observing How Others Relate
When you feel relatively safe and calm, take some time to observe other people's relationships, because this may offer you insights into effective (and ineffective) ways to deal with relationships. Notice how people relate

to each other, for example, by going to a restaurant or mall and just observing. Make sure you encourage all parts to watch and listen, so all parts of you can learn. Notice that many relationships are good, safe, and stable. Thus, not all relationships are dangerous or doomed to fail. Some people will have better skills than others, so pay close attention to those who seem content and relaxed. Make sure all parts of you notice what these people do differently in relating to others. This kind of observation, in addition to asking friends about their successes in relationships, is a good way to learn better relational strategies.

If some parts do not feel safe enough to watch, you (and other parts) can observe and report to them what you have learned, or they can watch from a distance. You might also want to do some reading about healthy relationships and encourage all parts of you to read along or listen. Spend time getting to know parts of you and their core beliefs about relationships and predictions about other people. Once you are more aware of these, you can begin to challenge them with empathy and respect.

Take a Time-Out

When you, or some parts of you, are triggered by a relational conflict, whether you are angry, hurt, afraid, or panicked, stop and give yourself a time-out. Or perhaps help parts of you take a time-out by going to their inner safe space. Inform the other person that you need to take a break and will come back to discuss the conflict at a later time on which you can both agree (from a few minutes to the next day or so). Set a firm time to come back to resolve the issue—do not continue to avoid it. When you take your time-out, go to a quiet place where you will not be disturbed, slow your breathing, talk inwardly to all parts to reassure them that you are safe, and help parts go to their inner safe places. You might want to take a short walk, lie down and imagine being in your safe place, or distract yourself until you calm down. Use your anchors to the present and make every effort to stay in the present and orient all parts to the here and now.

Reflect on Your Own and the Other Person's Intentions and Actions

Once you have calmed down, you can take time to reflect on what happened. One of the most important ways to cope with relational conflicts is to be able to reflect on the other person's possible motivations and intentions (see chapter 6 on learning to reflect). You then may be able to understand and empathize with, for example, a friend's abruptness because she did not feel well or was late to an appointment. And you can then relax because her abruptness was not meant as a personal snub of you. Help all parts of you be a part of this reflective time if possible. If not, ask parts who are upset to stay in a safe space while you (and perhaps other parts of you) reflect on the situation without such emotional intensity. Then return to those parts that have been triggered, help them calm down, and share your insights with them.

It is also important to reflect on your own reactions, including those of various parts of yourself. If you have been able to stop and take a time-out, you have already been able to notice that you needed to do so and have stopped your immediate reaction. It is essential to be able to step back and notice that you, or parts of you, are reacting, not responding, and to notice how you are reacting, rather than just continuing to be controlled by the reaction. For example, you might notice that when your friend was abrupt, you, or a part of you, immediately felt paralyzed and cold. Perhaps you immediately assumed she did not want to be with you, which terrified a part with phobia of attachment loss. Simultaneously, a part of you felt enraged, because you felt snubbed. You can begin by noting to yourself something like, *"I am frozen. This is a familiar experience. I need to step back and help myself get calm before I think or do anything else."*

Once you are aware of certain repetitive reactions you can begin to work to understand the parts that have those reactions, and how to help them be more aware of and open to the accurate perceptions of the here and now.

Orient Parts to the Present
Of course, many dissociative parts have a very restricted world, in which they reexperience the same awful feelings time and time again in relationships. It is vital that you become more aware of and empathic with these parts, helping them become ever more grounded and oriented in the present, where at least some of your experiences are indeed different and more positive than in the past.

Support Avoidant Parts to Deal with Conflict
Other parts may be so numb and shut down, or so rigidly attentive to non-relational activities such as work or solitary activities, that connection and disconnection seem to be of no importance. They have an extreme phobia of attachment. Such parts appear oblivious to your own and the other person's needs. When these parts function in daily life for extended periods, they can profoundly affect your relationships, which become ignored and neglected. This stance is of no help to you or your significant others. Again, empathy is sorely needed for these parts, because they are merely trying to go on with daily life as best they can by ignoring intense inner or relational chaos. Your task is to help these parts feel more secure in knowing that you can manage both daily life and your inner world to empathize with their experience; however, you also need to share your needs and desires with

them and begin to find common ground. Of course, this will be a work in progress, but every small step takes you further into healing.

Protect Vulnerable Parts of Yourself

If you know particular relational situations are likely to trigger parts of you, take the time beforehand to help these parts use their safe place(s), so they can begin to trust that there are parts of you that can handle these situations. For example, if your friend said something that was unintentionally hurtful, before you meet or speak again, talk inwardly to vulnerable parts, explaining that the hurt was unintentional, that she is your friend, that you are capable of working out conflicts with others, and that parts of you that are stronger will discuss the problem with her.

For many people with a dissociative disorder, a sexual relationship in the present may be a major trigger for vulnerable parts living in trauma-time. It may precipitate flashbacks and defensive reactions, especially freeze or collapse. Some people may be confused about the difference between emotional and sexual intimacy, which makes it difficult to accurately interpret the intentions of the other person. We will address this subject a little more in chapter 32 on boundaries, and we also advise that you discuss sexuality and sexual relationships with your therapist because these are important parts of your healing.

Calm and Contain Angry Parts of Yourself

A common and natural reaction to feeling hurt, rejected, or shamed is to react in anger. People may simply want to strike out verbally (or even physically) to make the other person back off. Or some parts may become obsessed with making the other person experience the same or worse, feeling justified in their actions (revenge). Behaving in disrespectful, hurtful, or shaming ways only increases relational conflicts and decreases trust; it does not help you heal or have the loving relationships that you need in your life.

Perhaps you are aware of parts of yourself that experience intense anger in conflicts, or perhaps you wish to avoid them. But it is essential to begin to empathize with the intense hurt and rage these parts of you feel. The sense of being heard and understood is already one step in the direction of becoming calmer. At the same time, you as a whole person must strive to set appropriate limits with these parts of yourself. The more you practice the skills in this manual, and particularly in this chapter, the more control you will have over explosive reactions or hurtful passive-aggressive behaviors, such as the "silent treatment," sulking, withholding love, or other underhanded ways of punishing the other person. The more you treat others in the way you wish to be treated, the more likely you will be to have better relationships. That said, of course, there are people who are truly dangerous and intentionally hurtful. You need to be able to identify and avoid such individuals.

Some additional ways to handle relational disruptions are found in chapter 32 on boundaries. And there are many readily available resources online and in books or classes that can help you learn to cope with relationships more effectively.

Homework Sheet 29.1
Using Conflict Management Skills

If you have a minor conflict during the coming week with another person, use as many of the skills listed in this chapter (and below) to cope. If you do not have a conflict during the week, describe one from the past and imagine using these skills to manage the conflict differently than you actually did. Then answer the questions below.

Skills

- Be present and focused on the here and now
- Orient parts of you to the present
- Reflect on your own and the other person's experiences and intentions
- Stay within your window of tolerance
- Take a time-out, or help parts of you go to an inner safe space
- Help numb or avoidant parts of yourself
- Help angry parts of yourself
- Protect vulnerable parts of yourself
- Be respectful of yourself and the other person
- Be willing to compromise

1. Which skills did you use or imagine using? Describe any difficulties you have with employing these skills.

2. Notice whether all parts of you can accept these skills as important and would like to learn them. Describe any fears or concerns of various parts about using these skills. Once you have described the fears and concerns, reflect on whether there are cognitive distortions or negative core beliefs at their roots.

Example: *"I am afraid I cannot protect myself if I am not angry."*

Reflection: *While it is important to protect myself, it is also important to consider the context and the intentions of the other person to determine to what degree I need protection. Perhaps the person did not mean to hurt me intentionally, but merely disagrees with my viewpoint, or said something that made me feel discounted, but was not meant to harm me. And there are many ways to protect myself during relational conflicts, not* *only by being angry. I can be assertive (see the next chapter) about what I need, rather than angry and aggressive. I can be present and realize I am not in danger and thus have more options to respond available to me. I can take a time-out and check in with all parts to reassure and orient them, to clarify inaccurate beliefs and perceptions.*

CHAPTER THIRTY

Coping With Isolation and Loneliness

AGENDA

- Welcome and reactions to previous session
- Homework discussion
- Break
- Topic: Coping With Isolation and Loneliness

  - Introduction
  - Understanding Isolation
  - Understanding Loneliness
  - Reflections on Your Experience of Isolation and Loneliness
  - Tips for Coping With Isolation and Loneliness

- Homework

  - Reread the chapter.
  - Complete Homework Sheet 30.1, Reflecting on a Time of Isolation and Loneliness.
  - Complete Homework Sheet 30.2, Skills to Resolve Isolation and Loneliness.

Introduction

In this manual we have discussed many reasons why people with a dissociative disorder might isolate themselves and feel lonely. Isolation is the state of being alone and separated from others. Loneliness is a sense of utter aloneness at a time when you most need someone to love or support you, and it can evoke panic and desperation. The fear or emptiness of being alone is a major precipitant of crises, including self-harm and suicide attempts. Even if you have friends or family, you may feel like an outsider who does not belong. Or you may experience relationships as exhausting, complicated, and frightening, and thus isolate yourself. Mistrust is a pervasive hindrance to feeling connected in the present with other people and a force that pushes you further into isolation. This type of isolation may breed loneliness. In this chapter we will discuss these feelings of isolation and aloneness, some of the factors that maintain them, and suggest some first steps to change patterns of isolation.

Understanding Isolation

In her classic book, *Trauma and Recovery*, Judith Herman (1992), one of the pioneers in the field of chronic childhood abuse, describes how trauma destroys bonds between the individual and his or her community. This is especially true when abuse or neglect involves trusted caregivers. Feelings of abandonment and betrayal, and a sense of alienation or disconnection, may interfere with subsequent relationships, regardless of the degree of closeness or distance of the other person. And of course, *feeling* isolated and *being* isolated may not be the same things. One can feel utterly isolated and alone even while he or she is surrounded by people.

Maintenance of Isolation

Social isolation may be maintained and reinforced by certain perceptions, predictions, emotions, and thoughts. Core beliefs, such as *"People can't be trusted"* or *"If anyone really knew me, they would be disgusted,"* support ongoing withdrawal from others. The fear and shame of "being found out" can be paralyzing if you think you are a bad person or if you are holding secrets that feel shameful to you, contributing to an increasing sense of isolation and disconnection. Mistrust is a major impediment to becoming less isolated. People with a dissociative disorder typically have many predictions about how people will betray, disappoint, or hurt them. Many find it difficult to take risks to be in relationships (see chapter 28 on phobias of attachment). And once inevitable conflicts occur, they are often quick to withdraw, expecting the worst (see chapter 29 on relational conflicts). Some people are isolated simply because they do not have adequate social skills to make friends and stay connected. But usually a lack of social skills accompanies the more complex inner experiences described earlier. Fortunately, social skills, like any other skill, can be learned.

Isolation Among Dissociative Parts

For those with a dissociative disorder, inner isolation of dissociative parts is a painful additional struggle. Some parts are stuck in a time of trauma during which they were isolated, feeling perpetually alone and in need. These parts feel alone no matter how much other parts may feel connected with some people. Other parts may have been "banished" from inner awareness out of shame, fear, or disgust, or are neglected behind inner barriers. The more inner disconnection among parts of the self, the more likely isolation and loneliness are problematic. These inner "barriers" between parts are maintained by ongoing shame, fear, and subsequent avoidance (see chapter 5 on the phobia of inner experience).

Isolation as a Reenactment of the Traumatic Past

Many traumatized individuals were quite isolated from supportive others during their childhoods. They typically endured the aftermath of abuse alone. On the one hand, this likely generated terrible loneliness, but on the other hand, isolation was also a signal that *"it's over now,"* that is, the abuse had ended. Thus, some people, or parts of themselves, automatically retreat to isolation to gain a sense of safety and relief. They may develop a habit of isolating when they are stressed in the present, often without even realizing what they are doing or why.

Isolation and Dysfunctional Boundaries

In chapter 32 you will learn about the disadvantages of lax or rigid personal boundaries. Both of these can lead to problems with isolation and loneliness. Lax boundaries mean that people can intrude into your life more than you want, and thus some parts of you may isolate to protect themselves from too many demands instead of setting appropriate and assertive limits with others. Rigid boundaries keep people out perhaps more than is helpful for you, leading to a self-imposed isolation that may result in profound loneliness. It is important to be able to identify your personal boundaries and how they affect your sense of isolation or loneliness.

Understanding Loneliness

Loneliness is a complex condition involving problems with social skills, difficulties with attachment, particular emotions, thoughts and core beliefs, situational issues, and sometimes, unrealistic expectations. Loneliness is not the same as being alone. We all have times when we are alone either due to circumstances or by choice. Alone time can be pleasant and rejuvenating when you choose it (see chapter 11 on using free time and relaxation). But when you do not want to be alone, when you are yearning to be with others, when you experience the need to be with others and are unable to soothe yourself, you will feel lonely. And as we mentioned earlier, you may feel lonely even though you are in the company of people, because you feel so disconnected. Loneliness can lead to further feelings of rejection, low self-esteem, shame, and even despair. In fact, loneliness can feel similar to intense grief following the death of a loved one, and it can be overwhelming in its unbearable sense of separateness.

Loneliness, Fear, and Shame

You, or some parts of you, may isolate because you feel afraid or overwhelmed by other people, and perhaps because you feel ashamed of who you are. On the one hand, you feel some relief that you are avoiding what you experience to be stressful and vulnerable situations. But on the other hand, you may feel lonely, because we are social beings at heart and have an innate drive to be with others.

Loneliness and the Phobias of Attachment and Attachment Loss

As you learned earlier in this manual, you, or parts of you, may have a phobia of attachment loss, that is, of separation, rejection, or abandonment, while other parts of you may be afraid to be connected with others (see chapter 28). Thus, you have a major conflict about being alone: Some parts wish to be alone and find safety in solitude, while other parts feel lonely and find safety in connection with others. It is important for you to acknowledge both and to resolve each side of this powerful conflict.

Loneliness as a Reenactment of the Past

People who were abused or neglected as children often experienced profound loneliness on top of lacking support for overwhelming feelings and experiences. This traumatic loneliness can be reexperienced in the present as a kind of flashback in which those feelings are relived. Because isolation and loneliness might have commonly followed on the heels of abuse, some people automatically isolate and feel lonely when something painful happens in the present. They are reenacting the lonely past.

Reflections on Your Experience of Isolation and Loneliness

- As always, the first step in overcoming a problem is to reflect on it. Take some time (with or without the help of your therapist) to have an inner meeting among parts to begin talking about isolation and loneliness instead of just experiencing them.
- Begin by asking all parts to participate, as they are able. Even if some

parts cannot, you may be able to sense or know something about how that part experiences and deals with isolation and loneliness.

- Notice conflicts among parts of yourself about being isolated or lonely.
- Are there parts of you that prefer to be alone? If so, do they enjoy alone time, or are they avoiding other people or stressful situations? Do they ever feel lonely? Are they aware of and attend to the needs of other lonely parts who may not want to be isolated? What do they feel and think about these parts of yourself? Is there any communication among these two types of parts?
- Are there parts of you that are very lonely and want to be with other people? If so, what keeps them from reaching out to others? Are they stuck in trauma-time, fearful of other people, socially anxious, lacking in social skills? Are they aware of parts of you that might prefer to have alone time or be isolated? Using an inner meeting space, try to encourage parts that isolate to communicate with parts that feel lonely without judgment, and visa versa. Can they find common ground; for example, is there agreement that it is good for all parts not to feel afraid, ashamed, or lonely?
- Notice what prompts you to isolate. Does it happen when you are stressed, after a hard therapy session, when you want to avoid a conflict, or when you feel ill? Are there other alternatives for you to take instead? For example, calling or e-mailing a friend about your stress or problems, being assertive in dealing with a conflict, asking someone to help you if you are ill. Notice any inner obstacles to making different choices than your usual ones.
- Pay attention to what you and all parts of you experience when you are isolated. Do you feel panic, disconnected, shameful, lonely, or numb?
- What happens in your body when you feel lonely; for example, do you feel tense, cold, paralyzed, or frenetic?
- Notice your thoughts and core beliefs.
- What do you expect if you reach out to others when you feel lonely? What do you expect if you are alone and cannot reach someone?
- Are parts of you able to empathize with each other in their need for isolation or their yearning not to be lonely? How might you and your therapist further facilitate and strengthen that empathy, which can lead to cooperation and resolution of the conflict?

Tips for Coping With Isolation and Loneliness

- Begin with grounding yourself, using the exercises in this manual and other ways you have learned to help yourself be in the present.

- Next, reflect inwardly (using the previous section as a guide, if you want) to determine your conflicts and what all parts of you need and want.
- First focus on *internal isolation and loneliness*. You may use all of the skills in this manual to support yourself and all parts inside in becoming less isolated and lonely internally: accepting and connecting with each other; reflecting; orienting parts to the present; helping parts develop empathy, communication, and cooperation; soothing and calming parts; developing safe places; developing pleasant or fun activities that all parts of you can enjoy as a whole person.
- The more you connect with all parts of yourself, the less overwhelmed you will be, which will help you feel more comfortable in connecting with others.
- The more you can accept yourself and all parts of you, the less ashamed and afraid you will be to connect with others.
- If you have severe problems connecting with others or making friends, begin with what is easiest. Is it easier to talk with one person, or with more than one? Does it help you to have a shared topic (such as volunteer work or a hobby)? You might consider taking a class to learn something new, where you will have a chance to meet new people, or volunteer where you will be with others.
- Some people with a dissociative disorder prefer to meet people on the Internet and chat or have a pen pal. This is not ideal, but it is a start.
- Some people find having a pet helps them to feel less isolated. And a friendly pet is a great source of conversation with other people if you go out for walks.
- Isolation can be a habit. Make an effort to get out or be with friends on a regular basis, even though it may be hard to do. If needed, encourage overwhelmed parts of you to stay in a safe space while you connect with others.
- Make necessary alone time pleasant (for example, with nice music, a good book or movie, healthy and tasty food, a walk, etc.) and productive (see chapter 11 on using free time).
- If you have religious or spiritual preferences, make use of mediation or prayer during your alone time to feel more connected to God or the universe. (You might reflect on whether your concept of God as loving or vengeful reflects your past experiences with other people.) And of course some people feel supported by attending the religious house of their preference or by spiritual meetings with others of like mind.
- Stay present so you can at least connect to the world around you. Walk outside and listen to the birds or look at the trees. There is life all around, and it will help if you can feel at least a little connection to it.

- Make an effort to reach out to others instead of waiting for them to call you.

Homework Sheet 30.1
Reflecting on a Time of Isolation and Loneliness

Choose a recent time when you felt isolated, lonely, or both and then answer the questions below.

1. Describe the situation in which you felt isolated and lonely.

2. Describe any specific triggers for you to isolate or feel lonely, if you are aware. Were any of these triggers present in the situation described above?

3. Describe any parts of you that might have been involved in isolating or feeling lonely. Describe any conflicts among parts that isolate and parts that feel lonely.

4. Describe your experience of being isolated or lonely (including the experience of various parts of yourself). You may include thoughts, feelings, sensations, perceptions, and predictions.

5. If someone had reached out to you, or you had reached out to someone, what would you have wanted from that other person in this situation? What kept you from reaching out?

6. List two or three small, manageable steps you could take to begin addressing your isolation and loneliness.

Homework Sheet 30.2
Skills to Resolve Isolation and Loneliness

Most of the skills you have learned in this manual can help you in some way to cope with and resolve your isolation and loneliness. Below you will find a number of these skills. Choose any four of the skills and describe one of the following next to each of the four skills:

- A situation in which you used the skill to cope successfully with isolation or loneliness. Describe what worked well.
- A situation in which you tried the skill but it did not help or you were not able to complete it. Describe what interfered or was too difficult.
- A situation in which you would like to try the skill.

Skills

1. Staying grounded and in the present.

2. Orienting parts of yourself to the present.

3. Reflecting on your experience of isolation or loneliness.

4. Using inner safe space.

5. Using alone time productively.

6. Being aware of and challenging core beliefs and thoughts.

7. Being aware of and regulating emotions.

8. Empathic communication with inner parts of yourself (including use of a meeting space).

9. Negotiating with parts phobic of attachment and those phobic of attachment loss.

10. Coping with a trigger for isolation or loneliness.

11. Regulating yourself within your window of tolerance.

12. Coping with fear or shame.

13. Being assertive.

14. Changing a dysfunctional personal boundary.

CHAPTER THIRTY-ONE

Learning to Be Assertive

AGENDA

- Welcome and reflections on previous session
- Homework discussion
- Break
- Topic: Learning to Be Assertive

  - Introduction
  - Basic Assertiveness Skills
  - Nonassertive Strategies: Appeasement, Avoidance, and Aggression
  - Problems With Assertiveness in People With a Complex Dissociative Disorder
  - Helping Parts of Yourself Cooperate in Being Assertive

- Homework

  - Reread the chapter.
  - Complete Homework Sheet 31.1, Identifying Inner Conflicts That Prevent Assertiveness.
  - Complete Homework Sheet 31.2, Using Assertiveness Skills: A Retrospective Look.
  - Complete Homework Sheet 31.3, Preparing to Be Assertive in an Upcoming Situation.

Introduction

Assertiveness is an essential interpersonal skill that involves being able to express your needs and desires in a confident manner that does not violate the rights of others and is not aggressive (Paterson, 2000; Phelps & Austin, 2002). It is active, not passive or forceful, and involves respect for self and others. It is a way to ask confidently for what you want, without harming anyone. Being assertive involves being able to know what you think, feel, need, and want, and then saying it clearly and respectfully. It also involves being able to set appropriate limits and boundaries without feeling guilty (see chapter 32 on boundaries; Adams, 2005; Dorrepaal, Thomaes, & Draijer, 2008; Linden, 2008). Assertiveness is always about clear, respectful communication between people.

In this chapter you will learn basic assertiveness skills and how to help different parts of yourself overcome obstacles that prevent you as a whole person to be more assertive. The chapter begins with some basic assertiveness skills, then discusses general difficulties with being assertive, and the special problems encountered by those with a complex dissociative disorder. Finally, we will share tips for helping all parts of you learn to be assertive together as a whole person.

Basic Assertiveness Skills

Assertive behavior offers people a number of important benefits. Assertive people tend to have fewer relational conflicts, and thus less overall stress. And because they have fewer conflicts, assertive people often have more stable and strong relationships with others. They get their needs met more consistently, and they can help others get their needs met as well, which further strengthens relationships.

How you view yourself and others is central to whether you are able to be assertive; thus, reflection is a major part of assertiveness skills. You must reflect on your own opinions, thoughts, feelings, needs, and also on those of other people. Assertiveness requires some self-confidence, but you can learn it with practice even when you do not yet feel completely at ease with yourself or others.

Assertiveness includes being able to do the following:

- Give and receive constructive criticism or feedback
- Ask for something; make a request
- Set clear limits by saying "no" or "not now"
- See both sides of an issue and negotiate on behalf of your viewpoint

There are a number of ways to express yourself and your position such that others will be more likely to listen to you.

- *Listen reflectively.* When another person is speaking to you, try not to formulate responses in your head. Instead, listen with an open mind and make sure you understand him or her. You can clarify by saying something like, *"Let me make sure I understand you,"* and then summarize what the person has said. Feel free to ask questions about what you do not understand, for example, *"I am not quite sure what you meant about . . . could you say more about it?"*
- *Use respectful humor,* when appropriate. Humor can lighten a situation and is a nice way to stay connected with another person.
- *Provide a context.* Briefly explain why you want something or why you disagree, so that people do not assume you are trying to hurt them. *"What you have to say is important to me, and I don't want to hurt your feelings, but I have to get off the phone now so I will get to my appointment on time."*
- *Be as specific and clear as possible.* Vague or tentative statements will likely lead to misinterpretation, for example, instead of *"I wonder what is playing at the movies? What do you want do to?"* say, *"I want to see a movie tonight. Would you like to go with me?"* The following statements are clear: *"I want. . . ." "I need. . . ." "I feel. . . ." "I don't want to. . . ." "I hear what you are saying, and can agree with you on . . . but disagree with you on. . . ."*
- *Ask for feedback and then listen carefully to the other person.* Ask the other person whether you are being clear and whether your position makes sense. Then ask for feedback, showing the other person that you are open to his or her opinions and needs as well, instead of just making a demand.
- *"Own" your message.* Use *"I"* statements instead of *"you"* statements (even when you have a dissociative disorder and use of the first person may be difficult at times). Acknowledge that what you are saying is yours and do not blame others, for example, *"I don't agree with you,"* rather than, *"You are wrong."* And when you criticize someone or give feedback, make it as specific and respectful as possible.
- *Make eye contact.* When you look directly at someone (not staring, but comfortably in visual contact), the person is more likely to be able to hear what you are saying.
- *Use your body language.* Turn toward the other person and face him or her. Stand or sit tall, not slumped down and not angry.
- *Be congruent.* Your facial expression and body language should match

what you are saying. Do not smile if you are angry or look afraid if you are trying to stand up for yourself.

- *Use a normal tone of voice.* Speak in your normal voice, not louder, timidly, quietly, or hesitantly. Pay attention to your tone, inflection, and volume and modulate them as you need.
- *Find the right time.* If you are able, the best way to deal with most situations is as they happen. But if you need to reflect in order not to make impulsive decisions, "buy" yourself some time. For example, you can say, "*I need to think about that. Let me get back to you.*" Then choose a specific time to have the discussion so it does not get avoided. Generally, the best practice is to respond in the moment. It will allow you to focus on your feelings at the time. However, it is never too late to return to a person at a later time to share your feelings about an interaction.

As you begin to practice, start with small steps, being assertive about minor issues. You are likely already familiar with many assertiveness skills. However, even though you may cognitively understand the value of being assertive, there are a number of reasons why it may be difficult. Next you will learn about common nonassertive strategies, why people use them, and how to change them.

Nonassertive Strategies: Appeasement, Avoidance, and Aggression

We each learned our patterns of expressing and negotiating our needs and wants in our families as we grew up. Some people may have had few opportunities to say "*No,*" or to ask for what they wanted, or they were punished if they did. Perhaps a family simply was not aware of assertiveness skills and did not know how to model and teach them. Other people learned to be especially aggressive, or that being aggressive was the only way to get what they needed. There are also learned cultural, religious, and gender role differences in assertiveness skills.

From these early experiences, we each develop core beliefs about assertiveness that affect how assertive we will or will not be, and in what situations we can be assertive. For example, "*I have no right to an opinion; I don't deserve to get what I need; Other people must be satisfied before I can get what I need; It's OK to ask for what I need; Needs are not nice to have; I can't get what I want; People will respect me when I speak up for myself; Men are supposed to take, while women are supposed to give; I should never say 'no' when someone asks a favor; It is important to take care of myself and be respectful of others; I can set boundaries with friends, but not with my family; in most cases, almost everyone can get what they need."*

Usually people who have difficulties being assertive will engage in appeasement, avoidance, or aggression when they need to make a choice or are in conflict with another person.

Appeasement

Some people are afraid they will anger or burden others with their needs, and they will then be rejected or harmed. These people are "people pleasers," so they put a lot of energy into appeasing behaviors, that is, making others happy and fulfilled at the expense of themselves. Even if they manage to be assertive, if the other person reacts strongly, they will back down and even apologize and feel they have done something wrong. They are generally passive and submissive, and they rarely show anger. However, they do experience resentment and anger that they do not show to others. They feel taken advantage of and underappreciated, and sometimes they expect that others should "know" what they need and want without having to say it. They view conflict in terms of *"I lose–you win, because your needs are more important, and I am afraid you will be angry or reject me if I ask for something, and besides you don't care about what I want."*

Avoidance

Some people have such a phobia of inner experience or are so confused internally that they completely avoid knowing their own needs or wants, and thus they are unable to articulate them. They appear to be appeasing because they generally go along with what others want, not out of conscious fear, but simply because they cannot find their own inner compass to direct them toward what they need. They view conflict as: *"You win because I don't know, it really doesn't matter to me, and I don't care."*

Aggression

Some people are convinced that the only way to get their needs met is to be forceful and aggressively fight for their rights, as others are only out to get what they want for themselves. These people do not understand the difference between aggression and assertiveness, quickly distrust the motives of others, are fearful that others will hurt or take advantage of them, have little empathy for what others may need, and are easily put on the defensive. They may come across as being entitled or bullying, and they view conflicts in terms of *"I win because I deserve to get what I need, even if I have to force you to give it to me—I don't really care if you lose. If you happened to win after I have fought as hard as I could, you have certainly taken advantage of me and greatly injured me."*

Examples

To explore how each of these behaviors might look, imagine you have a boss who asks you to work overtime during the weekend for the second time in a month. You had planned months ago an important weekend with your family or friends, you are all looking forward to it, and you have already worked extra during the week.

Appeasement. You say, "*Can't you find someone else?*" Your boss answers, "*No, I've already tried and no one else can do it.*" You feel pressured and are afraid your boss will be angry or even fire you, and say, "*Alright, I'll do it.*" But at the same time you feel enormous tension, and you become anxious as you envision the disappointment or anger from your family or friends. You resent being used and caught between the needs of your boss, your own needs, and the needs of your family or friends. You feel a terrible dilemma because you need to please your boss *and* your family or friends, and you have given in to the one who pressures you most in the moment. Your family and friends are disappointed and angry that you did not stand up to your boss. You feel helpless, hopeless, and resentful, and you are not very productive at work during the weekend.

Avoidance. You find it difficult to think clearly about whether you should work or keep your plans for the weekend. You feel muddled. On the one hand, it is good to do what your boss tells you; on the other hand, your friends are expecting you. Working is OK, and time with friends is OK. It is difficult to imagine how your boss or your friends will feel, or perhaps it does not occur to you to think about how they feel. It really does not matter to you, as you have no idea which choice is better or more important for you. It seems too hard to sort out, so you agree to work to avoid thinking about it anymore.

Aggression. You immediately become irritated or angry with your boss and say, "*That's your problem, not mine! You always ask me! Why don't you work yourself? This place is pathetic!*" You feel furious and used, and you feel that your boss does not appreciate your hard work at all, but only expects more of you. Then you walk away angrily. You fume the entire weekend about how unreasonable and mean your boss is and how he always picks on you. Your family or friends do not enjoy being with you, because you are so angry and upset. And you do not enjoy your weekend.

Assertiveness. You are thoughtful for a moment and then say, "*I'm sorry, I will be unable to work. I empathize with you that work needs to be done. However, this is my time off and I have plans for the weekend that I made some time ago with friends and family. My work is important to me, but time with friends and family is also important to me. And I value keeping my word and balancing my life. I am glad to discuss first thing next week how I can be of help, and how our team might better plan our work to be more efficient during the week in the future.*" You leave feeling satisfied that you offered a good compromise to your boss (regardless of whether he or she accepted it graciously), set a reasonable limit, said "no" to something you would have resented, and still have your weekend to which you look forward.

Problems With Assertiveness in People With a Complex Dissociative Disorder

Like many people in general, individuals who have a complex dissociative disorder often have difficulties with being assertive, engaging instead in some of the ineffective approaches described earlier. An additional complication involves unresolved conflicts among parts that make being assertive difficult. For example, an angry part may tend to be aggressive, while a fearful part might want to give in. The aggressive part then also becomes angry internally with the fearful part for being so passive, and in turn, the fearful part becomes more afraid. As a result, the person as a whole may be left feeling overwhelmed, caught up in inner turmoil, and wanting to avoid situations in which choices and assertiveness are needed.

As you can see from the previous example, dissociative parts are often not assertive with each other internally, employing aggression, avoidance, or appeasement instead. Thus, you are not only learning how to be assertive with other people, but each part of you is learning more about how to relate to other parts. Each dissociative part of you reacts to situations (and to other parts of yourself) according to the specific worldview of that part, which is often based in trauma-time. Thus, if a part has a tendency to engage in a particular behavior, for example, freezing, running away and avoiding, fighting and being aggressive, or submitting, that behavior may well be employed automatically, not only in situations in the present, but in reaction to other parts of yourself.

To understand the inner struggles you might have among various parts of yourself, return to the previous example of a boss who asks you to work overtime during the weekend when you already had plans. As soon as your boss approaches, even before he or she says anything, a child part of you is convinced that you are in trouble and you feel yourself freezing. A critical voice berates the younger part for being afraid, and it is ready to be aggressive with your idiotic boss. You are already primed for action, but it is action based on flight or fight, not on being present and assertive. Your boss then asks you to work over the weekend. The younger part immediately wants to say, "*Yes, I'll be glad to*" so as not to anger the boss, relieved that she is not in trouble yet, but still afraid. The angry part of you immediately wants to yell at the boss for his or her ridiculous demands. A part of you that dreads the time with friends because you are so uncomfortable around others breathes a sigh of relief that you now have an excuse not to go. Another part of you desperately wants some time off to play. You are able to consider being assertive, but you are so distracted by the inner conflict and activities among parts of yourself that you stand there with a confused look on your face and do not quite know what to do. In an extreme case, a person might switch to one of these parts to solve the conflict through control rather than assertiveness.

Next you will find some tips on how to work with parts of yourself to increase your ability to be assertive.

Helping Parts of Yourself Cooperate in Being Assertive

In this section you will find a series of steps that will help all parts of you become more willing to experiment with being safely assertive and become more proficient at it. These steps require time and practice and thus cannot always be used when a decision must be made in the moment. They are best used for times when you know you need to be assertive in an upcoming situation, and you have the time and willingness to prepare for it. But the more your practice these steps, the more quickly and automatically all parts of you will be able to be assertive when the situation calls for it.

- *Use your inner meeting room.* Gather all parts of you in your inner meeting room (see chapter 27), or use another way to have inner discussions that works best for you. Help all parts be as oriented to the present as possible, so you can have a dialogue about assertiveness and resolving the inner obstacles to it.
- *Engage in inner reflection.* Listen respectfully to all parts of yourself and learn more about what each part needs and wants, even if you do not agree. Notice how various parts of yourself react to situations in which being assertive would be helpful. And notice how parts react to each other.
- *Reflecting on inner conflicts.* When parts of you have differing opinions, emotions, and behaviors regarding a challenging situation, you may not yet be able to act assertively. However, in the meantime, such situations can be learning experiences upon which all parts can reflect in retrospect (see chapter 6 on reflection). For example, what did each part want or need at the time? What were their concerns or fears? What, if anything, triggered parts of you? What outcome did each part of you want? What did parts of you want to do at the time (whether they actually did something or not)? How did parts of you react to each

other during and after the situation? As you become more aware of the inner conflicts that prevent you from being assertive, you can begin the process of resolving them, using the steps that follow.

- *Challenge dysfunctional core beliefs and thoughts.* As you are aware of the beliefs and thoughts that support a particular reaction of a part of you, try to establish communication and have an inner dialogue about those beliefs, for example, *"I don't deserve to have anything; If I ask for anything, I won't get it, so I might as well take it (or give up)."*

- *Negotiate empathically.* Work toward inner agreements on how to act assertively in a certain situation that is coming up in the near future, and determine whether parts would be willing to compromise or delay getting what they want or need, if necessary. Find ways for all parts to feel satisfied with your decisions, as best you can (see chapter 27).

- *Agree on which parts of you deal with the situation.* Work toward obtaining sufficient inner cooperation so that more rational adult parts of you with relational skills can deal with a situation in which you need to be assertive. Prepare your message, so that you know exactly what you want to say. For example, *"I am not coming to visit you this week; I don't mean to hurt your feelings, but I have some obligations that I must take care of (or, I need some time to rest)."*

- *Help fearful, avoidant, or angry parts of yourself.* Certainly it takes time for angry or fearful parts of you to become more oriented and calm, and learn new skills. If parts of you are still quite reactive, you might try to help them go to an inner safe space during situations where you need to be assertive. This requires a level of inner agreement that assertiveness will be helpful for all parts and more likely to get their needs met. Begin by explaining why assertiveness is more effective, or by encouraging all parts of you to read the chapter together, or perhaps read it out loud to them (reading out loud helps you retain the content). Ask all parts whether they are willing to allow an "experiment" in which an adult and more rational part of you practices being assertive in a minor situation, while these parts remain in a safe place. Afterwards, bring all parts of you together to discuss how the situation turned out for you. Be sure to listen respectfully to feedback from all parts. Initially, it might be helpful to have fearful or very angry parts agree to stay in their inner safe places while the more cognitively inclined parts act assertively. Eventually, such parts could watch from behind an imaginary one-way screen or through a window, thus being at a safe distance and learning from the assertive behavior that other parts are able to model.

- *Use imaginal rehearsal.* Visualize yourself being successfully assertive (see chapter 15 for more on imaginal rehearsal). Also try to envision various responses of the other person and prepare yourself to deal with them. It also may be helpful to role play the situation with a trusted friend or partner, or your therapist. Gather all parts together and imagine they are supporting each other during this situation, so that you feel stronger and of one mind. You might also imagine a safe and trusted other person standing beside you to support you in the situation.

- *Blending.* Various forms of blending (which were discussed in chapter 25) can be useful in helping parts learn to be more assertive. As a first step, for example, a fearful part could look through the eyes of the adult part that is being assertive, to gradually become more familiar with the skills for and benefits of assertiveness. As you become more comfortable with blending, a more aggressive part might be willing to blend with parts that have better assertive skills, or even pair with a more fearful part to support that part in being stronger and more assertive. Check with your therapist to get help with blending, if needed.

- *Take a time-out.* When you are suddenly confronted with a situation where you immediately need to be assertive, you will not have much time for inner reflection and preparation. You may feel frozen or overwhelmed by inner turmoil in the moment. Always try to make time for yourself by telling the person you will respond to his or her request as soon as possible because you need to consider it first. You might even just take a quick bathroom break to think about if for a minute, saying, *"I'll be right back and respond then."* A time-out will give you and your parts inside a chance to "gather yourself together" and prepare for an assertive response that takes into account your needs, then the needs of the other person and the situation.

Homework Sheet 31.1
Identifying Inner Conflicts That Prevent Assertiveness

Choose a recent situation in which you wanted to be assertive but were not able to be. Using the steps provided in the previous section, use an inner meeting to identify reasons why being assertive was difficult; then answer the questions below.

1. Describe the situation.

2. Describe the reactions of various parts of yourself at the time and their concerns or fears.

3. If there were specific things that triggered you or parts of you during the situation, list them below, including your reaction to them.

4. What did each part of you want as an outcome of the situation? Is there inner agreement on the outcome or differences of opinion? If there were differences of opinion, describe the conflicts.

5. Describe how parts of you reacted to each other during and after the situation.

6. In retrospect, describe, as best you are able, a more effective way all parts might have dealt with the situation.

Homework Sheet 31.2
Using Assertiveness Skills: A Retrospective Look

1. Describe a recent situation in which you were able to be assertive, even if only partially so.

2. What skills were you able to use? Refer back to the beginning of the chapter for descriptions of these skills and check all that apply below.

- Listen reflectively.
- Use respectful humor.
- Provide a context.
- Be as specific and clear as possible.
- Ask for feedback and then listen carefully to the other person.
- Own your message.
- Make eye contact.
- Use your body language.
- Be congruent.
- Use a normal tone of voice.
- Find the right time.

3. If you had difficulties with some of the skills above, circle them and describe your difficulties below.

4. Did the difficulties you described in #3 involve inner conflicts among parts of yourself? If so, please describe the conflict(s).

5. Were all parts of you satisfied with the outcome of the situation? If so, describe how the needs of various parts of you were met. If not, describe why some parts of you were not satisfied, and what they would have wanted the outcome to be.

Homework Sheet 31.3
Preparing to Be Assertive in an Upcoming Situation

Choose an upcoming situation in which you need to be assertive. Choose a situation that reflects the level of challenge for which you feel ready.

1. Describe the upcoming situation.

2. What is the outcome you would like to occur?

3. Have an inner meeting in which you discuss the upcoming situation with all parts of yourself. Following the step-by-step approach in the section above on Helping Parts of Yourself Cooperate in Being Assertive and describe the responses of parts of yourself to each step.

   ○ Reflect on the needs and desires of parts of yourself regarding the situation and describe them below.

   ○ List any inner conflicts about the situation.

   ○ List any dysfunctional core beliefs or thoughts about the situation and how you respectfully challenged them.

   ○ Describe how you attempted to negotiate empathically with all parts about dealing with the situation, and their reactions.

○ Agree on which parts of you will deal with the situation and describe how parts of you reacted to this negotiation.

○ Help fearful, avoidant, or angry parts of yourself by orienting to the present, discussing their fears or concerns, taking into consideration their needs and wants, and offering an inner safe space during the situation. Describe what you were able to do, and how parts reacted.

○ Use imaginal rehearsal to envision a successful outcome of the situation. Enlist the help of a trusted other, including your therapist, if you need. Describe your experience of this exercise.

○ Practice forms of blending, if you are ready and able, before the situation, so that you will be ready to deal with the situation from a position of strength and confidence. Describe you experience of blending, if you were able to do so.

CHAPTER THIRTY-TWO

Setting Healthy Personal Boundaries

AGENDA

- Welcome and reflections on previous session
- Homework discussion
- Break
- Topic: Setting Healthy Personal Boundaries

  - Introduction
  - Healthy Boundaries
  - Unhealthy Boundaries
  - Problems With Boundaries for People With a Complex Dissociative Disorder
  - Helping Parts of Yourself Cooperate to Set Healthy Boundaries

- Homework

  - Reread the chapter.
  - Complete Homework Sheet 32.1, Identifying Your Personal Boundaries.
  - Complete Homework Sheet 32.2, Your Personal Space and Optimal Level of Closeness and Distance.
  - Complete Homework Sheet 32.3, Preparing to Set Boundaries in an Upcoming Situation.

Introduction

In the previous chapter you learned more about how to be assertive. Assertiveness skills are essential for setting your *personal boundaries*, which are your guidelines for reasonable and safe ways for other people to behave around you, and for how you will respond if someone crosses your boundaries (Adams, 2005). Boundaries help you stay both separate from and connected with others (Linden, 2008), including your comfort level with how emotionally and physically close or distant you are from people. Your boundaries are related to how close or distant you wish to be with other people. When you have a dissociative disorder, you often have conflicts not only about being assertive but also about the optimal emotional distance between you and another person (also see chapters 28 and 29 on relationships). You may feel confused about how to be separate from others but still close. Various parts of you may push people away, not wanting to be close, while other parts appease people to get closer or keep them from leaving or rejecting you, resulting in confusing and unclear boundaries. In this chapter you will learn more about different types of personal boundaries, how to set them, and how to help all parts of yourself negotiate reasonable boundaries.

Healthy Boundaries

Healthy boundaries help you protect and take care of yourself. They can be set respectfully, but firmly: Boundaries are not threats. They are clear communications about your limits and the consequences of crossing your limits when a person continues to do so. The other person has a choice about whether to continue his or her behavior; thus, the consequences of your limits are the result of the other person's behavior. Boundaries most often have to do with how much time you spend with a person, how much you do for that person, how much emotional energy you put into the relationship, and how other people treat you. And they sometimes involve issues about money, that is, how finances are managed, how much money you are willing to spend, and how much you are willing for your partner to spend.

Some people may be confused about whether setting boundaries is an attempt to control others. It is not; rather, it is a way to be responsible for ourselves and our lives. When we set a boundary, we let go of being invested in the outcome. This distinguishes boundaries from attempts to control. For example, if you are friends with a person who is drinking, and she calls you on the phone or shows up at your house drunk, you can set a boundary, but you have to be willing to accept the consequences of your limits. You can be clear and respectful by saying, "*I feel uncomfortable and disconnected from you when you are drinking. I value you, and our friendship, and miss connection with you, but I no longer want you to call me or come to my home if you have been drinking that day. If you do, I will not speak with you or let you in. And if you continue to call or come to my home when you have been drinking, I will have to reconsider what to do, including ending our relationship.*" In this case, you hope your friend will respect your limits and be willing to get help with her drinking. But those are her choices that you cannot control. You must be willing to follow through with what you said you would do and tolerate her reactions, and even risk losing the friendship in an extreme case.

Optimal Relational Closeness and Distance

As we have discussed earlier, every relationship has normal fluctuations in emotional (and physical) closeness and distance (see chapters 28 and 29 on relationships). And every person has his or her own preferences about what is too close or too distant, both in general and in specific situations. There is a wide range of what is normal, but typically people have a kind of balance where they are not intrusive or smothering of others and are not too distant or avoidant of contact. It is common for everyone to have some conflicts about closeness and distance from time to time. Your personal range is a subjective experience based on what you have learned, what you want, and what you are comfortable with. Many relational conflicts involve mismatches in how close or distant two people want and need to be at a given time and across the course of the relationship.

It is important to understand that most of the time when people want more distance, it is not because they do not care for you, but rather they are seeking what feels right at that moment for them, just like you ideally would do for yourself. And when people in the present want to be more close to you, usually they are not trying to smother, control, or hurt you. As we discussed previously, this might be difficult to comprehend if you have parts stuck in trauma-time that continue to think you always have to do what the other person wants or else you will get hurt.

Some major healthy personal boundaries follow, so you can begin to have a better idea of what to strive for in small steps that are right for you.

Healthy Personal Boundaries

- You are able to say "yes" or "no" to others.
- You are OK with someone saying "no" to you.
- You respect yourself.
- You share responsibility and power in a relationship. You are neither controlled nor controlling.

- You can identify or be receptive to hearing about your mistakes or role in a relational problem, and you take responsibility for them.
- You share personal information gradually in a mutually sharing and trusting relationship.
- You do not tolerate abuse or disrespect.
- You know your own wants, needs, and feelings.
- You communicate your wants, needs, and feelings clearly to the other person.
- You know your physical and sexual boundaries and are able to keep them.
- You are responsible for your own life, and you allow other adults to be responsible for theirs.
- You value your opinions and feelings and those of others.
- You respect the boundaries of other people and expect them to respect yours.
- You are able to ask for help when you need it and can manage on your own when appropriate.
- You do not compromise your values or integrity to avoid rejection.
- You are willing to follow through with consequences if a person continues crossing your boundaries.

Unhealthy Boundaries

Unhealthy boundaries are either too lax or too rigid. Lax or "collapsed" boundaries leave you at the mercy of other people's wants and needs. Rigid boundaries isolate you and prevent people from being close enough to have a significant relationship with you.

Next you will find basic characteristics of lax and rigid boundaries.

Lax or Collapsed Boundaries

- You cannot say "no," because you are afraid of rejection or abandonment or the anger or disappointment of others.
- You are so unclear about your own identity that you let others define who you are and what you do.
- You tend to be either overly responsible and controlling, or passive and dependent.
- You take on other people's problems and feelings as your own.
- You share too much personal information too soon in a relationship. You do not know how to pace personal sharing.
- You cannot say "no" to unwanted sexual contact; find yourself in sexual

relationships you do not really want; or think that it is OK to always agree to have sex if the other person wants it.

- You have a high tolerance for, or ignore, being abused or treated with disrespect.
- You have trouble identifying your needs, wants, and feelings.
- If you are able to identify them, your wants, needs, and feelings are almost always secondary to those of other people.
- You feel responsible for the happiness and well-being of other people, and you ignore your own.
- You rely on the help, opinions, feelings, and ideas of others more than your own.
- You rely on other people's boundaries instead of having your own.
- You compromise your values and beliefs to please others or to avoid conflict.
- If you do set a boundary, you back down if the other person pushes a little.

Rigid Boundaries

- You say "no" far more often than "yes," especially if the request involves close interaction.
- You avoid intimacy by failing to communicate, picking fights, working too much, and otherwise being unavailable.
- You have a phobia of attachment (getting too close) and perhaps of attachment loss (being rejected or abandoned), which keep you at a distance.
- You rarely share personal information and feel uncomfortable when you do.
- You have difficulty identifying your wants, needs, feelings, and in response, you distance yourself from others.
- You have few or no close relationships. You spend the majority of your free time alone.
- You rarely ask for help.
- You are not curious about or respectful of other people's boundaries if they do not fit with yours.
- You do not want to get involved with other people's problems.

Problems With Boundaries for People With a Complex Dissociative Disorder

For individuals with a dissociative disorder, each dissociative part likely has a different need and preference for particular boundaries and for relational closeness and distance. Some parts of you may have a profound desire to really belong with someone, to be connected, to be seen and appreciated, and to feel that the other person cares for you. Some parts experience themselves as young, overwhelmed, and incapable, and thus feel very dependent and needy of other people. These parts are often terrified of abandonment and have collapsed boundaries, willing to do whatever the other person wants, which makes you very vulnerable to being hurt further. Others parts despise dependency and do not want to get close to others at all, having built a high wall around themselves to keep people out. These parts pride themselves on being self-sufficient and independent. And some part(s) of you may have a much more adaptive balance. But it is likely that you experience serious inner conflicts about boundaries and optimal closeness and distance in relationships. Because of your painful experiences in the past, parts of you make extra efforts to avoid any potential for rejection, abandonment, or hurt, whether that is by giving in or keeping distance. In the maelstrom of all these contradictory wishes and emotions among parts, it can be difficult for you to know which boundaries are helpful and healthy.

Sexual boundary problems. People with a dissociative disorder may find it hard to set sexual boundaries, because they are afraid of violence, ridicule, or rejection if they do. Or they may compulsively have sex as a kind of re-enactment. Others set extremely rigid boundaries, excluding sex from their lives. Perhaps they, or parts of them, are ashamed of sexual feelings and may be unable to discuss sexual issues with their partner, for example, sharing what they do and do not like in a sexual encounter. Some dissociative parts may strongly influence sexual encounters with strangers or mere acquaintances, making themselves extremely vulnerable to danger. Other parts may believe that sex is the only way to get close to a person, so they have no sexual boundaries. Some parts do not feel anything at all, such that sex is irrelevant, while others feel pain and get triggered. Some parts might find sex disgusting or frightening. Finally, as we described in chapter 29, some parts are triggered by sex, which evokes painful memories. These parts may sometimes confuse the current partner with the original perpetrator.

Sexuality is often an issue that causes intense feelings and may be compulsive, shameful, or confusing for you or parts of you. If you experience problems in a sexual relationship with your partner, or you recognize any of the problems described, we encourage you to discuss it with your individual therapist and perhaps to read some of the helpful books on sexual relationships after sexual abuse (for example, Carnes, 1997; Graber, 1991; Maltz, 2001).

Next you will find tips to help you work with all parts of yourself on healthy boundaries. You will notice that the structure is the same as that from the previous chapter in which you worked with parts to become more assertive.

Helping Parts of Yourself Cooperate to Set Healthy Boundaries

- *Make a list of your current boundaries.* Once you have written them down, add additional ones you would like to have, even if there is inner disagreement.
- *Make a list of boundaries you would like to set but have not yet been able to.*
- *Use your inner meeting room.* Gather all parts of you in your inner meeting room (see chapter 27), or use another way to have inner discussions that works best for you. Help all parts be as oriented to the present as possible, so you can have a dialogue about boundaries and resolving the inner obstacles to them.
- *Engage in inner reflection.* Listen respectfully to all parts of yourself and learn more about what each part needs and wants about boundaries, even if you do not agree. Notice how various parts of yourself react to situations in which setting boundaries would be helpful. And notice how parts react to each other.
- *Understand inner conflicts about boundaries.* When parts of you have differing opinions, emotions, and behaviors regarding a particular boundary, it may be hard to find a balance. For example, some parts want to be touched and hugged, and others do not want to be touched or even close to another person. As a first step, acknowledge and respect both sides of the conflict, and find common ground (for example, all parts want to be safe and feel OK). As you become more aware of the inner conflicts that prevent you setting healthy boundaries, you can begin the process of resolving them, using the steps that follow.
- *Challenge dysfunctional core beliefs and thoughts.* As you become aware of the beliefs and thoughts that support a particular unhealthy boundary (too lax or too rigid), try to establish communication and have an inner dialogue about those beliefs, for example, *"I believe that if I share something vulnerable, people will use it against me, so I never share"* or *"I don't like being hit and called names, but you have to put up with a lot to get love."*
- *Negotiate empathically.* Work toward inner agreements on what boundaries to set in general, as well as in specific situations or with a certain person. Remember that some of your boundaries can be different with

various people. It is helpful to find boundaries that all parts can agree help you feel safe and respected.

- *Agree on which parts of you deal with boundary setting.* Work toward obtaining sufficient inner cooperation so that more rational adult parts of you with relational skills can set boundaries firmly but without being punitive. Prepare your message, so that you know exactly what you want to say. For example, *"I want you to stop yelling at me when we have an argument. If you yell, I will leave the room and do something else until you are calm enough to talk and stay connected. If you continue to yell, I will have to consider other options, including ending the relationship."*

- *Preparing parts of yourself to set boundaries.* Various parts of you will need time and attention in order to be ready to set some boundaries. Start where you can, and in the meantime, help all parts be oriented and calm; learn more about assertiveness skills to help you set boundaries, and more about healthy boundaries. If parts of you are still quite reactive, you might try to help them go to an inner safe space during situations in which you need to set boundaries. This requires a level of inner agreement that boundaries and limits will be helpful for all parts by keeping them safe. Begin by explaining why boundaries are effective, by encouraging all parts of you to read the chapter together, or perhaps read it out loud to them (reading out loud helps you retain the content). Ask whether all parts are willing to allow an "experiment" in which an adult and more rational part of you practices setting a small boundary in a minor situation, while these parts remain in a safe place. Afterward, bring all parts of you together to discuss how the situation turned out for you. Be sure to listen respectfully to feedback from all parts.

- *Use imaginal rehearsal.* Visualize yourself successfully setting healthy boundaries (see chapter 15). Also try to envision various responses of the other person and prepare yourself to deal with them. It also may be helpful to role play the situation with a trusted friend or partner, or your therapist. Gather all parts together and imagine they are supporting each other during this situation, so that you feel stronger and of one mind. You might also imagine a safe and trusted other person standing beside you to support you.

- *Blending.* Various forms of blending, which were discussed in chapter 25, can be useful in helping parts set clear and firm boundaries. More fearful parts could be supported by stronger parts, and perhaps temper the aggression of stronger parts.

Homework Sheet 32.1
Identifying Your Personal Boundaries

1. Make a list of your current personal boundaries and limits (different parts may have different boundaries and limits).

2. Try to determine whether these boundaries are healthy, lax, or rigid. On your list above, make a mark indicating the category of each boundary. If you are not sure, you might check with trusted others.

3. What helps you keep your boundaries? Are there parts of you that can help you set healthy boundaries? Please describe.

4. List any particular boundaries that you find especially hard to keep.

5. What makes it difficult to keep your boundaries? Are there parts of you that contribute to making certain boundaries hard to keep? Please describe.

6. Notice whether your boundaries are different than those of people around you. Describe how you deal with those differences.

7. Notice if there are conflicts among parts of you regarding particular boundaries, and describe the conflicts.

8. Make a list of healthy boundaries you would like to set but have not yet been able to. Describe what makes it difficult to set these new limits.

Homework Sheet 32.2
Your Personal Space and Optimal Level
of Closeness and Distance

1. Make a drawing or representation of yourself in the center of a sheet of paper. (It can be a stick figure. Your artistic ability is not important to this exercise.) Next, draw or represent the people who are important to you and label them by name. Indicate your current boundaries between yourself and these people by means of lines (thick, thin, absent, continuous, dotted, irregular) or representations (walls, gates, waterways, bridges, hedges, whatever you like) that express the degree of closeness or distance. Notice whether the general level of closeness and distance is something you want, or whether there is conflict about it among inner parts of yourself.

2. Draw an imaginary circle around yourself based on the distance for which it is comfortable for you to have other people near you. This is your "personal space." For most people it is around 2 feet, but it may be more or less, depending on the individual. Notice whether your circle is comfortable for all parts. If not, draw the circle wider until the part that needs the most space feels comfortable. Next, draw the circle closer until the part that wants to be closest to people feels comfortable. Notice the differences between the original circles and the wider and closer ones.

Homework Sheet 32.3
Preparing to Set Boundaries in an Upcoming Situation

Choose an upcoming situation in which you will likely need to set a boundary. Choose a situation that reflects the level of challenge for which you feel ready.

1. Describe the situation.

2. What is the outcome of the boundary you would like to set?

3. Have an inner meeting in which you discuss the upcoming situation with all parts of yourself. Following the step-by-step approach in the section above on Helping Parts of Yourself Cooperate to Set Healthy Boundaries and describe the responses of parts of yourself to each step.

   ○ Reflect on the needs and desires of parts of yourself regarding the boundary you want to set and describe them below.

   ○ List any inner conflicts about setting the boundary.

   ○ List any dysfunctional core beliefs or thoughts about the boundary and how you can respectfully challenge them.

○ Describe your attempts to negotiate empathically with all parts about setting a limit or boundary, and their reactions.

○ Agree on which parts of you will set the boundary and describe how parts of you reacted to this negotiation.

○ Help fearful, avoidant, or angry parts of yourself by orienting to the present, discussing their fears or concerns, taking into consideration their needs and wants, and offering an inner safe space during the situation. Describe what you were able to do, and how parts reacted.

○ Use imaginal rehearsal to envision yourself successfully setting the boundary.

○ Practice forms of blending, if you are ready and able, to help you set boundaries. Describe your experience of blending if you were able to do so.

PART SEVEN
SKILLS REVIEW

You have learned a number of skills in this section of the manual. Below you will find a review of those skills and an opportunity to develop them further. As you review, we encourage you to return to the chapters to read them again and repractice the homework a little at a time. Remember that regular, daily practice is essential to learn new skills.

For each skill set below, answer the following questions:

1. In what situation(s) did you practice this skill?
2. How did this skill help you?
3. What, if any, difficulties have you had in practicing this skill?
4. What additional help or resources might you need to feel more successful in mastering this skill?

Chapter 28, Finding Inner Common Ground About Relationships

1.

2.

3.

4.

Chapter 28, Your Experience of Secure and Insecure Relationships

1.

2.

3.

4.

Chapter 28, Balancing Auto- and Relational Regulation

1.

2.

3.

4.

Chapter 29, Using Conflict Management Skills

1.

2.

3.

4.

Chapter 30, Skills to Resolve Isolation and Loneliness

1.

2.

3.

4.

Chapter 31, Identifying Inner Conflicts That Prevent Assertiveness

1.

2.

3.

4.

Chapter 31, Preparing to Be Assertive in an Upcoming Situation

1.

2.

3.

4.

Chapter 32, *Identifying Your Personal Boundaries*

1.

2.

3.

4.

Chapter 32, *Your Personal Space and Optimal Level of Closeness and Distance*

1.

2.

3.

4.

1.

2.

3.

4.

PART EIGHT

Guide for Group Trainers

Guide for Group Trainers

AGENDA

- Introduction
- Trainer Qualifications and Guidelines
- Assessment and Diagnosis of Potential Course Participants
- Contact and Coordination With the Treating Therapist
- Conducting Course Sessions
- Understanding and Resolving Difficulties in the Group
- Using the Manual in Individual Therapy
- Using the Manual in Day-Treatment and Inpatient Groups

Introduction

In this chapter we provide guidelines for using the manual in an outpatient skills-training group, as well as in individual psychotherapy for those patients who are not able to participate in a group, or for whom a group is not available. A skills-training group is *not* a replacement for individual psychotherapy, which is the standard of care for those with dissociative disorders (ISSTD, in press). However, the group can be a helpful adjunct when it is highly structured and conducted by therapists who are experienced in treating complex dissociative disorders.

Trainer Qualifications and Guidelines

Trainers for the course should be licensed mental health professionals famil-iar with the current standard of care for dissociative disorders, and they should have several years of experience treating patients with complex dis-sociative disorders in individual therapy. They should be able to set and maintain firm but flexible therapeutic boundaries, maintain an empathic and nonreactive stance in the face of intense emotionality and relational disruptions with patients, and be willing to seek out consultation as needed. Trainers should be able to distinguish between skills-training and therapy-process groups, and they should maintain the structure of the skills-training course. Furthermore, they should be able to explain clearly the concept of dissociation and describe dissociative symptoms and disorders, based not only on theoretical knowledge but also on clinical experiences with pa-tients.

We recommend that each course be led by two trainers. If desired, a third mental health professional may serve as an assistant or observer as part of an effort to train additional group leaders. Such individuals may serve as a substitute in the absence of one of the main trainers.

Division of Group Tasks Among Trainers

We suggest that two trainers alternate roles in the group to familiarize them-selves with all aspects of guiding the group. For example, one trainer can discuss homework and exercises, while the other gives the lecture for the week, and then exchange roles the following week. Or perhaps trainers might choose to alternate roles each month. If there is a third trainer or ob-server, who is not actively engaged with the group in the moment, he or she may take notes during the session regarding difficulties and successes of group members with their homework and with group participation. In the beginning of the course, the division of roles is explained to all partici-pants.

Although this is not a therapy group, relational dynamics will invariably arise, and it is helpful for all participating trainers to be aware of and able to address them briefly and then redirect the group back to the course con-tent.

We encourage trainers to work collaboratively, including any observers. A silent observer may create a sense of unease and distrust among course participants; thus, they are encouraged to participate verbally, at least min-imally. Participation of all trainers and observers is generally welcomed by the group.

Assessment and Diagnosis of Potential Course Participants

Course participants should include patients who are in outpatient individual therapy and have been assessed for, diagnosed with, and in current treatment for DID or DDNOS. We do not recommend including individuals who have not received formal diagnostic assessments for these disorders.

Diagnostic Assessment for Complex Dissociative Disorders

Prior to the course, a thorough assessment for a dissociative disorder diagnosis should be conducted on any participants who have not yet received one. This prevents the inclusion of patients with a false-positive diagnosis who may not benefit from the course. It also may confirm the diagnosis in many individuals in whom it is suspected, and thus better guide their individual treatment. The diagnosis should be made by a trained therapist, using a structured clinical interview to assess the *DSM* dissociative disorders, even if the patient has been, or is currently in treatment for, the suspected disorder. Assessment may include the *Structured Clinical Interview for DSM-IV Dissociative Disorders, Revised* (SCID-D; Steinberg, 1994, 1995), the *Dissociative Disorders Interview Scale* (DDIS; Ross, 1989; Ross et al.,1989); the *Interview for Dissociative Disorders and Trauma-Related Symptoms* (IDDTS; Boon, Draijer & Matthess, 2006), or the *Multidimensional Inventory for Dissociation* (MID; Dell, 2002, 2006), along with additional extensive and careful clinical interviewing and observations.

A high score on the *Dissociative Experiences Scale* (DES; Bernstein & Putnam, 1986) is *not* sufficient for accurate diagnosis, because this is a screening instrument and includes many symptoms experienced by healthy populations and not unique to those with a dissociative disorder. The *DES-Taxon* (DES-T; Waller, Putnam, & Carlson, 1996) is helpful in identifying serious levels of dissociation, but it is not diagnostic either. The *Somatoform Dissociation Questionnaire* (SDQ-20; Nijenhuis, Spinhoven, Van Dyck, Van der Hart, & Vanderlinden, 1996) is another useful screening instrument that is a brief self-report test measuring somatoform dissociation.

Dissociative disorders should be distinguished from borderline, psychotic, and bipolar disorders and their potential comorbid existence. Additional psychological testing (for example, the MMPI, Rorschach, the *Schedler-Westen Assessment Procedure*–200 [SWAP] for personality disorders, and the *Structured Clinical Interview for DSM Personality Disorders* [SCID-II]) is helpful in determining comorbid disorders, but such testing is not specific for dissociative disorders. If there is uncertainty about the diagnosis, it is better to wait and allow the patient and therapist additional time in individual therapy to gain more clarity before participation in the course.

Inclusion Criteria for Participants

There are a number of inclusion criteria that should be met by participants. All persons must meet the following conditions:

- Have a confirmed diagnosis of DDNOS or DID
- Be in current treatment with an individual therapist who is addressing their dissociative disorder
- Understand the basic concept of dissociation and how the dissociative disorder affects their daily life
- Have sufficient realization of their dissociative disorder to be able to acknowledge they have dissociative parts
- Have a relatively stable therapeutic alliance with their individual therapist
- Be in the first phase of treatment, that is, stabilization, symptom reduction, and skills training
- Or, if patients have begun the second phase, treatment of traumatic memory, and have become overwhelmed, every effort should be made to contain the memories and restabilize the patient. At that point, patients may enter a skills group, but they must not be working actively on traumatic memories during this time, because the risk of destabilization is too great.
- Attend their individual therapy sessions regularly and exhibit a commitment to therapy
- Have clear goals in individual therapy regarding resolution of their dissociation
- Not be actively psychotic
- Not be sociopathic or so severely disordered as to be inappropriate for group therapy
- Be able to tolerate group interactions
- Be able to control switching during sessions, at least so it is not disruptive to the group
- Not have pseudo-epileptic seizures during group
- Be able to use the manual and complete homework assignments as tolerated

Additional Considerations for Choosing Participants

There are a number of other factors to consider when choosing course participants.

Inclusion of the trainer's patients in the course. Therapists who are competent, experienced, and willing to treat complex dissociative disorders are not always easy to come by. In many areas there are only a few to be found. Thus, it may not be uncommon for trainers to include some of their own patients in the group. As with any group, including your own patients has its pros and cons. The therapist is able to actively observe the patient's successes and difficulties with the material and can support him or her more effectively in individual therapy. In addition, any conflicts the patient has with other course members or group dynamics can be addressed more effectively when the therapist has his or her own experience of the course. The work done in group can be integrated into the work in individual sessions.

However, the potential for problematic transference and countertransference reactions is high. For example, the patient may want his or her therapist's exclusive attention, or a therapist may tend to favor his or her patient over other course members. "Sibling rivalry" transferences may arise more easily than when participants have individual psychotherapy elsewhere. There is also a risk that the therapist may inadvertently disclose information about the patient in the course that should have remained in individual therapy, thus breaching confidentiality.

Should any of these problems arise, they should always be discussed in individual therapy sessions, not in the course sessions. Some patients with intense and active transference may not be helped by participating in a course led by their therapists. Prior to the course, the individual therapist should always discuss with the patient possible (and understandable) difficulties that might rise from the therapist's and patient's different roles and relationships in individual therapy versus a skills-training group, and how both can best address the issues.

In individual therapy it is important to stress that feelings of wanting to be special in the group or be protected by the individual therapist are not bad or "crazy." The patient need not feel ashamed of these feelings and desires, which are important cues pointing to the need for the development of secure attachment. The therapist should explain that such feelings may be related to early attachment difficulties, and that it is best to deal with them in individual therapy rather than during course sessions. It should be clear that acting out those feelings is not appropriate in group.

Axis I comorbidity. Most patients with dissociative disorders have comorbid Axis I diagnoses. And some have a serious degree of comorbidity that complicates treatment and needs attention prior to participation in the course. For example, primary addictions, life-threatening eating disorders, or severe depression or anxiety may need medical and psychotherapeutic interventions before a patient is sufficiently stable to attend a group.

Axis II comorbidity. Because early childhood trauma and neglect affect the development of personality, many patients with a dissociative disorder have coexisting *DSM* personality disorders. These may be understood empathically as developmental adaptations to extreme situations, but there are times when some of the resulting behaviors may be inappropriate for a group setting. Individuals who are excessively demanding of attention and time during session, who easily regress, have intense transference enactments, or who cannot maintain the course ground rules might make better use of the manual in individual treatment. Individual therapy should not only address the dissociative disorder but also the personality disorder. It is imperative for course trainers to maintain limits and boundaries and not tolerate disruptive behaviors in session.

Timing of course participation. It is essential to consider the timing of the course in the context of the patient's current life situation. Sometimes current life issues demand all the energy available to an individual, and they may involve crises that preclude participation in the course for the time being. For instance, the presence of serious illness or loss; severe social, housing, occupational, or financial problems; or current abusive relationships may be indications that the timing of the group is not right for the individual.

Lack of control over severe dissociative symptoms. People who have no control over severe and disruptive dissociative symptoms, such as pseudo-epileptic seizures or uncontrolled switching to dysfunctional parts (for example, being in session as a child part and subsequently unable to drive home), need further stabilization prior to participating in the course. These behavioral symptoms are often a sign of severe inner conflict among parts. The demands of the course interactions and homework focused on dissociative parts may be too overwhelming to the individual, and the behaviors may be too disruptive for others in the course.

Dropping out and returning to the course at a later time. Occasionally, group participation may go well for a period of time, but an individual participant may eventually become overwhelmed. In such cases, it is best to allow the participant to drop out and restart a new course at a later time. For example, one individual began to realize after 14 sessions that she had more dissociative parts than she and her therapist had previously known. This realization, along with the intrusion of new traumatic memories, was overwhelming. The patient dropped out of the group, was restabilized, and returned a year later to participate successfully in a new course.

Repeating the course. As with other skills-training groups, some participants may find it useful to repeat the course in order to continue to practice essential skills. A number of patients to date have reported that a first group allowed them to become more familiar with the skills, and a second course supported more focused work as they overcame more of their avoidance. For those who have not had success, or had to drop out of a first group, the trainers and individual therapist should collaboratively assess whether a patient might benefit from a second try.

The Intake Session

Approximately 4 to 6 weeks prior to the start of the course, each potential participant should meet with one or both of the trainers for an intake assessment. If there are questions at that time about the diagnosis of a dissociative disorder, a diagnostic evaluation should be completed by a qualified clinician prior to the patient being accepted for group. If there remain questions about whether the group would be beneficial to the patient after an initial intake, a second session may be scheduled for further evaluation.

In addition to assessing the patient for group, the trainer describes the course, the format of each session, what is expected from participants, the role of trainers, and gives the patient a written copy of the ground rules (see appendix B). A *release of information form* should be signed in order for the trainer and therapist to speak together about the patient. If the course is part of a research study, participants must give informed consent according to the study protocol.

It is important to review the ground rules in detail with the individual and determine whether he or she understands and is willing to abide by them. The trainer explicitly states that the individual is expected to participate actively in sessions, and to complete and discuss homework assignments. If needed, the trainer can discuss the differences between a skills-training course and group psychotherapy, if the patient (or referring therapist) seems confused.

It is important to ascertain whether the patient feels he or she can arrive and leave each session safely and on time, and whether talking about homework during sessions is possible. The trainer should carefully explore the patient's expectations and concerns about the course. Unrealistic expectations and fears should be discussed. If the patient has been in other skills-training groups, for example, a dialectical behavior therapy (DBT) group, the trainer should inquire about the outcome, what was helpful, and what was difficult about the experience.

Potential problems that may emerge during the course can be evaluated and discussed with the participant. For example, if the patient has a history of switching to child or angry parts when stressed, the trainer emphasizes that an adult part must be present in the session and asks whether the patient feels it is possible to abide by this limit. Likewise, if a patient has pseudo-seizures, the therapist emphasizes that such episodes must not occur during the session, or the patient will have to stop the group. If there is any doubt about whether the patient has sufficient control, it is better to wait and reassess him or her for another course at a later time. The same decision might also be made if the patient is extremely fearful of participating in a group setting.

Optimal Group Composition

The optimal number of participants is eight, with a maximum of nine and a minimum of five per group. The majority of skills-based groups have one or two dropouts during the first 3 months. However, we do not advise beginning with 10 or more participants. Dropouts may be prevented most effectively by conducting a thorough assessment of potential participants and strictly adhering to the inclusion criteria.

In general, the professional literature tends to encourage a healthy balance among age, gender, sexual orientation, socioeconomic status, and life experiences among group members, but not to the degree that individuals might not fit in to a given group. For example, having only one older group member may be problematic in a group otherwise comprised of very young participants, or a single male may have difficulty in a group of all females, since life experiences may vary too widely for them to relate well to each other.

But beyond these well-known group composition issues, there are also special considerations specific to patients with dissociative disorders. First, we recommend a balance between participants who have DDNOS and those who have DID. There should at least be two, and preferably three, participants who have the less prevalent diagnosis in the group. For example, it may not be helpful for a single patient with DDNOS to be in a group of patients with DID, or vice versa. Although some experience of having parts is similar in both diagnoses, there are also significant differences in the interactions among parts in patients with DID, who may be far more invested in keeping parts separate.

Second, there should be some balance among participants in their degree of realization of the diagnosis and acknowledgment of dissociative parts, as well as of their ability to communicate with parts of themselves. For example, if the majority of patients avoid accepting the diagnosis and dissociative parts of themselves, the minority who has done so to a greater degree may feel they do not belong in the group, and that too much time in group is spent on acceptance of the diagnosis. Conversely, if a single patient has not accepted his or her diagnosis while the rest of the group is much farther along in their realization, this patient may feel like a failure and drop out of group, or even decompensate.

Finally, any one individual's level of functioning in the course and in daily life may affect the group as a whole. For example, a very high-functioning individual may not fit well with a group of otherwise low-functioning participants, and vice versa. Trainers may choose course participants on level of functioning, not pairing extremes. For example, a group of patients who function at an overall higher level should not include a very low-functioning individual, and vice versa. Adaptive group mixes might include higher and moderate levels of function, or moderate and lower functioning patients. Axis II problems should be taken into consideration as part of level of functioning. Patients who exhibit extreme avoidance, narcissism, and aggression, for example, are likely to disrupt and destabilize the group.

Contact and Coordination With the Treating Therapist

Regular and consistent coordination between trainers and the participants' individual therapists is essential, after appropriate informed consent has been obtained. The course work is demanding and challenging, requiring regular practice by patients and therapeutic troubleshooting by trainers and therapists to resolve impasses, and therapists are encouraged to work actively with their patients on the skills. Thus, participants need the coordinated support of both trainers and therapists. It is also imperative that splitting between trainers and therapists is prevented. We therefore recommend that regular contact between therapists and trainers be maintained. This may be done by telephone. Trainers are urged to update therapists every few weeks on the progress of their patients, at minimum, and most certainly should contact the therapist immediately should any crisis develop. Likewise, therapists should be asked to contact the trainers if any matter of importance develops that may affect the participant in group.

If at all possible, we recommend an educational meeting for therapists prior to the start of group to assist them in helping their patients gain maximal benefit from the course. During this meeting, trainers may hand out the dates of group meetings, a copy of the ground rules and participant contract, and their contact details. Likewise, trainers obtain contact information from the individual therapists. Therapists are encouraged to have a copy of the manual and to receive instruction on using it with their patients and on how to help patients resolve roadblocks to successful practice of the skills. Finally, they are given information on the structure of the group sessions. Depending on the therapists' skill level, educational material may also be given on dissociative disorders, including a copy of treatment guidelines for DID and DDNOS (ISSTD, in press), information on upcoming trainings in the field, and contact information for consultants and supervisors experienced in treating dissociative disorders. Time should be provided for any questions regarding the course, the manual, the structure of the group, and concerns about potential difficulties for individual patients in the group.

If desired, an additional meeting can occur midway through the course and even after the course is completed. In fact, we encourage therapists to get to know one another, and even meet together for peer consultation and learning opportunities. After all, treating patients with dissociative disorders is challenging and sometimes even isolating and overwhelming. When therapists feel supported by their colleagues, they are able to offer their best to their patients.

Motivations of Referring Therapists

While most therapists will make an appropriate referral to the skills group as an adjunct to an adequate individual psychotherapy, a few will refer for other reasons. The trainer must be attuned to these motivations and be able to address them. Some therapists who are novices in the treatment of dissociative disorders simply become overwhelmed in their good faith efforts to treat a patient and are looking for relief afforded by the group. As long as such a therapist is willing to continue with good training and supervision, this may not be a problem, but the therapist cannot abdicate the treatment to the course trainers.

However, as occasionally happens with referrals to specialty groups, therapists who do not have sufficient training in the specialty area (in this case, the treatment of dissociative disorders) may attempt to refer patients to the group in order to avoid treating the disorder. They may hold a mistaken belief that a patient's dissociative disorder may be treated separately from the rest of therapy. Nothing could be further from the truth: Chronically traumatized individuals need comprehensive, skilled, and integrated treatment. This type of referral can have a potentially disastrous outcome for the patient, who may be overwhelmed by material from the group and subsequently cannot get adequate help from the therapist. Therapists who lack training should be encouraged to obtain training and supervision or to refer the patient to another therapist who can treat appropriately. *A skills group should never be a substitute for comprehensive psychotherapy, and conversely, the individual therapist must agree to incorporate skills training and the group homework into the therapy.*

Some therapists insist that they do treat patients with dissociative disorders but work with dissociative parts as actual "people," overly focus on traumatic memories, or may be intensely overinvolved with the patient. While the patient of such a therapist may gain some helpful knowledge from the group, the likelihood of a misguided therapy creating chaos and crisis for the patient and splits between the trainers and therapist is great. Inclusion of patients from such a therapist may have a negative effect on the group and on the trainers.

Trainers should beware of attempting to "rescue" a patient from a therapist by inviting the patient to join the group, as the well-being of the group as a whole is a priority over the needs of any single participant. Both the individual therapist and the trainers should agree to abide by the most current treatment guidelines for dissociative disorders.

In short, the course trainers should develop an impression of the strengths and weaknesses of the potential group member independent of the individual therapist, while taking into account the many factors that may lead a therapist to refer a patient to the course.

Conducting Course Sessions

In this section, trainers will find material relevant to leading group sessions.

The Introductory Session

The introductory session (chapter 34) sets the stage for the course. We suggest the session begin with introductions and an ice breaker group exercise that is light, fun, and quick. For example, on a piece of paper, trainers and participants trace their hands with fingers spread. In one finger each, write in your age, hobby, music you like, favorite animal, and one free choice. Or each person can fill in the following sentence with a funny saying of a family member: "My *grandmother (or aunt, grandfather, brother, etc.) always said . . .*" (For example, "*My grandmother always said you should wear clean underwear in case you got in a car accident.*") During this session, the general format, the goals of the course and all ground rules (see appendix B) are discussed with the group. Explanation of the educational meeting for significant others (see section later in this chapter) is given. Participants sign their course contract (see appendix C) during this session and have time to ask questions about the course and ground rules.

Ground Rules

It is essential to set clear rules for the group and for all participants to understand them. These rules are discussed in the interview prior to being accepted for the course and are again discussed in this introductory session. Many difficulties encountered in groups are related to problems with ground rules and the course trainer's difficulties in maintaining them. The ground rules are found in appendix B.

One rule is important to mention here in more detail. During sessions participants are allowed to leave the room briefly and take a short time-out (maximum of 10 minutes), should they feel the need to do so in order to get grounded. They must announce to the group that they are taking a brief time-out rather than leave the room abruptly without notice. A trainer will *not* accompany them, and the group will continue. They are expected to return to group of their own accord within the 10-minute time frame. Should they decide that finishing the session is not in their best interest, they must at least return to the group to inform everyone that they are going home and can do so safely. If a participant is not grounded by the end of the session, the trainers should call an emergency contact to come get the patient, or in a worst-case scenario, emergency services can be contacted. It is essential that this rule is clear to all participants and that they know trainers will not follow them out of group, no matter how upset they may be. It can be difficult for both the trainers and the participants to maintain this limit, but it is essential for the ongoing stability of the group, and for patients to learn to take responsibility for themselves.

Format of Course Sessions

The skills-training course has a highly structured format, which is essential for the success of participants. Sessions should be held in a room of sufficient size, where participants can meet without undue interruptions. Sitting at a conference table is preferable to sitting in a traditional group circle, because the seating structure lends support to a training rather than a therapy format. Each session is 1 hour and 45 minutes long, with a 15-minute break between two 45-minute segments. The first segment begins with a brief check-in and any announcements, followed by a discussion of the homework and any questions about the topic from the previous session.

During the 15-minute break, trainers leave the room and have a chance to check in with each other about group process or any concerns about individual participants. Following the break, time is made for any questions about the previous part of the session. The next 45 minutes are dedicated to explaining and discussing the new topic and to practicing exercises, if applicable. Homework assignments are explained so that all participants have a clear understanding of what they need to work on during the week. The last few minutes of the session should be dedicated to a wrap-up with a check-out statement from each participant, or a short grounding exercise or ritual to ensure all participants are in the present and safe to leave. Trainers have the freedom to make small changes in the structure, for instance, practicing exercises before the break, but participants should be informed about changes. Sessions should begin and end on time. It is best not to wait to start the group if some participants are late.

Teaching the Skills Exercises

During the session, all exercises are explained and then practiced. Participants are invited to take part in the exercise, but they are never forced to do so, because pacing is essential. All participants are encouraged to practice exercises at home or during their individual therapy. They are supported in altering any exercise for a better individual fit or to find other exercises that have the same goal. Both trainers and participants should understand that what is helpful for one individual (or for certain inner parts) may not be helpful for another individual (or other inner parts). Thus, personal creativity and flexibility are important in using any exercises to learn skills. When participants are unable to practice an exercise, they should be encouraged to write about or articulate what makes it difficult for them and take those issues to individual therapy.

Teaching the Course Topics

After the mid-session break, one of the trainers discusses the new topic. Trainers are encouraged not to read the material out loud; rather, they should make the topic more relational and interactive. This teaching style requires memorization and familiarity with all aspects of the topic, and it will help participants remain more present and engaged. Trainers may discuss key concepts and ideas, and clarify details. The use of gentle humor, interesting anecdotes, slides, or short movie clips are great ways to make the topics more entertaining and thus better hold the attention of participants. Caution should be used in sharing anecdotes about other patients, because participants may feel it is a breach of confidentiality, thus affecting their trust in the trainers. Any case material should be discussed only in generic form.

It is important to create an atmosphere in which asking questions is safe, that is, where any question is allowed, as long as it is on topic. And even though the material is covered during session, it is especially important to encourage participants to read and reread the material themselves so they can better integrate it.

If trainers do not feel secure enough in their knowledge of the material, they may read out loud to the group from time to time. In that case they should stop after every paragraph or so and check to see whether participants are grounded and understand the material, inviting them to ask questions, make comments, or give their own examples. Listening to someone read can induce trance and can trigger dissociation, especially because there often is a phobia for the content of the topic. Therefore, this teaching method is not ideal, and trainers should make strenuous efforts to learn the material sufficiently to make discussions highly interactive.

Homework

Homework assignments are a central part of the training course, because consistent practice is the tried and true way to learn new skills. Although participants are asked and expected to complete the assignments in writing and bring them in for the next session as best they are able, there should not be negative consequences or punishments for failing to do so. Many traumatized individuals are afraid to fail and have long histories of severe punishments when they do not do as asked. There are many reasons why an individual may not complete homework. These include fear of the topic, shame, general avoidance, confusion, feeling overwhelmed, and occasionally, the homework topic may not be relevant to the person's experience. The reasons for not completing homework should be a topic of individual therapy, and if needed, course trainers may also help the participant overcome these obstacles. But failure to do homework should be addressed, because its completion is an expected part of participation, and avoidance is endemic in people with dissociative disorders. Regardless of whether a participant has done the homework, it is vital for him or her to participate actively during the sessions.

Each participant should share his or her homework assignments from time to time in group. For many, the very act of sharing is a frightening risk that can be safely taken during the course. Those who are highly avoidant and afraid to talk should receive support to overcome their phobia. Sharing is often minimal at first, but a gradually developed sense of safety and shared experiences supports more active participation on a regular basis. When a participant is chronically silent, tension builds within the group, and trust becomes an issue.

Educational Meeting for Significant Others

During the course, usually after eight or nine sessions, an educational meeting is organized for relatives, partners, or friends, that is, significant others of the participants. The purpose is for significant others to learn about complex dissociative disorders, and the goals of the course, and to have their general questions about the disorders answered. Thus, participants may receive more appropriate support in their relationships. Usually the meeting is held in the evening, or perhaps on a weekend, at a time when most people might be able to attend.

Prior to the meeting, trainers discuss the goals and contents of this meeting with all participants during a course session, invite them to mention themes they would like to have addressed during the meeting, and encourage them to discuss their expectations and concerns. For example, participants may want their partners to know how to respond appropriately when they are switching or are not grounded in the present. And trainers may want to explain, for example, that ongoing interactions with child parts without engaging adult parts of the person, or treating parts as though they are separate people, are detrimental to healing.

Although it is not obligatory, participants are strongly advised to attend the meeting with their significant others. Trainers state clearly that personal details will not be discussed and personal questions should not be asked: The content will remain general.

Ending the Course

The last two sessions of the course focus on leave taking and include a summary evaluation of the course by participants. In the first of these two sessions, participants discuss their homework from the previous session as usual before the break. Following the break, trainers support the group in developing their own leave-taking ritual. There are many options for rituals, limited only by the creativity and wishes of the group. For example, each participant might buy or make a card and write something for each group member on it. Each person in the group might say something positive about the other group members. Participants might write down or verbally share the most important things they will take away from the course and from being with others who have similar experiences. Each person might write a note to each individual, indicating their wishes for the future for him or her. Some might prefer to celebrate with food. The group trainers might give small colored stones or another meaningful memento to each participant. The first part of the last session is dedicated to the evaluation of the course, and during the second part of this session, participants have their leave-taking ritual and the group is ended.

If the trainers think it useful, they may schedule a follow-up session 8 to 12 weeks after the end of the group. During this session participants once more look back on the course and what they have learned, share how they have been able to use their skills in the past months, and garner support to continue work on the skills with which they still struggle. Trainers reinforce the need for regular practice of exercises and continued work until skills are mastered.

Understanding and Resolving Difficulties in the Group

Following are some common difficulties that arise during the group and which should be addressed directly. When problems in the group are left unacknowledged, tensions and mistrust build, so it is imperative to address them early and firmly.

Participants Who Talk Too Little or Too Much

In most groups there are participants who are relatively silent and find it painful to talk or discuss their homework. And there are other participants who talk too much, interrupting others, or losing themselves in prolonged, detailed, and off-topic ramblings. During the intake session, it is important to emphasize that everyone is expected to discuss homework and participate actively, and that there are time limits so that each participant can have a turn. But even when these guidelines have been emphasized, the issues of talking too little or too much inevitably arise during the course. Trainers should take an active role in ensuring that every participant is able to reflect on the quality of his or her own participation in the course, and to empathically but firmly set limits with those who cannot maintain themselves with the group guidelines. If a participant is talking too much or is too silent, and this behavior is disruptive to the group and cannot be changed, the individual therapist of the participant should be contacted to discuss whether the course is appropriate for the patient.

Participants Who Discuss Inappropriate Content

Even though group guidelines explicitly state that participants should avoid discussing material that is intense or provocative, invariably a participant will share a homework example or bring up a topic that is not appropriate for the group. This may lead to dysregulation in other course participants. Although the individual may not realize the effect of the content of his or her sharing on other participants, trainers should intervene immediately.

For example, a participant was discussing shame. She described how she had been very suicidal during the past week and had felt so ashamed that she had called her young adult son for help to prevent a suicide attempt. Tension in the participants rose not only because they were triggered as she shared her extreme suicidal tendencies but also because they were concerned for the young adult son upon whom they felt she relied inappropriately. Trainers intervened and told her that it was helpful for her to speak about her inner experience of feeling ashamed, but the content of the example was best discussed in her individual therapy, not in the session. Trainers also validated the experiences of the other participants and closed the discussion, advising all participants to take the subject to their individual therapy if they felt the need for further attention to the matter. In the next session the individual apologized, saying that she realized she should not involve her son in such situations and that she was developing better ways of coping with her individual therapist. The group was relieved and could move on.

Participants Who Are Unable to Stay Present

It is especially challenging for patients with a dissociative disorder to stay present while they are discussing their disorder and its consequences and implications. Thus, difficulties staying present are endemic to this course.

In particular, attention may lag during the second segment of the session following the break. This may be related to avoiding content but also because it is difficult for patients to maintain being present for long periods of time, and they easily tire after the first half of the group. In the beginning of the course, it is helpful for the trainers to explain this possibility and that they will offer a direct intervention once to help a participant get grounded in the present. However, if the participant continues to lose contact with the present, space out, or seems preoccupied internally after the intervention, the trainers should move on with the session, with the expectation that the participant will manage to return on his or her own. Episodes of not being fully present may last from several minutes to a greater part of the session. When this is a repeated issue during session, or if a participant is unable to be grounded enough to leave and go home at the end of session, the course trainers should contact the individual therapist to discuss whether the patient is able to continue with the course.

Participants Who Are Chronically Late

Chronic lateness may be the result of avoidance, dissociation, and inner conflict, or of executive dysfunction involving time management. Often it is a combination of all these factors. When a participant is late, the trainers should address it immediately and ask the individual to find a solution. If the problem is one of avoidance, the patient should work on a solution in individual therapy. One participant solved her lateness caused by severe inner conflict by having a friend drive her to session temporarily. There are a number of ways to learn to manage time more adequately (see chapter 10 on time management). If lateness continues to be a problem, the course trainers should discuss with the individual therapist whether the participant should leave the course.

Participants Who Must Drop Out Prematurely

It is never easy to make the decision for a participant to drop out of the course. However, it is essential to stick to the course guidelines and minimize disruptions during sessions. Patients should also be protected from overwhelming experiences in the group if they are ill equipped to handle them. A decision is ideally made jointly with the trainers in consultation with the individual therapist. When a decision has been made, the course trainers should speak to the participant privately, and in the next session, explain what has happened to the other participants. There may be times when it is appropriate for the participant to return briefly at the beginning of the next group to say goodbye, but this should not involve processing what happened.

The remaining participants may have strong feelings about the trainers' decision, ranging from relief to anger, from a feeling of being cared for, to betrayal. Although this is a training course, there should be at least some room for discussing these feelings in the group setting. However, the discussion should focus on group safety and moving forward. Once participants have had their feelings acknowledged, they should be asked to take the issue to their individual therapist, so the course can continue.

There are several common reasons for asking a group member to leave. These include seriously disruptive behaviors in session such as pseudo-seizures; uncontrolled switching; inappropriate anger outbursts or disrespect of trainers or group members; threat of violence to self or others; self-harm during sessions (for instance, head banging); inability to stay grounded and get home safely; attending group under the influence of drugs or alcohol; bringing a weapon to session; and prolonged absences (including hospitalization).

The longer a participant has been actively and cooperatively present as a group member the more difficult it is for all parties to accept a decision for him or her to leave the group, regardless of the rules. However, most participants are eventually able to acknowledge their relief that the trainers are protective of the group.

Participants Who Object to the Ground Rules

When a participant clearly and openly objects to ground rules in the intake session and is unwilling to sign the contract, he or she should not be included in the course. However, participants may challenge ground rules at some point during the course, and this must be addressed immediately. Often this revolves around episodes in which one or more participants feel the rules are too rigid or applied unfairly, or they should be excepted for a "special" circumstance. Although a degree of flexibility is important, it is equally important that course trainers maintain the frame of the group by keeping the ground rules. These guidelines have been developed over time and with experience, and they can be relied upon to be reasonable and effective.

As an example, a participant began a discussion about the rule that trainers do not follow a participant who leaves the session to take a time-out, no matter how upset the participant may be. This individual stated that if the trainers did not follow a participant, she would do so herself, because it was irresponsible to allow a person who was upset to leave the session by himself or herself. The course trainers explained that participants are responsible for themselves and that being overwhelmed or triggered is part of every participant's daily life, and thus it is a situation with which they have to learn to cope. The trainers also explained that they could not follow eight or nine participants if everyone decided to take a time-out simultaneously. All other participants understood this clearly. The participant who had brought up the issue was told that she could reconsider during the coming week whether she was able to participate with the ground rules as they stood, and if not, she should not continue. She decided to sign the contract and successfully completed the course.

Contact Between Sessions

There are several issues regarding contact between sessions. First, there is an expectation that participants in crisis should contact their individual therapist according to their set protocol, and not contact the group leaders. Either participants or trainers may initiate contact if there is an issue regarding the group that needs to be addressed outside the session. For example, one participant felt another was being too aggressive and asked for the help of trainers to set more limits. In turn, they helped her take a risk to be more assertive and speak up about the issue in group. Another was having severe flashbacks and needed a week to rest, and called to inform the trainers.

Contact among participants outside the course is not encouraged. There are situations in which patients with the same issues can be of support to one another, but the inherent risks often outweigh the benefits in the case of individuals with a dissociative disorder. They often have difficulties with setting appropriate boundaries and being assertive, are easily dysregulated, and have particular difficulties in managing relationships and relational conflicts. Cliques and interpersonal conflict among participants outside the group can be a destructive force within it.

Group trainers have the discretion to make course participation contingent on not having contact with other participants outside of group. Most trainers promote this stance. That said, some trainers do not make an issue of it, and participants do choose to have contact. If so, the possible ramifications should be discussed thoroughly both in their individual therapies and with the group, and the potential effect on the group explored extensively. Often contact is initiated before either participant has thought through the possible consequences: A discussion of the issue beforehand may lend a prudent cautiousness. Furthermore, the entire group of participants should know if some are having outside contact; otherwise it becomes a secret.

If contact between sessions leads to problems for one or more participants, they should take the issues to their respective therapists. If contact leads to group problems, it must cease immediately in all forms, that is, e-mail, texting, phone calls, social networking sites, and face-to-face meetings.

Using the Manual in Individual Therapy

The manual can be easily adapted to use in individual therapy when a patient is unable to take part in a group, or one is not available. The manual can be used in a highly structured format, such that therapy sessions are replaced by skills training for a period of time. However, most therapists will likely prefer a more unstructured approach, using it for periodic skills training, alternated with psychotherapy sessions. In this way, the manual can be helpful for patients in different phases of their individual therapy, not only in the stabilization phase. For instance, themes on emotions, anger, and shame can be revisited in all phases of treatment.

As with course participants, individuals should not use the manual unless they have been formally diagnosed with either DDNOS or DID. If the therapist is unsure, he or she should request a second opinion from an experienced colleague prior to using the manual with a patient. The manual should not be introduced immediately when a patient begins therapy. A stable alliance, establishment of safety, therapy frame, and treatment goals, in conjunction with thorough assessment, should occur first. Likewise, when a patient is first diagnosed with a dissociative disorder, he or she usually experiences a period of disequilibrium during which the manual should not be introduced. The patient and therapist must first explore thoroughly the meaning of the diagnosis to the patient and learn how the patient will cope. The patient should attend therapy regularly and should have a modicum of acceptance of the diagnosis and of dissociative parts before the manual is introduced.

Structured Use of the Manual

Once a reasonable therapeutic alliance is established and the patient regularly attends individual sessions, the manual can be used in a structured manner just as in the group. The therapist begins with the first theme (on dissociation) and systematically works through the entire manual with the patient, at his or her own pace. At home, the patient should read the topics, complete homework, and discuss successes and difficulties during individual sessions. This structured approach is recommended for those patients who are in greater need of skills in order to function in daily life.

The therapist may choose to alternate skills-training sessions with those focused on crisis intervention and stabilization, or the therapist may dedicate half of a session to skills training, while the other half is reserved for other issues. Some patients may find that two sessions a week are helpful, with one focused on skills and one on other issues. Beware of the situation in which a patient is in such chronic crisis that there is never time to discuss and practice skills. This is a trap for both patient and therapist, and it should be vigorously addressed and resolved.

Unstructured Use of the Manual

Higher functioning patients may not need the rigorous structure required by lower functioning individuals. They may choose chapters that are most relevant. Patient and therapist should discuss which topics are most helpful, and in what order. For instance, some patients are well aware of their dissociative symptoms and parts and thus have no need for the education offered in the first four chapters. Rather, they might better profit from learning how to improve sleep or cope with particularly difficult emotions. Virtually all patients will benefit from the chapters on learning to overcome the phobia of dissociative parts, learning to reflect, developing an inner sense of safety, and the window of tolerance.

Using the Manual in Day-Treatment and Inpatient Groups

Specific chapters of the manual may be used to organize short-term skills groups in day-treatment and inpatient programs. For example, a basic educational group could benefit from the first chapters on diagnosis and symptoms. A life-skills group could utilize the chapters on daily structure, healthy eating and sleeping, and use of leisure and free time. An emotion skills group could use the chapters on reflecting and the window of tolerance, and those on specific emotions. A cognitive-based group might use the ones on core beliefs and dysfunctional thoughts.

In conclusion, trainers will be most successful if they carefully select group participants, maintain the ground rules, and quickly address problems that may arise in the group. Trainers are encouraged to get regular consultation for themselves, because many complex issues are likely to arise over the course of the group, particularly regarding relational conflicts, boundaries, and impasses.

CHAPTER THIRTY-FOUR

Introductory Session

AGENDA

- Introduction of trainers and participants (use an ice breaker exercise of your own choosing and provide participants and trainers with name badges)

  - Explanation of Ground Rules (see appendix B)
  - How to Make the Most of the Skills-Training Course
  - Educational Meeting for Significant Others

- Signing of contracts (see appendix C)
- Questions
- Homework

  - Reread the chapter.
  - Read chapter 1.
  - Notice how you felt in this first session and whether you have any concerns. Feel free to bring up questions or concerns at the beginning of the next session.

Explanation of Ground Rules (Appendix B)

Trainers should cover the ground rules in detail. It is helpful to read them out loud and also make sure all participants have a written copy in addition to their skills training manual. All participants must agree to abide by these guidelines.

How to Make the Most of the Skills-Training Course

- *Make strong efforts to focus* on what is happening in each session. Concentrate on the present, not the past or future, and on the conversation, not what is going on in your head.
- *Take responsibility* for your own behavior, even though it may feel out of your control.
- *Encourage all parts of yourself to participate.*
- *Learn to listen* to others without interrupting. Let a person completely finish what he or she is saying before you begin to speak.
- *Be specific and give feedback directly to participants and trainers.* Describe what you observe and feel. Make "I" statements, rather than "you" statements (for instance, "*I feel confused by what you are saying,*" rather than "*You never make any sense*"). Avoid pointing fingers or the use of blaming or shaming statements. If you have a disagreement, please stay with the present topic. Avoid going back to discuss other issues from the past (for instance, "*I felt intimidated when you spoke so loudly and interrupted me just now*" rather than "*You are a bully. In the last two sessions you talked over other people*"). Also think about how you would want to be given the same feedback you are giving to others. The idea is to be constructive rather than hostile or rejecting.
- *Indicate you have heard feedback* that you receive from fellow participants or trainers (repeat what you have heard). Ask for clarification if there is something you do not understand. Do not try to defend yourself: Everyone is here to learn and to help each other in their learning. You do not have to agree with the feedback; just listen and think about it.
- *Experiment often with new behaviors* you have learned in the course. Practice is the one thing that helps most when learning new skills.
- *Regularly review your goals for taking this course.*
- *Be patient and do not lose heart!* A dissociative disorder is a chronic disorder; it takes time and hard work to change, and change will continue long after the final session if you are willing to continue practicing what you have learned. But most certainly, change can occur!

Educational Meeting for Significant Others

People with a complex dissociative disorder have a strong tendency to conceal their diagnosis and problems from others. They may actually have an inner prohibition about discussing the subject, or they may be deeply ashamed or afraid to talk about it. But it is difficult to change yourself alone. You need people who will help you to practice and strengthen the skills that you are learning, people you can trust to aid you in distinguishing which skill you need in a given situation. This may be a partner, a friend, a relative, or some other person you trust, at least to a degree.

You certainly do not need to share that you have dissociative problems with everyone, but we urge you to share important aspects of your current dissociative difficulties and what you are learning in this course with at least one person. Your individual therapist can help you decide what to share and the best way to do so. We recommend that you find at least one person with whom you can talk about what you are learning in this course and whom you would like to invite to the educational meeting. Again, this is strongly recommended, but not mandatory.

You may share manual materials regarding the skills with your support person if you choose. Together with the people who are important to you, you can work out how they may support you in putting these skills into practice and perhaps even help you to return to the present when you are spacing out or switching. It is important that you not feel so alone. And it can be of great help and relief for the people around you to understand a bit more about what happens for you.

You should not expect your support person(s) to have unlimited availability or to always take care of you in an emotional crisis. It is generally not desirable for them to become fascinated by various parts of you, treat them as separate people, or become especially attached to certain parts. Both you and your support person should treat you as a whole person as much as possible.

Please list the names of the people you would like to invite to the educational meeting. (This is just for you; you need not show it to anyone else.)

Name   **Telephone Number**

1. _____   _____

2. _____   _____

3. _____   _____

4. _____   _____

Leave-Taking Sessions

Leave-taking will begin in the second half of the session following chapter 32. Following the homework discussion and break, trainers will present a very short topic on the importance of saying goodbye, and the group will decide together on a leave-taking ritual.

In the final session, participants will partake in the leave-taking ritual and complete the course.

AGENDA

- Welcome and reflections on previous session (chapter 32)
- Homework discussion
- Break
- Short topic: Saying Goodbye

  - Introduction
  - Saying Goodbye
  - Leave-Taking Rituals
  - Evaluation of the Course

- Homework

  - Complete Homework Sheet 35.1, Saying Goodbye to the Group.
  - Complete Group Evaluation (optional; see appendix D).

Introduction

Saying goodbye, or leave taking, is an inevitable and normal part of life. But precisely because it is unavoidable, it is important to learn how to have a good experience in saying goodbye to someone else. Yet many people avoid it as much as possible because it does sometimes involve painful, sad, or disappointed feelings. You have been working hard to improve your ability to tolerate feelings and decrease your avoidance, so hopefully you are in a better position to cope with what comes up for you as you say goodbye to the participants and trainers. As you come to the end of this course, be sure to use the skills you have learned to help yourself. The importance of leave taking is discussed next.

Saying Goodbye

It is time to say goodbye. You have come to know other people in this group, some more and some less, but nevertheless, you have been united together in your struggle with difficult problems, with your suffering, and with your intentions to work toward healing. These are important commonalities, even though you each may be quite different from the other in many ways. You have risked sharing a bit more of yourselves with each other—not an easy feat! This has created a bond among you, even though you may have had conflicts or disagreements with each other from time to time. That is normal and part of growing relationships. You have worked hard to understand and empathize with each other. You should congratulate yourselves on this important work that you have accomplished as a group. And your sense of being connected with each other makes saying goodbye difficult.

The aim of this course was for you to learn new skills and information that will help you cope better in life, to deal with your problems more adaptively, and to develop more inner empathy, communication, and cooperation. But we also hope you have learned more about how you related to the different people in the group.

Although there is no one right way to say goodbye, there are some general guidelines that are helpful. For example, as you are saying goodbye, reflect on what you have received that is positive or growth-producing in the relationship (in this case, your relationship with the trainers and participants in the group). Even if every relationship is not the best, you likely learned some helpful things about yourself and other people along the way.

Consider what the course itself has meant to you. And you can be aware not only of the positive aspects of the group but also the negative or disappointing ones; after all, no one, and no group, is perfect. It is likely that you had hopes for this course that perhaps were not fully realized. These are important to acknowledge and accept. You can, if you like, share these positive and negative experiences with the group in a nonjudgmental way.

It will also be helpful to be aware of what you will miss about the group, and what various parts of you feel about leave taking. It is helpful if you reflect on ways to use your course experience to help yourself move forward into the future. Imagine taking in the group as an inner "cheering section" who encourages you in your mind as you continue to learn and practice new skills and work on your problems. Pay attention to what you have learned and what skills you wish to develop further, so you can continue your progress. It is important to find a balance between positive feelings and sadness or disappointment, and an understanding of how you might continue to make healing gains after the group has ended, taking what you have learned forward with you.

Most important, do your best to stay present and notice your inner experience as you engage in leave taking with the group. Perhaps you have never been able to experience a positive leave taking, or perhaps you have found it difficult to stay present in the past. Notice your thoughts, core beliefs, feelings, sensations, and urges. Each of these can help you learn more about how you and other parts of you react to saying goodbye. You can bring those issues to your individual therapy to get further help. In the meantime, savor your time with these people with whom you have walked side by side during part of your long journey.

Leave-Taking Rituals

You, along with your group, will decide what leave-taking ritual you prefer to use in your final session together next week. There are countless rituals, limited only by the constraints of your creativity and time. Perhaps some members in the group have some to propose. Next we offer a few suggestions, but you are not obligated to use them.

Suggestions for Leave-Taking Rituals

- You may consider (depending on the rules of the location in which you have group) bringing food to celebrate.
- You may bring music on which the entire group agrees.
- Bring in a memento of what the group has meant to you, for example, a stone, a small figure, a picture, a flower, or something else from nature. The group may decide to use the same kind of memento for each

person, which the trainers or a group member agrees to bring. Mementos should be small and very inexpensive, if they cost anything.

- Each person passes his or her memento around the group. Each person holds the memento in his or her hands, imbuing their good energy into the object for the other to take home. You may say something to the participant as his or her memento is passed around, or you may be silent. You may choose music for this part of the ritual, if you like.
- You may write a card for every group member and trainer with a personal note that you do not need to share in group.
- If you use flowers, each person can put his or hers into a single vase until all flowers together make a bouquet, representing the group, and also the increased cooperation and communication among all parts of each person present.

Evaluation of the Course

Trainers are encouraged to obtain feedback from group participants in order for group members to be heard, as well as to gather valuable suggestions to improve the next course. We have included an evaluation in appendix D. You may use it, or another one of your preference. The evaluation should be given out in this session and brought back the following session. Evaluations can certainly be anonymous if participants choose, or they are welcome to add their names. Trainers can learn much from the feedback they receive.

Homework Sheet 35.1
Saying Goodbye to the Group

During the week, take some time to write a short note to each member in the group, expressing something you appreciate about that person, and something you wish for him or her in the future. Bring in what you have written for the final session. You may make other remarks as well, if you like.

- What I especially appreciate about you is . . .
- My wish for you in the future is . . .
- Other remarks

Suggestions. You are encouraged to use your creativity to make this ritual fit your needs. Thus, you accomplish this project in the way that feels right for you. There is no right or wrong way to do it. Whether you use a simple piece of note paper or make something more elaborate, the details are not important; your sentiments and intentions are. If you do not feel you can write something, you might bring something that represents your thoughts and feelings, such as a picture or small memento. If you wish to do something more elaborate, you might consider the following:

- Drawing or painting something
- Making a collage
- Writing a poem or story
- Making a CD of music or songs
- Recalling a meaningful, warm, or funny moment you shared with the other person in group

Final Session

AGENDA
- Welcome
- Turn in evaluations (if used)
- Reflections on your experience in group and on moving forward
- Break (if needed)
- Leave-taking ritual
- Closing

There is no didactic portion of this ending session. Trainers and group members should structure it according to the desires and needs of the group as a whole. Some groups have brought in food or music, with a more celebratory feel to the session, while others have had a more somber, reflective session. Your group will decide together what is best.

Final Note From the Authors

We congratulate you for the hard work you have done over the course of this training. Please do not be discouraged if you did not accomplish everything you wished. The skills in this manual can be very difficult and time consuming to practice and learn. It is quite normal for you to need more time in therapy to continue on with what you have begun to grasp here. Dissociative disorders tend to be chronic and can take awhile to resolve. But each of us has seen many patients who have indeed healed and moved on to have fruitful and stable lives. We wish you all the best on your continued journey: strength, self-respect, courage, love, laughter, rest, and healing.

Suzette Boon
Kathy Steele
Onno van der Hart

Dissociative Identity Disorder (DID)

A. The presence of two or more distinct identities or personality states (each with its own relatively enduring pattern of perceiving, relating to, and thinking about the environment and self).

B. At least two of these identities or personality states recurrently take control of the person's behavior.

C. Inability to recall personal information that is too extensive to be explained by ordinary forgetfulness.

D. The disturbance is not due to the direct physiological effects of a substance (e.g., blackouts or chaotic behavior during Alcohol Intoxication) or a general medical condition (e.g., complex partial seizures). *Note:* In children, the symptoms are not attributable to imaginary playmates or other fantasy play. (APA, 1994, p. 487)

Dissociative Disorder Not Otherwise Specified (DDNOS), Subtype 1b

This category is included for disorders in which the predominant feature is a dissociative symptom (i.e., a disruption in the usually integrated functions of consciousness, memory, identity, or perception of the environment) that does not meet the criteria for any specific dissociative disorder. DDNOS, Subtype 1b is described as follows:

1. Clinical presentations similar to Dissociative Identity Disorder that fail to meet full criteria for this disorder. Examples include presentations in which a) there are not two or more distinct personality states, or b) *amnesia for personal information does not occur* [italics added]. (APA, 1994, p. 490)

Posttraumatic Stress Disorder (PTSD)

A. The person has been exposed to a traumatic event in which both of the following were present:

   (1) the person experienced, witnessed, or was confronted with an event or events that involved actual or threatened death or serious injury, or a threat to the physical integrity of self or others

   (2) the person's response involved intense fear, helplessness, or horror.

Note: In children, this may be expressed instead by disorganized or agitated behavior.

B. The traumatic event is persistently reexperienced in one (or more) of the following ways:

(1) recurrent and intrusive distressing recollections of the event, including images, thoughts, or perceptions. *Note:* In young children, repetitive play may occur in which themes or aspects of the trauma are expressed.

(2) recurrent distressing dreams of the event. *Note:* In children, there may be frightening dreams without recognizable content.

(3) acting or feeling as if the traumatic event were recurring (includes a sense of reliving the experience, illusions, hallucinations, and dissociative flashback episodes, including those that occur on awakening or when intoxicated). *Note:* In young children, trauma-specific reenactment may occur.

(4) intense psychological distress at exposure to internal or external cues that symbolize or resemble an aspect of the traumatic event

(5) physiological reactivity on exposure to internal or external cues that symbolize or resemble an aspect of the traumatic event

C. Persistent avoidance of stimuli associated with the trauma and numbing of general responsiveness (not present before the trauma), as indicated by three (or more) of the following:

(1) efforts to avoid thoughts, feelings, or conversations associated with the trauma

(2) efforts to avoid activities, places, or people that arouse recollections of the trauma

(3) inability to recall an important aspect of the trauma

(4) markedly diminished interest or participation in significant activities

(5) feeling of detachment or estrangement from others

(6) restricted range of affect (e.g., unable to have loving feelings)

(7) sense of a foreshortened future (e.g., does not expect to have a career, marriage, children, or a normal life span)

D. Persistent symptoms of increased arousal (not present before the trauma), as indicated by two (or more) of the following:

(1) difficulty falling or staying asleep

(2) irritability or outbursts of anger

(3) difficulty concentrating

(4) hypervigilance

(5) exaggerated startle response

E. Duration of the disturbance (symptoms in Criteria B, C, and D) is more than 1 month.

F. The disturbance causes clinically significant distress or impairment in social, occupational, or other important areas of functioning. (APA, 1994, pp. 427–429)

Complex Posttraumatic Stress Disorder (CPTSD) or Disorders of Extreme Stress Not Otherwise Specified (DESNOS)

This proposed disorder is not included in the *DSM-IV*. However, some of its symptoms are included in the *DSM-IV* under "Associated descriptive features and mental disorders" of PTSD (APA, 1994). The *DSM-IV* states that this "constellation of symptoms may occur and are more commonly seen in association with an interpersonal stressor (e.g., childhood sexual abuse or physical abuse, domestic battering, being taken hostage, incarceration as a prisoner of war or in a concentration camp, torture)" (APA, 1994, p. 435).

A. Alterations in regulating affective arousal
   (1) chronic affect dysregulation
   (2) difficulty modulating anger
   (3) self-destructive and suicidal behavior
   (4) difficulty modulating sexual involvement
   (5) impulsive and risk-taking behaviors
B. Alterations in attention and consciousness
   (1) amnesia
   (2) dissociation
C. Somatization
D. Chronic characterological changes
   (1) alterations in self-perception: chronic guilt and shame; feelings of self-blame, of ineffectiveness, and of being permanently damaged
   (2) alterations in perception of perpetrator: adopting distorted beliefs and idealizing the perpetrator
   (3) alterations in relations with others:
      (a) an inability to trust or maintain relationships with others
      (b) a tendency to be revictimized
      (c) a tendency to revictimize others
E. Alterations in systems of meaning
   (1) despair and hopelessness
   (2) loss of previously sustaining beliefs (Herman, 1992; Van der Kolk, 1996)

Note: The *Diagnostic and Statistical Manual of Mental Disorders* (*DSM*) is continually evolving. A new *DSM-V* edition is slated to be published in 2013. The criteria for dissociative disorders and PTSD will likely change at that time, at least to a degree.

- ***Regular attendance is essential*** for you to gain the greatest benefit from the sessions. If for some reason you cannot be present, call (phone #) _____ as soon as possible and ask for your trainer, leave a message with the secretary, or leave a voice mail. You are not obliged to give a reason for your absence but we would appreciate it if you did. *If you miss three consecutive sessions or five sessions in total, you cannot continue in the course.*
- ***Complete your homework assignments for every session*** so you can participate in sessions and learn the skills offered in this course. Please complete them in writing, using the spaces provided in your manual and bring them to each session. Your assignments will not be read by others in the course unless you choose to share, and they will remain your personal property.
- ***This course is designed to help you master specific skills. It is not a substitute for individual therapy***. This course has two objectives: (1) to educate you about dissociation and other trauma-related problems; (2) to help you learn skills that will improve your ability to handle your difficulties. Thus, it is not a goal of this course to explore your personal past and the causes of your dissociative disorder. We expect participants to avoid discussing details of their past or details of their therapy work with other participants, whether inside or outside session, because such information may be upsetting to others, and/or to you. Continue to work in your therapy as usual during the course and feel free to take issues from the course to discuss with your therapist.
- ***The role of the trainers is to teach*** and help you with skills, not to act as your therapists.
- ***All sessions are confidential*** so that every participant can feel comfortable and safe. Do not reveal the names or any other identifying information of other participants. Any discussions with outsiders about the course should be strictly limited to your own experience and the skills you are learning. However, you may speak openly and freely with your individual therapist, because what you discuss with him or her is confidential.
- ***Contact among participants outside sessions is discouraged***, as you should not have to feel responsible for the needs or crises of other participants. At times, outside contact can create conflicts among group members that affect the sessions. As per your agreement to keep confidentiality, do not discuss others in the group or their problems with any participant (or anyone else). If you do have contact with other participants outside of session, we ask that you not to talk about others or their problems.

- *Active participation in each session is expected* because it will help you learn more effectively, even when you feel intense. Participation also helps you stay more present and focused.
- *Time-outs of up to 10 minutes may be taken during a session* should you have need to compose and ground yourself. You are requested to inform the trainers that you are taking a break, rather than just leaving without saying anything. You are also requested to return to the session on your own accord within 10 minutes. If at all possible, try to stay in the session, where it might be easier for you to get yourself grounded and calmer. If you cannot, then take the break. If you feel you cannot return to group after 10 minutes, inform a trainer that you are going home and are safe. If you cannot control your behavior or manage your feelings such that you can participate in group, it is likely that the course is too overwhelming for you. In addition, uncontained behaviors such as unrelenting crying, screaming, switching to disruptive parts of yourself, or hurting yourself are upsetting to other participants. Therefore, if you are unable to control your behaviors, you will be asked to withdraw from the course until you are better able to remain present and in control.
- *Trainers or other participants will <u>not</u> follow you if you take a time-out; they will continue on with the session.* There are no exceptions to this policy. You are expected to be responsible for yourself during sessions, as well as for arriving and leaving safely and in a timely manner.
- *Never leave a session abruptly without saying anything*. If you decide during a session, or while you are taking a break that you are unable to continue with the session, always inform the trainers, assuring them that you can get home safely.
- *Physical or verbal intimidation or abuse is not acceptable.* Any such behavior will lead to your immediate termination from the course. You are expected to be able to remain in an adult state and be respectful of yourself and others. If you feel angry or frustrated during a session, please remain in your seat. Do not raise your voice, scream, or curse. Do not make threatening physical movements or gestures toward others, or throw objects of any kind.
- *Weapons or instruments of self-harm of any kind are not allowed in sessions*, even if they are kept in a covered or sealed bag. Each participant, including you, deserves and needs to feel safe.
- *The use of alcohol and drugs is prohibited during sessions*. If you come to a session under the influence of alcohol or drugs, you will be immediately terminated from the group. You may then sign up for the next course if you are able to abstain from using.
- *If you require psychiatric hospitalization or have any other prolonged absence* during the training course that lasts longer than 3 weeks (three course sessions), you must drop out. However, you may sign up for the next available course if you are stable enough. In case of a hospitalization that is less than 3 weeks, a meeting with your trainers, your therapist, and you will determine whether you are able to continue in the course. It is important that you learn to find the pace of learning and challenges that are right for you. If you miss

five sessions during the course, you will need to drop out, and can repeat the group next time.

- *If you have questions about the course, ask them during sessions.* Other participants often have the same or similar questions, so your questions are welcomed in the sessions and are usually helpful to others. However, there may be times when the trainers may postpone a particular question until a later time, depending on how it fits with the current topic.
- *Please refrain from discussing any problems or matters that are not related to what you are learning in the course.* These should be discussed with your personal therapist, not in the sessions.
- *If one of the trainers is also your personal therapist*, he or she will be as discreet as possible with regard to your personal information from your individual sessions. It is wise to discuss ahead of time with your therapist what should and should not be shared in the training course.
- *You must sign a release of information* if your personal therapist is not one of the trainers, so that the trainer and your therapist can communicate and coordinate for your benefit. You cannot attend the course unless you are willing to sign a release, as treatment coordination is essential for your well-being.
- *An educational meeting will be held* for people who are important to you, for example, a partner, close friend, or family member. During the meeting general facts about dissociation and complex dissociative disorders and about the skills-training topics will be discussed. No personal information about you or other participants will be disclosed or discussed by the trainers, your significant others, or you. You may submit a list of questions or issues you would like for your support person(s) to know more about. We ask that you bring at least one person to this meeting with you, but we realize that you may not have such a support person, so it is not mandatory. Regardless of whether you bring someone, we strongly encourage you to attend.

APPENDIX C
PARTICIPANT CONTRACT FOR A
SKILLS-TRAINING GROUP

1. I understand that it is important to attend every session, both for my own sake and for the success of the training course. Therefore, I hereby commit to attending every session unless I am prevented by circumstances beyond my control. If I cannot attend, I will inform the trainers as soon as possible, with the understanding that it is a courtesy for the trainers and participants to know who will be absent.

2. I understand that I will be obliged to leave the course if I miss more than three consecutive sessions or a total of five sessions over the course of the group, including for reasons of prolonged hospitalization or illness. I understand I will be allowed to sign up for the next course, if I am ready.

3. I agree to complete my homework assignments and bring them to sessions, and to practice the skills to the best of my ability.

4. I agree to participate verbally in sessions to the best of my ability.

5. I will respect the confidentiality of all course participants and of matters that come up in the course. I will not discuss personal information about fellow members outside the course.

6. I agree to abstain from alcohol or drugs (other than those prescribed, which I will take according to the prescribed dose and time) for at least 24 hours prior to and following sessions.

Printed Name_____

Address_____

_____

Phone

  Day   (_____)_____

  Evening   (_____)_____

  Cell   (_____)_____

Best number to reach me is: _____day   _____evening   _____cell phone

E-mail: _____

_____   _____

Signature   Date

Name of individual therapist_____

Phone number of individual therapist_____

E-mail of individual therapist (if available)_____

APPENDIX D
SKILLS-TRAINING GROUP FINAL EVALUATION

1. What was your experience of participating in the course?

2. What was the most important thing you, or parts of you, learned in this course?

3. Describe ways in which the group felt safe or unsafe to you, or parts of you.

4. What goals did you set for yourself during the course? Did you meet (some) of them?

5. What, if any, positive changes have you noticed in yourself or other parts of you?

6. What, if any, negative changes have you noticed in yourself or other parts of you?

7. Did you find it difficult to participate in group at times? If so, what was difficult for you? Was there something that the group trainers or participants might have done differently to help you?

8. On average, were you able to use the topics and homework exercises to benefit yourself? If so, give an example. If not, please elaborate.

9. List any imagery or relaxation exercises you found particularly helpful in the manual, and note what was helpful about them.

10. Which parts of this course have helped you most? Order them from the most helpful to the least helpful by ranking them 4 (most helpful) to 1 (least helpful).
_____Homework
_____New topics and facts
_____Exercises
_____Sharing with other participants
Comments:

11. Which topics were most helpful to you? Least helpful?

12. During the course a lot of attention was paid to improving inner empathy, communication, and cooperation among parts of yourself. What in the course was most helpful for you in this regard? Least helpful? Were you able to improve your inner empathy, communication, and cooperation? If so, please describe. If not, do you have some ideas about what might have been more helpful?

13. What do you think of your own participation during the course? (for example, satisfied for the most part, did better than I expected, was harder than I thought)

14. What was your experience of the contributions of other group members (for example, helpful, boring, hard to follow, too long, not enough participation). Please elaborate, if you are able.

15. On average, how would you rate the helpfulness of the homework?
    ○ Excellent
    ○ Good
    ○ Fair
    ○ Poor
    ○ Inconsistent
    Comments:

16. On average, how would you rate the difficulty of the homework?
    ○ Beyond my abilities
    ○ Difficult but manageable most of the time
    ○ Just about right
    ○ Easy
    ○ Too simplistic
    Comments:

17. How would you rate the expertise and professionalism of the trainers?

Name of trainer_____   Name of trainer_____
- ○ Excellent   ○ Excellent
- ○ Good   ○ Good
- ○ Fair   ○ Fair
- ○ Poor   ○ Poor
- ○ Inconsistent   ○ Inconsistent

Comments: Comments

18. How would you rate the helpfulness of the trainers?

Name of trainer_____   Name of trainer_____
- ○ Excellent   ○ Excellent
- ○ Good   ○ Good
- ○ Fair   ○ Fair
- ○ Poor   ○ Poor
- ○ Inconsistent   ○ Inconsistent

Comments: Comments

19. Suggestions for the manual or future courses.

REFERENCES

Adams, J. (2005). *Boundary issues: Using boundary intelligence to get the intimacy you want and the independence you need in life, love, and work.* New York: Wiley.

Allen, J. G., Fonagy, P., & Bateman, A. W. (2008). *Mentalizing in clinical practice.* Washington, DC: American Psychiatric Publishing.

American Psychiatric Association. (1994). *Diagnostic and statistical manual of mental disorders* (4th ed.). Washington, DC: Author.

Artigas, L., & Jarero, I. (2005). El abrazo de la mariposa [The butterfly's embrace]. *Revista de Psicotrauma para Iberoamérica, 4*(1), 30–31.

Bandler, R., & Grinder, J. (1975).*The structure of magic.* Palo Alto, CA: Science and Behavior Books.

Beck, A. T. (1975). *Cognitive therapy and the emotional disorders.* Madison, CT: International Universities Press.

Bernstein, E., & Putnam, F. (1986). Development, reliability, and validity of a dissociation scale. *Journal of Nervous and Mental Disease, 174,* 727–735.

Blum, N., St. John, D., Pfohl, B., Stuart, S., McCormick, B., Allen, J., et al. (2008). Systems Training for Emotional Predictability and Problem Solving (STEPPS) for outpatients with borderline personality disorder: A randomized controlled trial and 1-year follow-up. *American Journal of Psychiatry, 165,* 468–478.

Boon, S. (1997). The treatment of traumatic memories in DID: Indications and contraindications. *Dissociation, 10,* 65–79.

Boon, S. (2003). Directieve en hypnotheraputische interrenties als onderdeel van een fasengerichte behandeling voor vroeger seksueel misbruik. In N. Nicolaï (red.), *Handbook Psychotherapie na seksueel misbruik* (pp. 209–224). Utrecht: De Tijdstroom.

Boon, S., & Draijer, N. (1993). *Multiple personality disorder in the Netherlands.* Amsterdam: Swets & Zeitlinger.

Boon, S., & Draijer, N. (1995). *Screening and diagnostiek van dissociatieve stoornissen* [Screening and diagnostics of dissociative disorders]. Lisse, The Netherlands: Swets & Zeitlinger.

Boon, S., Draijer, N., & Matthess, H. (2006). *Interview voor dissociatieve stoornissen en traumagerelateerde symptomen (IDSTS).* Eerste versie, uitgave in eigen beheer. [Interview for Dissociative Disorders and Trauma-related Symptoms (IDDTS)]. Unpublished manuscript. (Available from Suzette Boon, PhD, at s.boon@altrecht.nl; or Suzette Boon, PhD, Brinkveld TRTC, Oude Arnhemse Weg 260, 3705BK, Zeist, The Netherlands.)

Boon, S., & Van der Hart, O. (1991). De behandeling van de multiple persoonlijkheidsstoornis. In O. van der Hart (red.), *Trauma, Dissociatie & Hypnose* (pp. 159–187). Lisse: Swets & Zeitlinger.

Bos, E. H., Van Wel, E. B., Appelo, M. T., & Verbraak, M. J. (2010). A randomized controlled trial of a Dutch version of systems training for emotional predictability and problem solving for borderline personality disorder. *Journal of Nervous and Mental Disease, 198,* 299–304.

Bowlby, J. (1973) *Attachment and loss: Volume 2. Separation: Anxiety and anger.* New York: Basic Books.

Brand, B. L., Classen, C. C., Lanius, R., Loewenstein, R. J., McNary, S. W., Pain, C., et al. (2009). A naturalistic study of Dissociative Identity Disorder and Dissociative

Disorder Not Otherwise Specified patient treatment by community clinicians. *Psychological Trauma: Theory, Research, Practice, and Policy, 1*, 153–171.

Brand, B. L., Classen, C. C., McNary, S. W., & Zaveri, P. (2009). A review of dissociative disorders treatment studies. *Journal of Nervous and Mental Disease, 197*, 646–654.

Braun, B. G. (Ed.). (1986). *Treatment of multiple personality disorder*. Washington, DC: American Psychiatric Press.

Brown, D., Scheflin, A. W., & Hammond, D. C. (1998). *Memory, trauma treatment, and the law*. New York: Norton.

Burns, D. D. (1999). *Feeling good: The new mood therapy* (rev. ed.). New York: Harper.

Carnes, P. (1997). *Sexual anorexia: Overcoming sexual self-hatred*. Center City, MN: Hazelden Publishing.

Chu, J. A. (1998). *Rebuilding shattered lives: The responsible treatment of complex posttraumatic and dissociative disorders*. New York: Wiley.

Cloitre, M., Cohen, L. R., & Koenen, K. C. (2006). *Treating survivors of childhood abuse: Psychotherapy for the interrupted life*. New York: Guilford Press.

Coons, P. M., & Milstein, V. (1990). Self-mutilation associated with dissociative disorders. *Dissociation , 3*(2), 81–87.

Courtois, C. A. (1999). *Recollections of sexual abuse: Treatment principles and guidelines*. New York: Norton.

Dell, P. F. (2002). Dissociative phenomenology of dissociative identity disorder. *Journal of Nervous and Mental Disease, 190*, 10–15.

Dell, P. F. (2006). A new model of Dissociative Identity Disorder. *Psychiatric Clinics of North America, 29*(1), 1–26.

Dorrepaal, E., Thomaes K., & Draijer, N. (2006). Stabilisatiecursus als antwoord op complexe posttraumatische stress-stoornis [Stabilization course as an answer to complex post-traumatic stress disorder. Diagnosis, treatment and research in women abused in childhood with a complex post-traumatic stress disorder]. *Tijdschrift voorPsychiatrie, 48*, 217–222.

Dorrepaal, E., Thomaes, K., & Draijer, N. (2008). *Vroeger en verder: Cursus na een geschiedenis van misbruik of mishandeling* [Earlier and further: Stabilization course as an answer to complex PTSD]. Amsterdam: Pearson Assessment.

Eysenck, M. W. (1992). *Anxiety: The cognitive perspective*. Hove, England: Erlbaum.

Fine, C. G. (1988). Thoughts on the cognitive perceptual substrates of multiple personality disorder. *Dissociation, 1*(4), 5–10.

Fine, C. G. (1996). A cognitively based treatment model for DSM-IV dissociative identity disorder. In L. Michelson & W. J. Ray (Eds.), *Handbook of dissociation: Theoretical, empirical, and clinical perspectives* (pp. 401–411). New York: Plenum Press.

Fine, C. G., & Comstock, C. (1989). Completion of cognitive schemata and affective realms through temporary blending of personalities. In B. G. Braun (Ed.), Dissociative Disorders 1989--Proceedings of the 6th International Conference on Multiple Personality/Dissociative States (p. 17). Chicago: Rush University.

Fonagy, P., Gergely, G., Jurist, E., & Target, M. (2002). *Affect regulation, mentalization, and the development of the self*. New York: Other Press.

Fonagy, P., & Target, M. (1997). Attachment and reflective function: Their role in self-organization. *Development and Psychopathology, 9*, 679–700.

Follette, V. M., & Pistorello, J. (2007). *Finding life beyond trauma: Using acceptance and commitment therapy to heal from posttraumatic stress and trauma-related problems*. Oakland, CA: New Harbinger Publications.

Ford, J .D., & Russo, E. (2006). Trauma-focused, present-centered, emotional self-regulation approach to integrated treatment for posttraumatic stress and addiction: Trauma Adaptive Recovery Group Education and Therapy (TARGET). *American Journal of Psychotherapy, 60*, 335–355.

Fraser, G. (1991). The dissociation table technique: A strategy for working with ego states in dissociative disorders and ego-state therapy. *Dissociation, 4*, 205–213.

Fraser, G. (2003). Fraser's Dissociative Table Technique revisited, revised: A strategy for working with ego states in dissociative disorders and ego-state therapy. *Journal of Trauma and Dissociation*, 4(4), 5–28.

Goodwin, J. M., & Attias, R. (1993). Eating disorders in survivors of multimodal childhood abuse. In R. P. Kluft & C. G. Fine (Eds.), *Clinical perspectives on multiple personality disorder* (pp. 327–341). Washington, DC: American Psychiatric Press.

Graber, K. (1991). *Ghosts in the bedroom: A guide for partners of incest survivors*. Dearfield Beach, FL: Health Communications.

Gratz, K., & Walsh, B. (2009). *Freedom from selfharm: Overcoming self-injury with DBT and other skills*. Oakland, CA: New Harbinger Publications.

Harris, M. (1998). *Trauma recovery and empowerment: A clinician's guide for working with women in groups*. New York: Free Press.

Hayes, S. C., Folette, V. M., & Linehan, M. M. (Eds.). (2004). *Mindfulness and acceptance: Expanding the cognitive-behavioral tradition*. New York: Guilford.

Hayes, S. C., Wilson, K. G., Gifford, E. V., & Follette, V. M. (1996). Experiential avoidance and behavioral disorders: A functional dimensional approach to diagnosis and treatment. *Journal of Consulting and Clinical Psychology*, 64, 1152–1168.

Herman, J. L. (1992). *Trauma and recovery*. New York: Basic Books.

Horevitz, R., & Loewenstein, R. J. (1994). The rational treatment of multiple personality. In S. J. Lynn & J. W. Rhue (Eds.), *Dissociation: Clinical and theoretical perspectives* (pp. 289–316). New York: Guilford Press.

International Society for the Study of Trauma and Dissociation (ISSTD). (in press). Guidelines for treating dissociative identity disorder in adults, 3rd revision. *Journal of Trauma and Dissociation, 12*.

Jacobson, E. (1974). *Progressive relaxation: A physiological and clinical investigation of muscular states and their significance in psychology and medical practice* (3rd ed.). Chicago: University of Chicago Press.

Janoff-Bulman, R. (1992). *Shattered assumptions: Towards a new psychology of trauma*. New York: Free Press.

Kashdana, T. B., Barrios, V., Forsyth, J. P., & Steger, M. F. (2006). Experiential avoidance as a generalized psychological vulnerability: Comparisons with coping and emotion regulation strategies. *Behaviour Research and Therapy*, 44, 1301–1320.

Kluft, R. P. (Ed.). (1985). *Childhood antecedents of multiple personality*. Washington, DC: American Psychiatric Press.

Kluft, R. P. (1987). First-rank symptoms as a diagnostic clue to multiple personality disorder. *American Journal of Psychiatry*, 144, 293–298.

Kluft, R. P. (1993). Clinical approaches to the integration of personalities. In R. P. Kluft & C. G. Fine (Eds.), *Clinical perspectives on multiple personality disorder* (pp. 101–133). Washington, DC: American Psychiatric Press.

Kluft, R. P. (1999). An overview of the psychotherapy of dissociative identity disorder. *American Journal of Psychotherapy*, 53, 289–319.

Kluft, R. P. (2006). Dealing with alters: A pragmatic clinical perspective. *Psychiatric Clinics of North America*, 29, 281–304.

Kluft, R. P. (2007). Applications of innate affect theory to the understanding and treatment of dissociative identity disorder. In E. Vermetten, M. J. Dorahy, & D. Spiegel (Eds.), *Traumatic dissociation: Neurobiology and treatment* (pp. 301–316). Arlington, VA: American Psychiatric Publishing.

Kluft, R. P., & Fine, C. G. (Eds.). (1993). *Clinical perspectives on multiple personality disorder*. Washington, DC: American Psychiatric Press.

Krakauer, S. Y. (2001). *Treating dissociative identity disorder: The power of the collective heart*. Philadephia: Brunner-Routledge.

Lanius, R. A., Vermettcn, E., Loewenstein, R. J., Brand, B., Schmahl, C., Bremner, J. D., et al. (2010). Emotion modulation in PTSD: Clinical and neurobiological evidence for a dissociative subtype. *American Journal of Psychiatry*, 167, 640–647.

Lehrer, J. (2009). *How we decide*. New York: Houghton Mifflin Harcourt.

Linden, A. (2008). *Boundaries in human relationships: How to be separate and connected*. Williston, VT: Crown House Publishing.

Linehan, M. M. (1993). *Skills training manual for treating borderline personality disorder*. New York: Guilford Press.

Loewenstein, G. F., Weber, E. U., Hsee, C. K., & Welch, N. (2001). Risk as feelings. *Psychological Bulletin, 127*, 267–286.

Loewenstein, R. J. (1991). An office mental status examination for complex chronic dissociative symptoms and multiple personality disorder. *Psychiatric Clinics of North America, 14*, 567–604.

Lynd, H. (1958). *On shame and the search for identity*. New York: Harcourt.

Maltz, W. (2001). *The sexual healing journey: A guide for survivors of sexual abuse* (2nd ed.). New York: Harper Collins Publishers.

Mann, L., & Tan, C. (1993). The hassled decision maker: The effects of perceived time pressure on information processing in decision making. *Australian Journal of Management, 18*, 197–209.

McCullough, L., Kuhn, N., Andrews, S., Kaplan, A., Wolf, J., Hurley, C. L., et al. (2003). *Treating affect phobia: A manual for short-term dynamic psychotherapy*. New York: Guilford Press.

McLean, P. D., (1985). Brain evolution relating to family, play, and the separation call. *Archives of General Psychiatry, 42*, 405–417.

Michelson, L., & Ray, W. J. (Eds.). (1996). *Handbook of dissociation: Theoretical, empirical, and clinical perspectives*. New York: Plenum Press.

Miller, D. (1994). *Women who hurt themselves: A book of hope and understanding*. New York: Basic Books.

Najavits, (2002). *Seeking safety: A treatment manual for PTSD and substance abuse*. New York: Guilford Press.

Nathanson, D. L. (1992). *Shame and pride: Affect, sex, and the birth of the self*. New York: Norton.

Nijenhuis, E. R. S., Spinhoven, P., Van Dyck, R., Van der Hart, O., & Vanderlinden, J. (1996). The development and psychometric characteristics of the Somatoform Dissociation Questionnaire (SDQ-20). *Journal of Nervous and Mental Disease, 184*, 688–694.

Ogden, P., Minton K., & Pain C. (2006). *Trauma and the body: A sensorimotor approach to psychotherapy*. New York: Norton.

O'Shea, K. (2009). EMDR friendly preparation methods for adults and children. In R. Shapiro (Ed.), *EMDR solutions II: For depression, eating disorders, performance, and more* (pp. 289–312). New York: Norton.

Panksepp, J. (1998). *Affective neuroscience: The foundations of human and animal emotions*. New York: Oxford University Press.

Paterson, R. J. (2000). *The assertiveness workbook: How to express your ideas and stand up for yourself at work and in relationships*. Oakland, CA: New Harbinger Publications.

Pelcovitz, D., Van der Kolk, B. A., Roth, S., Mandel, F., Kaplan, S., & Resick, P. (1997). Development of a criteria set and a structured interview for the disorders of extreme stress (SIDES). *Journal of Traumatic Stress, 10*, 3–16.

Phelps, S., & Austin, A. (2002). *The assertive woman*. San Luis Obispo, CA: Impact Publications.

Putnam, F. W. (1989). *Diagnosis and treatment of multiple personality disorder*. New York: Guilford.

Putnam, F. W. (1997). *Dissociation in children and adolescents: A developmental perspective*. New York: Guilford Press.

Ross, C. A. (1989). *Multiple personality disorder: Diagnosis, clinical features, and treatment*. Toronto, Canada: Wiley.

Ross, C. A. (1997). *Dissociative identity disorder: Diagnosis, clinical features, and treatment*. New York: Wiley.

Ross, C. A., Heber, S., Norton, G. R., Anderson, B., Anderson, G., & Barchet, P. (1989). The Dissociative Disorders Interview Schedule: A structured interview. *Dissociation, 2*, 169–189.

Rothbaum, B., Foa, E., & Hembree, E. (2007). *Reclaiming your life from a traumatic experience: A prolonged exposure treatment program workbook*. New York: Oxford University Press.

Schmidt, S. J. (2009). *The Developmental Needs Meeting Strategy: An ego state therapy for healing adults with childhood trauma and attachment wounds*. San Antonio, TX: DNMS Institute.

Schore, A. (2001). The effects of a secure attachment relationship on right brain development, affect regulation, and infant mental health. *Infant Mental Health Journal, 22*, 7–66.

Siegel, D. J. (1999). *The developing mind: Toward a neurobiology of interpersonal experience*. New York: Guilford Press.

Slade, A. (1999). Attachment theory and research: Implications for the theory and practice of individual psychotherapy with adults. In J. Cassidy & P. R. Shaver (Eds.), *Handbook of attachment: Theory, research and clinical applications* (pp. 575–594). New York: Guilford

Steele, K., Dorahy, M., Van der Hart, O., & Nijenhuis, E. R. S. (2009). Dissociation versus alterations in consciousness: Related but different concepts. In P. F. Dell & J. A. O'Neil (Eds.), *Dissociation and the dissociative disorders: DSM-V and beyond* (pp. 155–170). New York: Routledge.

Steele, K., & Van der Hart, O. (2009). Treating dissociation. In C. A. Courtois & J. D. Ford (Eds.), *Treating complex traumatic stress disorders* (pp. 145–165). New York: Guilford Press.

Steele, K., Van der Hart, O., & Nijenhuis, E. R. S. (2001). Dependency in the treatment of complex posttraumatic stress disorder and dissociative disorders. *Journal of Trauma and Dissociation, 2*(4), 79–116.

Steele, K., Van der Hart, O., & Nijenhuis, E. R. S. (2005). Phase-oriented treatment of structural dissociation in complex traumatization: Overcoming trauma-related phobias. *Journal of Trauma and Dissociation, 6*(3), 11–53.

Steinberg, M. (1994). *Structured clinical interview for DSM-IV dissociative disorders, revised*. Washington, DC: American Psychiatric Press.

Steinberg, M. (1995). *Handbook for the assessment of dissociation: A clinical guide*. Washington, DC: American Psychiatric Press.

Tomkins, S. S. (1963). *Affect/imagery/consciousness: Vol. 2. The negative affects*. New York: Springer.

Tracy, J. L., Robins, R. W., & Tangney, J. P. (Eds.). (2007). *The self-conscious emotions: Theory and research*. New York: Guilford Press.

Van Derbur, M. (2004). *Miss America by day: Lessons learned from ultimate betrayals and unconditional love*. Denver, CO: Oak Hill Ridge Press.

Van der Hart, O. (2009, November). *Haunted and harassed: Perception, memory, and decision-making in the dissociative patient: The 2009 Pierre Janet Memorial Lecture*. Paper presented at the International Society for the Study of Trauma and Dissociation 26th Annual Conference, Washington, DC.

Van der Hart, O., & Boon, S. (1997). Treatment strategies for complex dissociative disorders: Two Dutch case examples. *Dissociation, 10*, 157–165.

Van der Hart, O., Boon, S., Friedman, B., & Mierop, V. (1992). De reactivering van traumatische herinneringen. *Dth, 12*(1), 12–55.

Van der Hart, O., Steele, K., Boon, S., & Brown, P. (1993). The treatment of traumatic memories: Synthesis, realization, and integration. *Dissociation, 6*(2/3), 162–180.

Van der Hart, O., Nijenhuis, E. R. S., & Solomon, R. (2010). Dissociation of the personality in complex trauma-related disorders and EMDR: Theoretical considerations. *Journal of EMDR Practice and Research, 4,* 76–92.

Van der Hart, O., Nijenhuis, E. R. S., & Steele, K. (2005). Dissociation: An under-recognized feature of complex PTSD. *Journal of Traumatic Stress, 18,* 413–424.

Van der Hart, O., Nijenhuis, E. R. S., & Steele, K. (2006). *The haunted self: Structural dissociation and the treatment of chronic traumatization.* New York/London: Norton.

Van der Hart, O., & Steele, K. (1997). Time distortions in dissociative identity disorder: Janetian concepts and treatment. *Dissociation, 10,* 91–103.

Van der Hart, O., Van der Kolk, B. A., & Boon, S. (1998). Treatment of dissociative disorders. In J. D. Bremner & C. R. Marmar (Eds.), *Trauma, memory, and dissociation* (pp. 253–283). Washington, DC: American Psychiatric Press.

Van der Kolk, B. A. (1996). The complexity of adaptation to trauma: Self-regulation, stimulus discrimination, and characterological development. In B. A. van der Kolk, A. C. McFarlane, & L. Weiseath (Eds.), *Traumatic stress: The effects of overwhelming experience on mind, body, and society* (pp. 182–213). New York: Guilford Press.

Vanderlinden, J., & Vandereycken, W. (1997). *Trauma, dissociation, and impulse control in eating disorders.* Bristol, PA: Brunner/Mazel.

Vermilyea, E. G. (2007). *Growing beyond survival: A self-help toolkit for managing traumatic stress.* Baltimore, MD: Sidran Press.

Waller, N. G., Putnam, F. W., & Carlson, E. B. (1996). Types of dissociation and dissociative types: A taxonomic analysis of dissociative experiences. *Psychological Methods, 1,* 300–321.

Westen, D., Novotny, C. M., & Thompson-Brenner, H. (2004) The empirical status of empirically supported psychotherapies: Assumptions, findings and reporting in controlled clinical trials. *Psychological Bulletin,130,* 631–663.

Williams, M. B., & Poijula, S. (2002). *The PTSD workbook: Simple, effective techniques for overcoming posttraumatic stress symptoms.* Oakland, CA: New Harbinger Publications.

Wolfsdorf, B. A., & Zlotnick, C. (2001). Affect management in group therapy for women with posttraumatic stress disorder and histories of childhood sexual abuse. *Journal of Clinical Psychology, 57,* 169–181.

World Health Organization. (1992). *The ICD-10 classification of mental and behavioural disorders.* Geneva: Author.

Wright, P. (1974). The harassed decision maker: Time pressures, distractions, and the use of evidence. *Journal of Applied Psychology, 59,* 555–561.

Zlotnick, C., Shea, T. M., Rosen, K., Simpson, E., Mulrenin, K., Begin, A., et al. (1997). An affect-management group for survivors of sexual abuse with PTSD. *Journal of Traumatic Stress, 10,* 425–436.

INDEX

abandonment, 169, 366

absences, skills-training group and, 430, 447

abuse, 139, 266, 366

    see also child abuse; sexual abuse; trauma

acceptance

    of dissociation, 76

    of parts of self, gradual acknowledgment and, 73

acceptance and commitment therapy (ACT), xii

activity, balanced distribution of, 112

adaptive decisions, 324

adaptive guilt, pervasive guilt vs., 293

addictions, xi, 141. *see also* substance abuse

affect, in complex PTSD and alterations in regulation of, 44

affect phobia, xi

aggression, as nonassertive strategy, 380, 381. *see also* anger

alcohol

    sleep problems and, 100

    traumatized people and self-medication with, 141–42

alienation from self, dissociative disorder and symptoms of, 16–17

alienation from surroundings, dissociative disorder and symptoms of, 17–18

all-or-nothing thinking, 237

alone time

    loneliness vs., 367–68

    pleasant experiences during, 370

altered physical sensations, dissociation and, 139–40

amnesia, 15–16, 248, 282, 315

anchors, 19–20, 47, 101, 104, 105, 180–81

anger

    agenda on coping with, 263

    common inaccurate beliefs about, 264–65

    complex dissociative disorder and, 266–68

    coping with, 263–76

    dissociative parts and avoidance of, 30, 267–68, 271, 273–76, 334, 361–62

    dissociative parts fixated in, 267–68

    expressions of, 265

    in people with complex dissociative disorder, 266–68

    personality parts imitating people who hurt you and, 30

    physical signs of, 269

    resolving, challenging core beliefs and using reflection for, 272

    as substitute for other emotions, 265

    time outs from, 270, 272

    tips for coping with, 269–71

    understanding your experience of, homework, 273–74

angry dissociative parts of self

    calming and containing in relational conflicts, 361–62

    understanding and coping with, homework, 275–76

    understanding and coping with, skills review, 334

anniversary dates, difficult feelings and triggers related to, 190, 191

"anniversary reactions," 169

antidepressants, 142

anxiety, xi

    chronic, 278

    eating problems and, 150

    fear vs., 279

    healthy, 279–80

    holidays and, 190

    perception, judgment and effects of, 328

    posttraumatic stress disorder and, 35, 36

    self-medicating with substances and, 141

    time pressure and, 327

appeasement, 380, 381, 382

appointments

    current daily structure and, 119–20

    realistic and healthy daily structure and, 121–22

arousal and window of tolerance, 214–17

    auto- and relational regulation, 215–16

    avoidance of emotion, 216–17

    lack of reflection and, 216

ashamed parts of personality, 31

assertiveness

    basic skills for, 378–80

    benefits of, 378

    complex dissociative disorder and problems with, 383–84

    defined, 378

    example of, 382

    identifying inner conflicts and in the way of, 387–88, 408

    identifying inner conflicts preventing, skills review, 408

    inner cooperation and, 384–86

    learning about, 377–91

    personal boundary setting and, 393

    preparing for, in upcoming situation, 390–91, 408

    preparing for, in upcoming situation, skills review, 408

    using skills: retrospective look at skills, 389

attachment. *see* abandonment; phobia of attachment; phobia of attachment loss; relationships

attention, complex PTSD and changes in, 40, 44

attention-deficit disorders, 189

attention problems, identifying, homework, 40
autobiographical memory, traumatic memory
        and, 166
automatic thoughts, 229, 247
auto-regulation, 215–16, 346, 406
avoidance, 35, 36, 40, 53, 216–17, 290, 292–93,
        380, 381, 429
avoidant parts, support for, in dealing with rela-
        tional conflict, 360–61
awareness, 18–19, 76
Axis I comorbidity, in patients with dissociative
        disorders, 417
Axis II comorbidity, in patients with dissociative
        disorders, 417–18

balance in daily structure, finding, 113
bedtime routine, 110, 158
bedwetting, 98, 99
behaviors, feedback loops of, 205–6
being in the present, 84
beliefs, realistic, developing, 252–53
betrayal, 366
bingeing, 151, 154
bipolar disorders, dissociative disorders vs., 415
birthdays, 191
blending of parts, 307–9, 337, 386, 391, 399
body awareness, 138–41
body language, assertiveness, 379
body perceptions, 138–39
borderline personality disorders, xiii
        dialectical behavior therapy for, xi
        dissociative disorders vs., 415
boundaries, 345, 393–98, 399, 403–4, 410
breathing, 6
breathing exercises, 104

calming and soothing yourself, 219–20, 255
calmness, 84, 181–82
care of self. see physical self-care
CBT. see cognitive-behavioral therapy (CBT)
child abuse, 9, 138
childhood traumatization, 8
child parts
        blending and, 308–9
        experience of, 302–3
        phobic avoidance of, 303
        working with, 305–7
chores
        communicating about, 115
        current daily structure and, 119–20
        realistic and healthy daily structure and,
                121–22
chronic dissociation, origins of, 9
chronic lateness, 429
chronic reactions to an emotion, 61
cognitive-behavioral therapy (CBT), xii
cognitive errors, 236–40, 242–44, 246, 258
        see also core beliefs
collapsed boundaries, 395–96
collapse mode
        dissociative parts of self and, 347
                fear and, 279
        relationships, dissociative parts of self and, 347
        shame and, 288

communication
        forms of, 72–74
        inner meetings, 75
        with parts of yourself, 73–74
        talking inwardly, 75
        written forms of, 74–75
complex dissociative disorder
        anger and, 266–68
        assertiveness problems and, 383–84
        avoidance of emotion and, 216–17
        blending and, 308–9
        boundary problems and, 396–98
        decision-making problems and, 326
        diagnostic assessment for, 415
        eating problems and, 151–52
        executive functioning problems and, 189
        exploring thoughts and, 248–49
        fear and, 277, 278, 280–82
        inner chaos, confusion, and, 188
        negative core beliefs and, 229–31
        planning issues for people with a, 188–89
        priority setting and, 189
        problems with daily structure and, 112–13
        problems with emotions and, 206–8
        problems with free time and relaxation and,
                124–25
        problems with reflection and, 59–61
        resolving relational conflicts and, 358–62
        sleep problems and, 98
        time management difficulties and, 189
complex posttraumatic stress disorder (CPTSD),
        xii, 35, 38, 43, 44, 45, 444–45
concentration difficulties, 19, 40
confidentiality issues, 417, 446
conflicted emotions, 84–85
conflict management skills, 363–64, 407
        relational conflicts and, homework, 363–64
        using, skills review, 407
conflicts in relationships, 356–64
conscious avoidance, 53
conscious decisions, 330
consciousness, 44
contact between sessions, 431, 446
containment, 219, 255
control, fearing loss of, 71
cooking, 113, 150, 151, 152, 153, 154, 155
cooperation, inner, 181–82
core beliefs
        agenda on challenging of, 245
        agenda on understanding of, 227
        assertiveness and challenging of, 385
        automatic thoughts and, 247
        challenging, reflections for understanding,
                248–49, 250–51, 258, 272
        challenging, skills review, 258
        challenging, to resolve anger, 272
        healthy boundary setting and, 398
        identifying negative, homework, 232–33
        inaccurate, challenging, homework, 250–51
        maintenance of isolation and, 366
        negative, 229–31
        origins of, 228–29
        realistic and healthy, 231, 234–35, 257
        understanding, 228
        see also cognitive errors
counter-phobic dissociative parts, 282

countertransference issues, 417
course participants
    assessment and diagnosis of, 415–21
    choosing course participants, 416–18
    diagnostic assessment for complex dissociative
        disorders, 415
    inclusion criteria for, 416
    intake session, 419
    optimal group composition, 420–21
course participation
    dropping out, 418
    repeating course and, 418
    timing of, 418
cutting behaviors, 316

daily structure, 112–13, 119–20, 159
day-treatment, 433
DBT. *see* dialectical behavior therapy (DBT)
DDNOS. *see* dissociative disorder not otherwise
        specified (DDNOS)
"death feigning," in animals, 37
decision making
    complex dissociative disorder and problems
        with, 326
    conscious, 330
    creating inner meeting space for, 330–31
    of daily living, 324
    examining pros and cons in, 329–30
    improving, 323–39
    rating system for, 330
    time pressure and, 327–28
    understanding, 324–25
deep breathing, 220
defense reaction, triggers and, 167
defensive fight mode, 267
dental appointments, 144, 191
depersonalization, 16–17
depression, xi
    eating problems and, 150
    holidays and, 190
    posttraumatic stress disorder and, 35
    self-medicating with substances and, 141
derealization, 17–18
DES. *see Dissociative Experiences Scale* (DES)
DES-Taxon (DES-T), 415
detachment, 35
Developmental Needs Meeting Strategy, 306
diagnosis, of dissociative disorders, 9–11
*Diagnostic and Statistical Manual of Mental Disor-
        ders* (*DSM*)
    dissociative disorder not otherwise specified,
        subtype 1b criteria, 443
    dissociative disorders classifications and, 10
    dissociative identity disorder diagnostic crite-
        ria, 443
    posttraumatic stress disorder criteria, 443–44
diagnostic assessment, of complex dissociative
        disorders, 415
dialectical behavior therapy (DBT), xi, 419
diary, tracking time in, 115
DID. *see* dissociative identity disorder (DID)
difficult times
    agenda on planning for, 187
    holidays and other special times, 190–92
    how to plan for, 188–89, 192–94

preparing for, homework, 196–98
    reflections to help with planning for, 193
    strategic skills review for, 200
    when obligations to others conflict with your
        needs, 194–95
disgust
    body perceived as object of, 138–39
    phobia of inner experience and, 52
disorders of extreme stress not otherwise speci-
        fied (DESNOS), criteria for, 444–45
disruptions, minimizing during group sessions,
        429
dissociation
    agenda for session on, 3
    alienation or estrangement from self or body
        and, 16–17
    alienation or estrangement from your sur-
        roundings and, 17–18
    altered physical sensations and, 139–40
    chronic, origins of, 9
    defined, 8
    depersonalization and, 16–17
    derealization and, 17–18
    dissociative amnesia and, 15–16
    experiencing too little: apparent loss of func-
        tions with, 15
    experiencing too much: intrusions and, 18
    other changes in awareness with, 18–19
    problems with identity or sense of self and,
        14–15
    reflecting on what you learned about, 12
    reflective functioning impeded by, 60–61
    stages of awareness and acceptance of, 76
    symptoms of, 13–19
        agenda for, 13
    time distortions and, 16
    understanding, 6–8
dissociative amnesia, 15–16
dissociative disorder not otherwise specified
        (DDNOS), xi, xii, xiii, xiv, xvii, 10
    basic functions of parts of personality and, 26
    as complex posttraumatic stress disorder, 38
    manual use and formal diagnosis of, 432
    parts of personality with functions in daily life
        for people with, 26, 29
    subtype 1b, *DSM-V* diagnostic criteria, 443
dissociative disorders
    body perceptions and, 138–39
    diagnosis of, 9–11
    diagnostic assessment for, 415
    experiencing fear without knowing why and,
        280–81
    intense emotions and, 206–7
    remaining stuck in trauma-time and, 84
    sexual boundary problems and, 397–98
    time management problems and, 115–16
    time pressures and, 327
Dissociative Disorders Interview Scale, 415
Dissociative Experiences Scale (DES), 415
dissociative identity disorder (DID), xi, xii, xiii,
        xiv, xvii, 8, 10
    basic functions of parts of personality in and
        people with, 26
    as complex posttraumatic stress disorder, 38
    DSM-V diagnostic criteria, 443
    executive control and, 27

dissociative identity disorder (DID) (*continued*)
  failure of parts to accept the body as their own, 140
  manual use and formal diagnosis of, 432
  struggle for time among dissociative parts and, 100
dissociative individuals, inner world of, 25–28
dissociative intrusions, 18
dissociative parts of the personality, 8
  agenda on beginning work with, 70
  avoidance of anger and, 268
  awareness of parts for each other, 26
  counter-phobic, 282
  as "decision-making centers," 326–27
  elaboration and autonomy of parts, 28
  fixated in anger, 267–68
  identifying and coping with, 43–45
  images of "inner world" of, 25
  influence of parts on each other, 26–27
  isolation among, 367
  negative judgments of emotions among, 207
  number of parts, 28
  relational models and, 344
  self-harm and, 317
  struggle for time among, 100
  understanding, agenda for, 24
dissociative parts of yourself
  first steps in working with, 72
  initial dilemmas in working with, 71
  recognizing, homework, 33, 77
  reflection used with, 61–62
dissociative symptoms
  identifying, homework, 32
  recognizing, 21–22
dissociative table technique, 330–31
  see also inner meeting room
distraction, 218–19, 255
doctor
  appointments, 144
  fear of, 141
driving, automatic, dissociation and, 19
dropouts, optimal outpatient skills-training group and, 420
drugs, sleep problems and, 100
DSM. see Diagnostic and Statistical Manual of Mental Disorders (DSM)
dysfunctional boundaries, 367
dysfunctional thoughts 245, 250–51

eating
  with complete attention, 208–9
  many meanings of, 150
  tips for resolving inner conflicts about, 152–54
  see also meals
eating habits
  healthy, developing, 149–61
eating problems
  complex dissociative disorder and, 151–52
  improving, plan for, 156–57, 161
  self-harm and, 316
educational meetings for significant others, 426–27, 435–36, 448
emotional intimacy, 361
emotional pain, abuse and, 139

emotional reasoning, 238–39
emotional signals, difficulty attending to, in the present, 207–8
emotion dysregulation, lack of reflection and, 216
emotion regulation, xi, xii
  healing and, 214
  impulse regulation and, xiii
emotions
  agenda on understanding of, 203
  avoidance of, 216–17
  basic, and their functions of, 204–6
  core beliefs and, 228
  decision making and, 325
  identifying, skills review, 255
  identifying and understanding, homework, 210–11
  intense, relationships and, 344
  judging, 204–5
  meeting our needs with, 205
  mindfulness exercise and, 208–9
  negative judgments of, among dissociative parts, 207
  self-conscious, 205
  sensory experience of, homework, 212
empathic acceptance, 220
empathic understanding, reflection and, 58–59
empathy
  healthy personal relationships and, 345
  toward yourself, 64–65, 92
estrangement from self or body, 16–17
estrangement from surroundings, 17–18
European Society for Trauma and Dissociation Web site, xiv
evaluation of course, 440
executive control, 27–28
executive functioning, 189
exercises
  creating inner meeting space for decision making, 330–31
  expansion of learning to be present: finding your anchors to the present, 19–20
  experiencing an inner sense of safety, 87
  finding common ground about relationships, 349–50
  Healing Pool, 129
  learning to be present, 5–6
  mindfulness, 208–9
  necklace of positive experiences, 240–41
  store, 171–72
  stress reduction and healing, 38–39
  tree, 128–29
experiential avoidance, 52

facial expressions, 243
family time
  current daily structure and, 119–222
  realistic and healthy daily structure and, 121–22
fatigue, 142
fear
  about relationships, 347
  anxiety vs., 279
  body perceived as object of, 138–39
  chronic, 278

collapse mode and, 279
  healthy, 279–80
  inappropriate, 281
  of inner experiences, 279
  loneliness and, 368
  of losing control, 71, 207
  perception, judgment and effects of, 328
  physiological reactions to, 278
  posttraumatic stress disorder and, 35
  reckless actions without, 282
  reflecting on inner experience of, skills review,
      335
  reflecting on your experience of, 285–86
  tips for coping with, 283–84
feedback
  assertiveness and, 379
  from group participants, 440
feedback loops, 205–6, 246–48
fight parts of personality, 30–31
final evaluation, 451–54
flashbacks, 18, 166, 167, 216
  during nighttime, 98, 99
  holidays and, 190
  identifying, homework, 40
  nighttime, 98, 99
  posttraumatic stress disorder and, 35, 36
  prolonged, healthy daily structure and reduc-
      tion in, 112
  self-harm and, 319
  self-medicating with substances and, 141
  shame and, 288–89
  as you fall asleep, 99
flight-or-fight reaction, 278
food
  eating with complete attention, 208–9
  many meanings of, 150
food restriction, 151
forgetfulness, dissociative amnesia vs., 15
free time
  complex dissociative disorder and problems
      with, 124–25
  managing, tips for, 126–27
  resolving inner conflicts about, 125–26
freezing
  fear and, 283
  relationships and, 347
  shame and sense of, 288, 295
friends
  current daily structure and, 119–20
  realistic and healthy daily structure and,
      121–22

goodbyes. see leave-taking session
grounding, coping with hyperarousal through,
    220–21
ground rules, 424, 430–31, 434, 446–48
group composition issues, 420
group difficulties, 427–31
  contact between sessions, 431
  participants who are chronically late, 429
  participants who are unable to stay present,
      428–29
  participants who discuss inappropriate content,
      428

participants who must drop out prematurely,
    429–30
  participants who object to ground rules, 430–31
  participants who talk too little or too much,
      427–28
  understanding and resolving, 427–31
group trainer's guide, 413–33
  assessment and diagnosis of potential course
      participants, 415–21
  conducting course sessions, 423–27
  contact and coordination with treating thera-
      pist, 421–23
  trainer qualifications and guidelines, 414
  understanding and resolving difficulties in
      group, 427–31
  using manual in day-treatment and inpatient
      groups, 433
  using manual in individual therapy, 432–33
guilt
  agenda on coping with, 287
  childhood trauma and feelings of, 44
  chronic, 289, 295
  coping with, homework, 299–300
  coping with, skills review, 336
  coping with, tips for coping with, 293–96
  realistic, 295–96
  self-harm and reduction of, 316
  understanding, 288, 293

hallucinations
  posttraumatic stress disorder and, 36
  as you fall asleep, 99
hate
  body perceived as object of, 138–39
  feelings of, 264
head banging, 316, 430
healing
  emotion regulation and, 214
  free time and, 124
  working with inner experiences and, 54
  work/life balance and, 117
Healing Pool exercise, 129–30, 159, 180
healthy boundaries
  agenda on setting, 392
  characteristics of, 394–95
  description of, 393–95
  setting, cooperating with yourself and, 398–99
healthy core beliefs, 231
  developing, about self, about others, and about
      the world, 234–35
  developing, skills review, 257
healthy daily structure, 111–22
  agenda on establishing, 111
  establishing, 111–22
  new, reflections on developing, 117–18
  realistic, developing, 121–22
  reflections on developing, 113–14
healthy eating habits
  developing, 149–61
  resolving inner conflicts about, tips for, 152–54
healthy relationships, 344–46
helper parts of personality, 30
here-and-now awareness, 4–6
"highway hypnosis," 19

hobbies, 118, 119–20, 121–22
  current daily structure and, 119–20
  realistic and healthy daily structure and,
    121–22
holidays, managing, 190–91
home, creating safe spaces in, 86
humiliation, 169
humor, 379
hunger, 142, 152
hyperarousal, 36–37, 40, 214, 217–21, 225–26,
    255, 279
hypoarousal, 37, 41, 221–23, 215, 221, 225–26,
    255, 283

*ICD. see International Classification of Diseases
    (ICD)*
identity, 14–15
illicit drugs, 141–42
illusions, 99
imagery-based inner experiences, 306
imaginal rehearsals, 179–80, 195, 385–86, 391,
    399
imaginary inner safe places, 84–86
imaginary rehearsals, 195
inaccurate thoughts, challenging, skills review,
    258
inner awareness, forms of, 72–74
inner child parts of self, 301–11, 336
inner communication 73–75, 78–81, 91
inner cooperation, 312–13, 323–39, 384–86
inner deliberation, time for, 114
inner empathy, xiii
inner experiences
  avoiding, becoming aware of, 55–56
  defined, 51
  fear of, 279
  noticing without judgment, 64
  reflecting on, 68–69, 91
inner meeting room, 384, 398
  see also dissociative table technique
inner meetings, 75, 330–31, 332, 338, 390–91
inner orientation, 181–82, 186
inner reflection
  current daily structure and, 119–20
  realistic and healthy daily structure and,
    121–22
  time for, 118
inner safe places, 195
  angry parts in, 271
  imaginary, examples of, 85–86
inner sense of safety
  developing, 83–86, 93
  developing, homework, 88–89
  experiencing, exercise for, 87
  relaxation and, 127–28
inner voices, various dissociative parts of the self
    and, 73
inner world of dissociative individuals
  awareness of parts for each other, 26
  basic functions of parts of the personality,
    25–26
  elaboration and autonomy of parts, 28
  executive control, 27–28
  images of "inner world" of dissociative parts, 25
  influence of parts on each other, 26–27
  number of parts, 28
inpatient groups, 433
insecure relationships, 352–53, 406
intake session, 419
integration, 7
intense emotions, dissociative disorder and,
    206–7
interactive regulation, 215
internal triggers, 170
International Classification of Diseases (ICD), 10
International Society for the Study of Trauma and
    Dissociation (ISSTD), xi, xiv
*Interview for Dissociative Disorders and Trauma-
    Related Symptoms*, 415
introductory session, 434–36
intrusions, 18, 27, 36, 40
  dissociation and, 18
  identifying symptoms of, homework, 40
  posttraumatic stress disorder and, 36
involuntariness, 14
isolation, 36, 40, 115, 290–92, 365–76, 407
  see also loneliness
ISSTD. *see* International Society for the Study of
    Trauma and Dissociation (ISSTD)
"I" statements, 379

judging emotions, 204–5
judgment, effects of fear and anxiety on decision
    making and, 328

lax boundaries, 367, 395–96
learning to be present, 4–6, 11, 19–20, 46
leave-taking rituals, 427, 439–40
leave-taking session, 437–42
  educational meeting for significant others,
    435–36
  evaluation of course, 440
  explanation of ground rules, 434
  final session agenda, 441
  leave-taking rituals, 439–40
  making the most of skills-training course, 435
  saying goodbye to group, 438–39
  saying goodbye to group, homework, 441–42
  see also introductory session; training course
    sessions
leisure time, 112, 119–22, 124–25, 135–36
  balanced distribution of, 112
  complex dissociative disorder and problems
    with, 124–25
  current daily structure and, 119–20
  exploring inner obstacles to, 135–36
  realistic and healthy daily structure and,
    121–22
liquid nutritional supplements, 154
listening, reflective, assertiveness and, 379
lists, 116
loneliness, 141, 190–92, 365–76, 407
  agenda on coping with, 365
  coping with, 365–76
  coping with, tips for, 369–71
  coping with difficult times and, 191–92
  defined, 365–66

dysfunctional boundaries and, 367
fear, shame, and, 368
holidays and, 190
as reenactment of the past, 368
reflecting on a time of, homework, 372–73
reflections on your experience of, 368–69
resolving, homework skills for, 374–76
resolving, skills review, 407
self-medicating with substances and, 141
understanding, 367–68
see also isolation
losing control, fear of, 207
lost time, complex dissociative disorder and,
    189

magnification, 238
meals, 119–22, 150–55
see also eating
meaning, 45
medical appointments, 191
medical problems, 45
meditation, 370
mementos, for leave-taking rituals, 439–40
memories, 15–16
see also traumatic memories
menstruation, 170
mental filtering, 238
mentalization, xiii, 58
mindfulness, xiii
mindfulness exercise, 208–9, 254
mindfulness and mentalization based treatments,
    xi–xii
mistakes, 346
mistrust, 366
Multidimensional Inventory for Dissociation, 415
music, calming and soothing yourself with, 220

"necklace of positive experiences" exercise,
    240–41, 257
negative core beliefs, 229–33, 256
negative feedback loops, 246
neglect, 138, 366, 417
negotiation
    assertiveness and, 385
    healthy boundary setting and, 398–99
nightmares, 35, 36, 98, 99, 104–5
nonverbal parts, 307
numbness, 17, 35, 36, 40, 139–40, 214, 222–23,
    281
nutrition, 150–55

obesity, 150
optimal level of closeness and distance, 402, 409
overgeneralizing, 238
overwhelming emotions, 188, 208

pain sensitivity, 139
panic, 26, 36, 98, 99, 279, 327
partial intrusion, 26
participant contract, for skills-training group,
    449–50

parts of the personality, 29–31
    see also dissociative parts of the personality
passive influence, 26
past, distinguishing from the present, 180–81
perceptions, 205–6, 228, 328
perpetrators, 267–68
personal boundaries, 392–410
personality
    basic functions of parts of, 25–26
    dissociative parts of, 8, 14–15
    integration and, 7
personal organizers, 115
personal reflection, 114
personal space, optimal level of closeness and
        distance and, 402, 409
pets, 101, 113, 370
phobia of attachment
    development of, 346
    difficulties with regulation and, 346–48
    isolation and, 366
    loneliness and, 368
    relational conflict and, 358
    rigid boundaries and, 396
phobia of attachment loss
    development of, 346
    difficulties with regulation and, 348–49
    loneliness and, 368
    relational conflict and, 358
    rigid boundaries and, 396
phobia for dissociative parts of the personality,
    31, 71
phobia of inner experience
    becoming aware of avoiding inner experience,
        55–56
    developing, 53–54
    overcoming, 90
    physical self-care as trigger of, 140
    skills review, 90–93
    understanding, 52–53
phobias
    common perceptions of, 52
    relational, 346–49
physical energy, 142
physical examinations, fear of doctors or, 141
physical exercise, 114–15, 118
physical relaxation, 130
physical self-care, 137–48
physiological arousal, 214
physiological dysregulation, 35
planning, effective, tips for, 193–94
positive experiences, triggers for, 170
positive triggers, 176
posttraumatic stress disorder (PTSD), 10, 40–42,
        345–98, 443–44
predictions, core beliefs and, 228
premature (arbitrary) conclusions, 238
prereflective reaction, 59
prescription medications, 141–42
present moment
    anchors to, 19–20
    being in, 4–5
    difficulty attending to emotional signals in,
        207–8
    distinguishing the past from, 180–81
    inner sense of safety and, 84

present moment (*continued*)
  orienting to, skills review, 255
  overwhelming feelings in, 188
  safe anchors to, 23
primary care physicians, choosing, 141
priority setting, 189
progressive muscle relaxation, 131–32, 159
protective imagery, 186
pseudo-seizures, 430
psychiatric medications, 142
psychotic disorders, dissociative disorders vs., 415
PTSD. *see* posttraumatic stress disorder (PTSD)
purging, 151

rage, 30, 169, 264
rape victims, 35
reactivated traumatic memories, 166
  see also traumatic memories
realistic core beliefs, 231, 234–35, 257, 259
realistic positive thoughts and beliefs, 252–53
reassurance, 220–21
reckless actions, 282
reflection
  on anger, 270, 272
  assertiveness and, 384–85
  automatic thoughts and, 247
  complex dissociative disorder and problems
    with, 59–61
  developing new healthy daily structure and,
    117–18
  emotional dysregulation and lack of, 216
  empathic understanding of yourself and others
    through, 58–59, 62–63
  on experiences of isolation and loneliness,
    368–69
  healthy boundary setting and, 398
  on inner experience, 68–69, 91
  learning about, 57–69
  problems with, 59–61
  time for, 114
reflective functioning, 58, 59
reflective listening, 379
reflective skills, to identify and explore cognitive
    distortions, 239–40
reflective skills development, 63–65
regulation
  phobia of attachment and difficulties with,
    346–498
  phobia of attachment loss and difficulties with,
    348–49
rejection, 169
rejuvenation, 124
relational closeness and distance, optimal, 394
relational conflicts
  basic skills for resolving, 357–58
  calming and containing angry parts of yourself,
    361–62
  conflict management skills and, homework,
    363–64
  observing how others relate, 358–59
  orienting parts to the present, 360
  protecting vulnerable parts of yourself, 361
  reflecting on your own and other person's in-
    tentions and actions, 359–60

  resolving, 356–64
  supporting avoidant parts to deal with conflict,
    360–61
  time-outs from, 359
relational models, 344
relational phobias, 346
relational regulation, 215–16, 346, 354–55, 406
relational triggers, 169–70
relationships
  complex PTSD and changes in, 45
  finding inner common ground about, 349–51,
    405
  interpersonal trauma and effect on, 346
  see also healthy relationships
relaxation, 47, 84, 114, 124, 125–28, 135–36, 144
relaxation exercises, 128–31
  Healing Pool exercise, 129–30, 159
  physical relaxation exercise, 130
  progressive muscle relaxation technique,
    131–32, 159
  Tree exercise, 128–29, 159
relaxation kit, 133–34, 160, 191, 217
release of information, 419, 448
respect, 345
rest, 142, 144, 220
  see also sleep
retrospective reflection
  with chronic reaction to an emotion, 61
  with dissociative part of yourself, 61–62
revenge, feelings of, 264
rigid boundaries, 367, 396, 397
risky behaviors, 316
routine, 115

safe places
  developing sense of, 93
  developing sense of, homework, 88–89
  imagery of, 83
safe present, anchors to the present and, 19–20
safe relationships, 345
safety, xi
  see also inner sense of safety
Schedler-Westen Assessment Procedure-200 for per-
    sonality disorders, 415
SCID-II. *see Structured Clinical Interview for DSM
    Personality Disorders*
SDQ-20. *see Somatoform Dissociation Questionnaire*
    (SDQ-20)
seasons, difficult feelings and triggers related to,
    190, 191
secure relationships, 352–53, 406
self, sense of, 7–8
self-awareness, 58
self-conscious emotions, 205
self-harm, xi, 314–22, 337, 338, 366
self-loathing, 150
self-medication, 141–42
self-perception, 44
self-regulation, 346, 354–55
sense of self, 7–8, 14–15
sensory awareness, 220
sensory triggers, 170
severe dissociative symptoms, 418
sexual abuse, 139, 397

sexual boundary problems, 397–98
sexual intimacy, 361
shame, 44, 52, 138–39, 150, 169, 216, 264, 288–96, 316, 335, 347, 368
shame scripts, 290–93
    attack others, 290, 291–92
    attack self, 290, 291
    avoidance of inner experience, 290, 292–93
    withdrawal from others (isolation), 290, 292
shopping, 113
    fear around, 281
    for food, 151, 152, 153, 155, 156–57
    lists for, 116
"should/ought to" statements, 239
"sibling rivalry" transferences, 417
skills-training group
    final evaluation, 451–54
    ground rules for, 446–48
    participant contract for, 449–50
skills-training manual
    development of, xiii–xiv
    introductory session, 433
    use in day-treatment and inpatient groups, 433
    use in individual therapy, 432, 433
sleep, 97, 101–2, 144
sleep apnea, 98
sleep disorders, 98
sleep kit, 101, 109, 158
sleep medication, 105
sleep problems, 99–105
sleep quality, improving, 100–102
sleep record, 106–7
sleep routine
    addressing obstacles to, 110
    establishing, 102
sleepwalking, 98, 99
social anxiety, xi
socializing, 115, 121–22, 118
somatic symptoms, 45
somatoform dissociation, measuring, 415
Somatoform Dissociation Questionnaire (SDQ-20), 415
spacing out, 19
startle reflex, 35
"start-stop" behavior, 113
STEPPS. *see* systems training for emotional predictability and problem solving
Store exercise, 171–72, 180, 186, 199
stress ball, 38, 47
stress reduction, 38-9, 47
structure, 115
Structured Clinical Interview for DSM-IV Dissociative Disorders, Revised, 415
Structured Clinical Interview for DSM Personality Disorders, 415
substance abuse, 35, 141-42, 316, 347, 430
suicidal behavior, 318
suicide, loneliness and, 366
support, inner, 181–82
survival mechanisms, 53
switching, 27, 28, 303–4, 403
sympathetic nervous system, 278
systems training for emotional predictability and problem solving (STEPPS), xi, xiii

"talking inwardly," 75
tardiness, 429
TARGET. *see* trauma adaptive recovery group education and therapy (TARGET)
tasks, 119–22
teaching
    course topics, 425
    skills exercises, 424–25
telephone contact between sessions, 431
therapeutic alliance, 432
therapists
    referrals to skills group and motivations of, 422–23
    trainer contact and coordination with, 421–22
thirst, 142, 152
thoughts
    challenging, reflections for understanding, 248–49
    core beliefs and, 228
    decision making and, 325
    exploring, when you have complex dissociative disorder, 248–49
    feedback loops of, 205–6
    inaccurate, challenging, homework, 250–51
    realistic, developing, 252–53
threatening situations, failure to feel fear in, 281–82
thrill seeking, 214
time, keeping track of, 115–16
time distortions, 16, 19
time loss, 16, 189
time management, 189
time-outs
    from anger, 270, 272
    assertiveness and, 386
    conflict management skills and, 363
    relational conflicts and, 359
    skills-training group and, 447
time pressure, decision making and, 327–28
time-related triggers, 169
tiredness, 98
tobacco use, 100
trainers
    contact and coordination with treating therapist, 421–22
    division of group tasks among, 414
    qualifications and guidelines for, 414
    role of, 446
training course sessions
    conducting, 423–27
    educational meeting for significant others, 426–27
    ending the course, 427
    format of, 424
    ground rules, 423–24
    homework, 425–26
    introductory session, 423
    teaching course topics, 425
    teaching skills exercise, 424–25
    see also introductory session; leave-taking session
trance-like behavior, 19
transference issues, 417
trauma
    dissociation and, 8
    healthy eating and healing from, 149–61

trauma (*continued*)
  isolation as reenactment of, 367
  relationships and effect of, 346
  sleep problems and, 99–100
trauma adaptive recovery group education and
    therapy (TARGET), xii
traumatic memories
  autobiographical memories and, 166
  avoiding situations or experiences related to,
    26
  PTSD and intrusion of, 35
trauma-time, 26, 31, 230, 237,358
traumatizing experiences
  ashamed parts holding onto, 31
  fight parts holding onto, 30–31
  helper parts holding onto, 30
  parts imitating people who hurt you holding
    onto, 30
  parts of personality holding onto, 29–31
  young parts holding onto, 29–30
Tree exercise, 128–29, 159, 180
triggers
  agenda on coping with, 177
  agenda on understanding, 165
  of anger, 270–71
  anticipating, 179
  conflicts in relationships and, 358
  coping with, 177–85
  distinguishing the past from the present,
    180–82
  eliminating or avoiding, 178
  of fear, identifying, 283
  identifying, 173–74
  identifying and coping with, 183–84
  identifying and coping with, skills review, 200
  imaginal rehearsal, 179–80
  neutralizing effects of, 180
  overwhelming emotions evoked by, 208
  positive, identifying, 176
  for positive experiences, 170
  posttraumatic stress disorder and, 36
  recognizing, 167–68
  recognizing options to, 180
  reflecting on reactions to, 175

  removing from bedroom, 101, 108
  self-harm and, 318, 319
  sexual, 397
  skills to cope with, 185–86
  store exercise and coping with, 171–72
  types of, 168–70
  understanding, 166–67
  vulnerability to, 168
trust problems, 346

unconscious avoidance, 53
understanding other people through reflection,
  62–63
unhealthy boundaries, 395–96

volunteering, 113, 192
vulnerable parts of yourself, protecting, in relational conflicts, 361

weekends, difficult feelings and triggers related
  to, 190
weekly structure, 112
well-being, 84
WHO. *see* World Health Organization (WHO)
window of tolerance, 214–17
withdrawal from others, shame script and, 290–92
work, 112, 113, 119–20, 121–22
work habits, healthy, 116–17
World Health Organization (WHO), 10
written forms of communication, to yourself,
  74–75

young parts of self
  goals for working with, 304–5
  holding traumatizing experiences, 29–30
  problems related to switching to, in daily life,
    303–4
  understanding, 302–4
  working with, 305–7
"you" statements, 379

The Norton Series on Interpersonal Neurobiology

Louis Cozolino, PhD, Series Editor

Allan N. Schore, PhD, Series Editor, 2007–2014

Daniel J. Siegel, MD, Founding Editor

The field of mental health is in a tremendously exciting period of growth and conceptual reorganization. Independent findings from a variety of scientific endeavors are converging in an interdisciplinary view of the mind and mental well-being. An interpersonal neurobiology of human development enables us to understand that the structure and function of the mind and brain are shaped by experiences, especially those involving emotional relationships.

The Norton Series on Interpersonal Neurobiology provides cutting-edge, multidisciplinary views that further our understanding of the complex neurobiology of the human mind. By drawing on a wide range of traditionally independent fields of research—such as neurobiology, genetics, memory, attachment, complex systems, anthropology, and evolutionary psychology—these texts offer mental health professionals a review and synthesis of scientific findings often inaccessible to clinicians. The books advance our understanding of human experience by finding the unity of knowledge, or consilience, that emerges with the translation of findings from numerous domains of study into a common language and conceptual framework. The series integrates the best of modern science with the healing art of psychotherapy.